NON-INVASIVE
DIAGNOSTIC TECHNIQUES
IN CARDIOLOGY

NON-INVASIVE DIAGNOSTIC TECHNIQUES IN CARDIOLOGY

Alberto Benchimol, M.D.

Director, Institute for Cardiovascular Diseases
Good Samaritan Hospital
Phoenix, Arizona

The Williams & Wilkins Company
BALTIMORE

Made in the United States of America

Library of Congress Cataloging in Publication Data

Benchimol, Alberto.
    Non-invasive diagnostic techniques in cardiology.

    Bibliography:
    Includes index.
    1. Cardiovascular system—Diseases—Diagnosis. 2. Cardiography. I. Title.
       [DNLM: 1. Heart diseases—Diagnosis. WG141 B457n]
RC669.B38   616.1'2'0754   76-4843
ISBN 0-683-00525-1

Composed and printed at the
Waverly Press, Inc.
Mt. Royal and Guilford Aves.
Baltimore, Md. 21202, U.S.A.

Dedication

To my wife Helena, our sons Nelson and Alex, my beloved father Isaac, my mother Nina, and my sisters and brothers.

Introduction

This book represents the author's 14 years of experience analyzing phonocardiograms, pulse waves, and other non-invasive techniques in patients with a variety of cardiovascular diseases. In addition, experience gained from the analysis of over 2,000 echocardiograms during the past 2 years is included.

The text is divided into 13 chapters. Chapter 1 describes basic principles involved in auscultation and phonocardiography, with emphasis on instrumentation, recording techniques, personnel and laboratory requirements.

Knowledge of the fundamental principles of cardiovascular physiology is of great importance in understanding abnormalities of heart sounds and murmurs, and, whenever appropriate, they are discussed.

Chapter 2 outlines the principles of ultrasound and its application for clinical cardiology. Special reference is made to the principles of echocardiography and the Doppler flowmeter technique used for transcutaneous, non-invasive evaluation of blood velocity over various superficial arteries and veins. A discussion of instrumentation is included, with a description of a normal echocardiogram and normal phasic blood velocity over various vascular beds in man.

In Chapter 3 the mechanisms of normal heart sounds involving pulse wave production and heart murmurs are described, as well as a discussion of systolic time intervals and their value in the non-invasive evaluation of cardiovascular functions.

Specific pathologic states are described in Chapters 4 through 11. Each chapter covers most of the non-invasive techniques used to evaluate patients with aortic, mitral, and tricuspid valvular disease; coronary artery disease; congenital heart disease; and myocardial and pericardial disease. The values and limitations of phonocardiograms, carotid and jugular venous tracings, apexcardiograms, and echocardiograms are placed together. Correlation with invasive techniques from the author's experience with over 5,000 cardiac catheterizations is made in some instances.

Chapter 12 is a discussion of other non-invasive techniques used to evaluate patients with cardiovascular diseases such as kinetocardiography, radarkymography, isotope techniques, vectorcardiography, and others.

In Chapter 13 the use of non-invasive techniques in a number of disease states not covered in previous chapters are illustrated. The illustrative material is correlated with clinical problems and electrovectorcardiographic, hemodynamic, and angiographic findings.

The book is clinically oriented and purposely avoids areas of major controversy. However, observations on some controversial findings are emphasized. The author did not intend to review all of the literature available. A list of references is found at the end of each chapter for those who want a more detailed exposure and statistical data confirming the findings summarized in the text.

A book of this size covers a very broad area and suffers from the omission of some important non-invasive techniques such as electrocardiography, exercise stress testing, vectorcardiography and others which have been mentioned only briefly.

The book is intended for physicians and students who want a close exposure to the values and limitations of non-invasive techniques in the evaluation of patients with cardiovascular diseases.

Acknowledgments

I am very grateful to Dr. E. Grey Dimond for the stimulation and support received during my postgraduate training at the University of Kansas School of Medicine, Kansas City, Kansas, and later as his associate at Scripps Clinic and Research Foundation in La Jolla, California. The experience gained during those years working with Dr. Dimond and his encouragement to pursue academic and teaching opportunities made this book possible.

The assistance of postgraduate trainees, technicians, nurses and secretaries who have worked in the cardiac catheterization and non-invasive laboratories of The Institute for Cardiovascular Diseases at Good Samaritan Hospital, Phoenix, Arizona, has been invaluable. I especially want to acknowledge the cooperation of Jenny Goff, Carol Graves, Bonnie Griner, Frances Maldonado, Bettie Jo Massey, Karen Mc-Cullough, Della Olsen, and Connie Sheasby. Sydney Peebles prepared most of the illustrations shown and I am greatly indebted to her. I want to express my sincere appreciation to Carole Crevier for her outstanding efforts during preparation of the manuscript and for editing and indexing this book.

Foreword

The pleasure in writing this foreword is manyfold but the real satisfaction comes in knowing that the author is thoroughly competent and personally experienced in all areas covered in this book. The reader can be assured that Alberto Benchimol has utilized the full range of techniques and has wisdom gained from personal involvement is subsequent clinical decisions.

And of course, the other private pleasure is in watching the full development of the talent that joined our laboratory eighteen years ago. The progress from Manaus, Brazil to the authorship of this book is a reminder that young people with capacity and energy are not handicapped by problems of language, culture, distance, etc. Real talent succeeds. A good training program perhaps helps but the natural ability of the individual is the key ingredient.

E. Grey Dimond, M.D.
Distinguished Professor of Medicine
University of Missouri
Provost—Health Sciences
University of Missouri—Kansas City

Contents

chapter 1

Basic Principles of Auscultation and Phonocardiography

BASIC PRINCIPLES OF SOUND AND WAVE FORMATION

Heart sounds and pulse waves basically follow the physical principles of a wave, which is defined as periodic disturbance or vibratory motion which takes place in the vectorial direction as it moves through a medium. Heart sounds originating from the cardiac structures move toward the chest wall through the air-lung structures. These waves compress and rarefy gas molecules in the direction in which they vibrate forward and backward. Heart sounds and pulse waves, as heard with the stethoscope and recorded on a phonocardiogram, follow the concept of longitudinal wave production. Heart sounds and murmurs are composed of a multiple series of waves. A primary vibration is always present in various components of the recorded heart sounds and murmurs. Each particle of any given matter vibrates about its normal resting position and propagates along the longitudinal axis. All particles surrounding these structures participate in this type of wave motion with the exception of the progressive change in the quality of the vibratory motion. As a result, particles complete the cycle of reaction at a subsequent time. The strongest vibrations of heart sounds and murmurs cause an upward deflection in the baseline of the recording; the smallest vibrations are recorded as a downward defelection. The number of vibrations per unit of time is defined as wave frequency. Frequency characteristics of the heart sounds and murmurs are of importance in ausculation and phonocardiography because their variation in frequency have diagnostic implications. One complete wavelength is the result of the contraction rarefaction per complete cycle. The number of wave frequencies per unit of time represents the number of complete wave cycles and

1

FREQUENCY

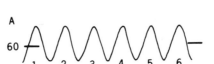

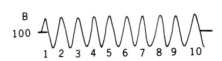

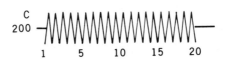

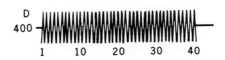

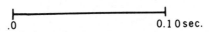

.0   0.10 sec.

Fig. 1.1. Diagrammatic representation of pulse waves. Intensity of the waves is represented by the height of the oscillation. Frequency of the waves corresponds to the number of oscillations per unit of time. On *line A*, 6 oscillations are present for a period of $\frac{1}{10}$ sec which corresponds to 60 cycles per second; *line B*, 10 oscillations per $\frac{1}{10}$ sec; *line C*, 20 oscillations per $\frac{1}{10}$ sec; *line D*, 40 oscillations per $\frac{1}{10}$ sec, corresponding to 100, 200 and 400 cycles per second, respectively.

by definition determines whether a murmur would have low frequency characteristics such as we see in patients with mitral stenosis or high frequency such as in patients with aortic insufficiency. In figure 1.1, diagram *A* and *B* have a small number of completed vibratory waves and result in low frequency murmurs as seen in patients with mitral or tricuspid stenosis; examples *C* and *D* contain a greater number of completed vibratory waves, ordinarily causing high frequency murmurs of the type seen in patients with aortic or pulmonic stenosis or insufficiency. Every sound has four major characteristics: (1) time, (2) frequency, (3) amplitude or intensity and (4) quality. Time and frequency have been described above. Amplitude or intensity, as defined by magnitude of the vibrations of a sound or murmur, is ordinarily expressed in ausculation by grading the murmur, from Grade I to VI (Levine classification). Quality is a derived characteristic from the combination of time, frequency and magnitude. Musical sounds or murmurs are composed of vibrations which are perfectly regular in frequency. Each component of a perfectly regular sine wave is defined as a harmonic. Therefore, in musical murmurs, such as those observed in patients with calcific aortic stenosis, rupture of the aortic cusps in patients with bacterial endocarditis, etc., there are multiple vibrations of different magnitude and the small number of sine waves are single multiples of the lowest vibration.

Propagation of sound from the heart to the chest wall is a function of the various structures which are interposed between them. Air is a poor conductor of sound; therefore, the interposition of large masses of lung tissue would result in attenuation of the propagated waves. This is commonly seen in patients with chronic lung disease in which the heart sounds and murmurs are markedly diminished as detected over the precordium.

In phonocardiography, the one vibration occuring per unit of time is defined as a completed cycle per second. One complete frequency cycle is also defined as Hertz. Throughout this book, all illustrations indicate the setting of the band pass filter system used in the phonocardiographic amplifier and they are defined as cycles per second (CPS) or Hertz (Hz). Vibrations which have low intensity and frequency are called infrasonic or low frequency vibrations. It is difficult for an untrained ear to hear them, e.g., third and fourth heart sounds. In many patients these vibrations are best appreciated by careful palpation of the precordium with the patient in the left lateral decubitus position. Fortunately most heart sounds, clicks and murmurs are within the range of the threshold of human hearing with vibrations in the range of approximately 30 to 2,000 CPS.

The unit which defines wave intensity is called a decibel. This is important in phonocardiography because most phonocardiographic amplifiers have a band pass filter which amplifies the vibrations caused by the cardiac contraction, valve motion and murmurs by using decibels. In phonocardiography, the qualification of these vibrations is expressed as one tenth of a unit or bell-decibel. Qualification of heart sounds and murmurs is very complex. In order to define sound pressure per unit of sound intensity, one uses dyne per square centimeter, which is defined as a microbar. The microbar represents one atmosphere (14.7 pounds per square inch—10^6 dynes per square centimeter). For the purpose of simplification, to define the threshold of audibility of heart sounds or murmurs, decibels are used. The decibel scale follows the logarithmic on a base of 10, or the duration of acoustic power.

Heart sounds, caused by valvular structures, or by rapid acceleration and deceleration of blood within the intracardiac cavities, are of short duration. They are also called transients. A transient is a sound of short duration such as the first, second, third and fourth heart sounds, opening snaps and clicks. Heart murmurs are vibratory waves of longer duration and varying frequency. The vibrations within a murmur have varying frequency characteristics. Most phonocardiographic amplifiers record these vibrations within a wide range of frequencies.

The main purpose of filtering the vibrations is to attempt to simulate what is heard with the stethoscope. When the recorder is set for a stethoscopic recording, the high frequency vibrations are filtered using a band pass filter with a flat frequency response between 100 and 500 CPS. Frequencies above those limits are attenuated at a rate of 6 decibels per octave. On a logarithmic recording, the vibrations are attenuated at the rate of 12 decibels per octave and log-logarithmic recordings are attenuated at a rate of 18 decibels per octave as shown in figure 1.2.

EQUIPMENT FOR PHONOCARDIOGRAPHY AND PULSE WAVE RECORDINGS

The most common type of microphone used for clinical phonocardiography employs piezoelectric crystals. Piezoelectric crystals, usually made of barium titanate, are sensitive to changes in the surrounding pressures which will deform the molecular structure of the crystal causing them to vibrate. Other types of microphones used in phonocardiography include condensor, capacitor and contact microphones. Although they have theoretical advantages over the crystal barium microphone, they are much more difficult to use for routine clinical evaluation. All microphones are very sensitive to artifacts and great care must be exercised in the interpretation of phonocardiograms. A minimum of four consecutive cardiac cycles should be obtained and configuration, amplitude and frequency characteristics of heart sounds, and murmurs should be identical in all cycles if the patient is in sinus rhythm. In patients with cardiac arrhythmias, a larger number of cardiac cycles should be recorded since rhythm abnormalities affect heart sounds and murmurs significantly, depending on the disease state which is being analyzed. These changes will be described in detail in subsequent chapters. The advantage of the contact microphone is that there are no air conduction delays, air leaks or movable parts and they have a higher frequency response. A disadvantage of piezoelectric crystal microphones is that they are sensitive to fluctuations in environmental humidity which changes their frequency characteristic response, and they are

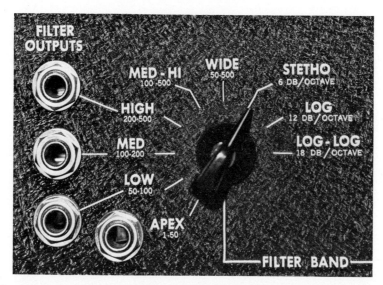

Fig. 1.2. Electronics for Medicine phonocardiographic amplifier showing the various band pass filter settings for stethoscopic, logarithmic and log-logarithmic recordings. Stethoscopic recordings are made with filtering at 6 decibels (DB) per octave, logarithmic at 12 DB per octave and log-logarithmic at 18 DB per octave.

susceptible to fractures if a unit is accidentally damaged. The crystals should be replaced at fairly frequent intervals particularly in geographical areas which have a high humidity atmospheric pressure. However, for most practical uses, piezoelectric crystal microphones are quite suitable and easy to use. Other types such as electromagnetic or dynamic microphones use a movable coil located in the range of a magnetic field. Unfortunately, they are not sensitive to low frequency vibrations as the piezoelectric microphone is and are not suitable for pulse wave recordings.

Microphones used in clinical phonocardiography should accurately record sound vibrations with a frequency as low as 0.2 to 0.4 CPS or Hz without significant loss of amplitude. The frequency response of the transducer is extremely important in phonocardiography and pulse wave recordings. These transducers should faithfully reproduce vibrations with a long range frequency which is defined as a time constant. The time constant of a transducer which is less than 3 seconds lacks the required electronic characteristics to obtain tracings which are free of artifacts. The time constant of a capacitor circuit in the transducer is defined as the length of time, in seconds, required for the output voltage to reach 63% of the applied input voltage (fig. 1.6). This indicates that transducers with a long time constant should record longer plateaus

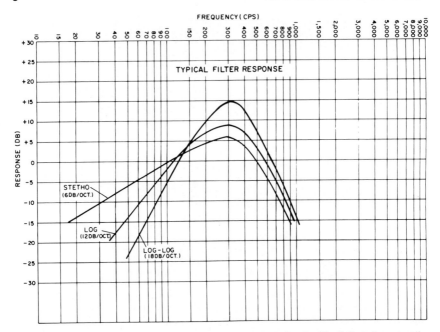

Fig. 1.3. Diagrammatic representation of the Electronics for Medicine phonocardio-graphic amplifier showing the typical filter response for various filters used. (From Electronics for Medicine, Inc., White Plains, N.Y., with permission.)

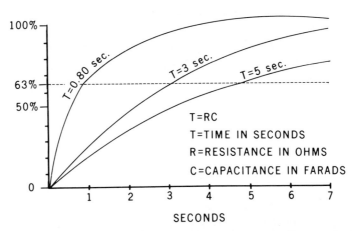

Fig. 1.4. Diagrammatic representation of the time constant of a transducer used for recording phonocardiograms, pulse waves, mechanical and electrical signals generated by the heart. The time constant of any resistor-capacitor (RC) is defined as the length of time, in seconds, required for the output voltage to reach 63% of the applied input voltage.

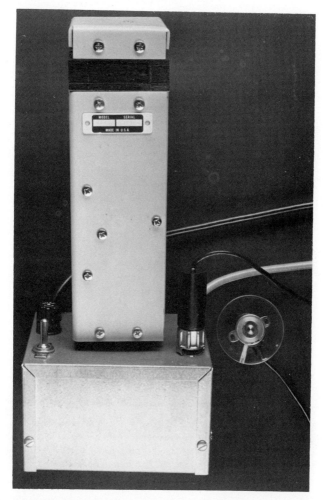

Fig. 1.5. APT-16 differential transformer transducer currently used in our laboratory to record carotid pulse tracing, venous pulse tracing and apexcardiograms. This transducer is manufactured by Hewlett-Packard.

without decay at the time a specific phenomenon is being recorded. This is quite important in recording the apexcardiogram, precordial motion, carotid pulse tracing or jugular venous tracing. Therefore, pulse tracings recorded with transducers having a long time constant will record a deflection which should be held below or above the resting baseline without decay below 63% of the supply of the input voltage and without returning to the baseline. For the past several years, we have been using a transducer which is a differential transformer. This unit eliminates air

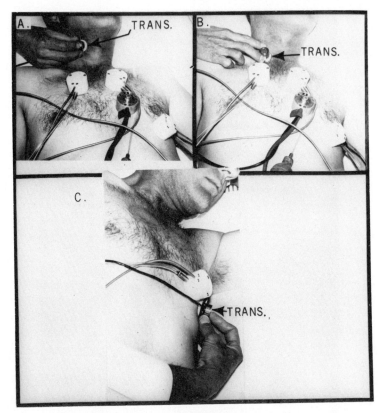

Fig. 1.6. Positioning of the four microphones in the precordial areas. *Panel A* indicates the proper position of the transducer to record carotid artery tracings. *Panel B* shows position of the transducer for recording jugular venous tracings. *Panel C* shows position of the transducer to record the apexcardiogram.

leaks, one of the major problems with crystal transducers; furthermore, it has a long time constant and thus eliminates artifacts.

After microphones are properly placed on the chest wall, the signal is amplified on the phonocardiographic amplifier. The amplifier is a matching device which converts volts to watts (electromotive force to power). The tracing is displayed on an oscilloscope for photographic recording and recorded on magnetic tape or some form of direct writing unit. Most recording units employ a cathode ray tube for photographic recording or a galvanometer for direct writing -recording. A galvanometer is a moving coil which oscillates in response to electrical impulses. A disadvantage of the galvanometer for direct writing-recording is that it has significant inertia which limits the recording of high and low frequency vibrations. However, recent direct writing-recorders are adequate for clinical phonocardiography because of significant electronic improvements which result in better frequency response. Direct writer-recorders must have a flat frequency response to a minimum of 10 or 20 cycles to 200–500 CPS or Hz without causing significant loss of amplitude of the vibratory waves, or elimination of vibrations above that range. Some galvanometers can be equipped with a mirror connected to a photographic unit so that high frequency vibrations are properly recorded.

Recording devices which use a cathode ray tube are the most popular and probably represent the best unit available for recording phonocardiograms and pulse waves. These units amplify the input signal into electrical energy causing the electronic beam on the oscilloscope to be deflected. This deflection is proportional to the strength of the wave. Since they use a photographic recording unit, the frequency response is quite high. Attachments for rapid processing are available for immediate analysis of the records. However, for better quality records, the standard processing method for photographic paper is needed. Most of the tracings illustrated in this book were recorded on an Electronics for Medicine DR-8 oscilloscopic photographic recorder. The transducer used for recording the carotid artery pulse, jugular venous pulse and apexcardiogram is the Hewlett-Packard APT-16 differential transformer. Leatham microphones manufactured by Cambridge Company were used to record phonocardiograms.

LABORATORY REQUIREMENTS FOR RECORDING NON-INVASIVE TRACINGS

Adequate non-invasive evaluation of a patient with cardiovascular disease should include phonocardiograms at multiple precordial areas recorded simultaneously with a carotid pulse tracing, jugular venous tracing and apexcardiogram. Techniques such as the electrocardiogram at rest, stress exercise electrocardiogram and others will be summarized. We record simultaneous phonocardiograms with one or two pulse waves such as the carotid or jugular venous pulse tracings and apexcardiogram. A large number of measurements from various components of the cardiac cycle can be derived from these recordings at rest or during maneuvers, exercise and administration of pharmacologic agents. Laboratories for non-invasive examinations should also have the capability of obtaining vectorcardiograms, echocardiograms and other non-invasive techniques such as the use of radioisotopes, kinetocardiogram, etc (see Chapter 12). A non-invasive technique which is gaining increasing popularity is the use of high frequency ultrasound with the transcutaneous Doppler flowmeter. This will be described in Chapter 2.

For proper recording of a phonocardiogram, a quiet atmosphere such as a soundproof room is desirable. It is important that the microphones have good contact with the skin which requires shaving the chest in male patients. This is a routine procedure in our laboratory.

A good phonocardiographic unit should have at least two phonocardiographic amplifiers and be equipped with a band pass filter system to provide the capability for stethoscopic and logarithmic recording. One of the pulse waves (carotid, jugular venous pulse or apexcardiogram) and one lead of the electrocardiogram should be recorded simultaneously. The advantage of a multiple system recording is that it allows precise measurement of the systolic and diastolic intervals. It is helpful to have the phonocardiographic unit connected to an oscilloscope for visual display which allows for recognition of artifacts. The unit should also have the capability of multiple speed recordings. Phonocardiograms recorded at a speed of 75 mm/sec or greater are quite satisfactory in the majority of patients to record heart murmurs and abnormal heart sounds. For measurements of systolic and diastolic time intervals, in addition to the 75 mm/sec tracing, another recording should be taken at a paper speed of 100 or 150 mm/sec. Slower paper speed is also important in patients with prosthetic cardiac valves for good reproducibility of prosthetic valve sounds in a great number of cardiac cycles. A speed of 25 or 50 mm/sec is important to record heart sounds during inspiration and expiration, maneuvers and administration of drugs.

TECHNIQUES FOR RECORDING CAROTID PULSE TRACING

The transducer can be placed over the right or left common carotid arteries, although most commonly it is placed over the right carotid artery, 1–2 inches below the jaw. For a short recording, the transducer can be held by hand with slight pressure applied over the area. The best recording is obtained over the right carotid artery when the patient's head is turned slightly to the left and the neck is slightly hyperextended. For recordings of the left carotid artery pulse tracing, the patient's head should be turned slightly to the right. This maneuver has the advantage of bringing the carotid artery closer to the skin and moving the sternocleidomastoid muscle away from the carotid artery. At times, recording over the suprasternal notch in the area overlying the aortic arch can be suitable for analysis. A normal carotid pulse is shown in Chapter 3.

Another technique for recording the carotid pulse is to attach the transducer to a cuff placed around the neck. There is no particular advantage to this technique for short records, but it would be advantageous if records are to be obtained continuously or intermittently for prolonged periods of time.

JUGULAR VENOUS PULSE RECORDING

The ability to make good recordings of the jugular venous pulse requires practice and experience. The best anatomical area to record this pulse wave is over the supraclavicular area near the manubrium or the anatomical area 2–3 cm below the jaw. The transducer should be held by hand with very slight pressure applied over the skin. The patient should be turned on the left side with slight hyperextension of the neck. The head should be elevated slightly with a pillow placed under the neck and head making an angle of about 30–50 degrees. This moves the sterno-cleidomastoid muscle away from the junction of the jugular and subclavian veins. The tracing should be monitored on the oscilloscope for recognition of the two most important waves on this tracing (A and V waves) as shown in Chapter 3. A technically satisfactory jugular venous pulse tracing can be obtained in most patients with cardiovascular diseases and a large number of normal subjects. However, technically satisfactory recordings cannot be obtained in approximately 5–10% of subjects.

APEXCARDIOGRAM RECORDING

Recordings of the precordial pulsations have gained increasing popularity because of their value in timing the various events of the cardiac cycle, clicks and opening snaps, etc. In order to obtain a technically satisfactory apexcardiogram, it is important that proper techniques be applied. The transducer should fulfill the electronic characteristics described earlier in this chapter. Several techniques for recording precordial pulsations have been given different names by different investigators. The one which has gained popularity for clinical use is the apexcardiogram. Other techniques which are valuable but a little more complex include the kinetocardiogram, vibrocardiogram, ballistocardiogram and acceleration tracings (accelerogram) of the precordial pulsations. Some of these techniques will be described in Chapter 12.

For a good recording of the apexcardiogram, the patient must be turned in a left lateral decubitus position with the left arm placed behind the head. It is important for the patient to be relaxed, and it is quite helpful to place a pillow behind the patient's back. The tracing should be continuously displayed on the oscilloscope in order to recognize artifacts and the reproducibility of the various components of the apexcardiogram. The point of maximal cardiac impulse must be carefully palpated by hand. Subsequently, one should identify the center of the maximal cardiac impulse that is represented by the most forceful contraction of the heart against the chest wall. The transducer is then placed in the center of the maximal impulse and held by hand or rubber straps. We prefer to hold the transducer by hand unless the recording will be done for a prolonged period. The patient is instructed to take a short inspiration followed by a short held expiration. Adequate, reliable and reproducible tracings can be obtained in approximately 90% of patients with cardiovascular disease and in most normal subjects. Our earlier work in this field was done utilizing a transducer bell connected by rubber tubing to a piezoelectric crystal. However, we have abandoned the use of this transducer because of problems with poor frequency response, short time constant and air leaks. The transducer which we are currently using is a differential transformer (Hewlett-Packard APT-16) which fulfills most of the electronic requirements outlined earlier in this chapter. It is desirable to obtain a simultaneous recording of the phonocardiogram at the mitral and tricuspid areas.

Other recordings of precordial motion such as in patients with right ventricular hypertrophy can be made by placing the transducer along the left sternal border at the third or fourth intercostal space or over the subxyphoid area. Other anatomical locations for recording the apexcardiogram over the point of cardiac impulse, such as in patients with coronary artery disease and left ventricular aneurysm, and others, will be discussed in subsequent chapters.

PERSONNEL

Only the highly skilled technician, well versed in characteristics of heart sounds and murmurs and the techniques for recording them, will be able to obtain good tracings. A physician must be present during maneuvers or administration of pharmacological agents used to induce changes in cardiac function which may be important in differential diagnosis.

REFERENCES

1. Aronow, W. S.: Effect of position on the resting and post-exercise phonocardiogram. Chest, *61:* 439, 1972.
2. Barker, L. F.: Electrocardiography and phonocardiography. Bull. John Hopkins Hosp., *21:* 358, 1910.
3. Battaerd, P. J. T. A.: Further graphic researches on the acoustic phenomena of the heart in normal and pathological conditions. Heart, *6:* 121, 1915.
4. Bekkering, D. H., and Weber, J.: Standardization of phonocardiography efforts in the Netherlands. Am. Heart J., *54:* 316, 1957.
5. Bertrand, C. A., Miline, I. G., and Hornick, R.: A study of heart sounds and murmurs by direct heart recordings. Circulation, *13:* 49, 1956.
6. Blumgart, H. L., Gargill, S. L., and Gilligan, D. R.: Studies on the velocity of blood flow; XIII. The circulatory response to thyrotoxicosis. J. Clin. Invest., *9:* 69, 1930.

7. Bramwell, C.: Use of the phonocardiograph in clinical cardiology. Br. Heart J., *10:* 98, 1948.
8. Braunwald, W., Fishman, A. P., and Cournand, A.: Time relationship of dynamic events in the cardiac chambers, pulmonary artery and aorta in man. Circ. Res., *4:* 100, 1956.
9. Burger, A. C., Koopman, L. J., and Overeem, A. P. T.: On the analysis and the origin of heart sounds (II). Acta Cardiol., *5:* 1, 1950.
10. Burton, A. C.: Improvement in construction of apparatus for demonstration of turbulence. J. Appl. Physiol., *6:* 719, 1954.
11. Cabot, R. C.: *Physical Diagnosis.* William Wood Co., New York, 1926.
12. Carstensen, E. L., Kam, L., and Schwan, H. P.: Determination of the acoustic properties of blood and its constituents. J. Acoust. Soc. Am., *25:* 286, 1953.
13. Churcher, B. G., and King, A. L.: Measurement of noise. Nature, *138:* 329, 1936.
14. Coulter, N. A. Jr., and Pappenheimer, J. R.: Development of turbulence in flowing blood. Am. J. Physiol., *159:* 401, 1949.
15. Cowen, E. D. H., and Parnum, D. H.: The phonocardiography of heart murmurs; I. Apparatus and technique. Br. Heart J., *11:* 356, 1949.
16. Dimond, E. G., and Benchimol, A.: Phonocardiography. Calif. Med., *94:* 139, 1961.
17. Effert, S., Gross-Brockhoge, F., and Loogen, F.: Intracardiac phonocardiography. Ger. Med. Mon., *7:* 9, 1962.
18. Emerson, C. P.: The effect of pressure on the stethoscope on the intrathoracic sounds. Bull. John Hopkins Hosp., *19:* 49, 1908.
19. Erlanger, J.: Relation of longitudinal tension of an artery to the preanacrotic phenomina. Am. Heart J., *19:* 398, 1940.
20. Fletcher, J., and Munson, W. A.: Loudness, its definition, measurement, and calculation. J. Acoust. Soc. Am., *5:* 82, 1933.
21. Foulger, J. H., Smith, P. E., Jr., and Fleming, A. J.: Cardiac vibrational intensity and cardiac output. Am. Heart J., *35:* 953, 1948.
22. Foulger, J. H., Smith, P. E. Jr., and Fleming, A. J.: Changes in cardiac vibrational intensity in response to physiologic stress. Am. Heart J., *34:* 507, 1947.
23. Garb, S.: The relationship of blood viscosity to the intensity of heart murmurs. Am. Heart J., *28:* 568, 1944.
24. Grant, R. P.: Architectonics of the heart. Am. Heart J., *52:* 944, 1956.
25. Groedel, F. M., and Miller, M.: The influence of the chest wall on the heart sounds. Exp. Med. Surg., *2:* 328, 1944.
26. Groom, D., and Boone, J. A.: The recording of heart sounds and vibrations; II. The application of an electronic pickup in the graphic recording of subaudible and audible frequencies. Exp. Med. Surg., *14:* 255, 1956.
27. Hale, J. G., McDonald, D. A., and Womersley, J. R.: Velocity profiles of oscillating arterial flow, with some calculations of viscous drag and the Reynolds number. J. Physiol., *128:* 629, 1955.
28. Hartman, H.: Differentiation between the influence of the right and left ventricle in the phonocardiogram, with the aid of pulsation curves (Abstracts of papers, p. 127). Second European Congress of Cardiology, 1956.
29. Hartman, H.: Simultaneous recordings of the phonocardiograms, venous and arterial pulses. Arch. Inst. Cardiol. Mex., *31:* 39, 1961.
30. Hillard, J. K., and Fiala, W. T.: Condenser microphones for measurement of high sound pressures (mimeograph). Altec Lansing Corporation, 9356 Santa Monica Blvd., Beverly Hills, California.
31. Hillard, J. K., and Noble, J. J.: The "Lipstik" condenser microphone system. *Proceedings of the Institute of Radio Engineer Professional Group on Audio*, Vol. AU-2 (No. 6), 1954.
32. Holldack, K., Luisada, A. A., and Ueda, H.: Standardization of phonocardiography. Am. J. Cardiol., *15:* 419, 1965.
33. Huggins, W. H.: A phase principle for complex frequency analysis and its implications in auditory theory. J. Acoust. Soc. Am., *24:* 582, 1952.
34. Kelly, J. J. Jr.: Symposium on cardiovascular sound. Circulation *16:* 270, 1957.

35. Kotis, J. B.: The value of the ultrasonic Doppler method and apexcardiography as reference tracing in phonocardiography. Am. Heart J., *84:* 634, 1972.
36. Leatham, A.: Phonocardiology. Br. Med. Bull., *8:* 333, 1952.
37. Leech, G.: Measurement problems in external pulse recording. Annual meeting of the Laenaec Society of the American Health Association, Anaheim, Calif., 1971.
38. Lewis, D. H., Deitz, G. W., Wallace, J. D., and Brown, J. R. Jr.: Intracardiac phonocardiography. Prog. Cardiovasc. Dis., *2:* 85, 1960.
39. Luisada, A. A., and Gamna, G.: Clinical calibration in phonocardiography. Am. Heart J., *48:* 826, 1954.
40. Luisada, A. A., Richmond, L., and Aravanis, C.: Selective phonocardiography. Am. Heart J., *51:* 221, 1956.
41. McKusick, V. A., Jenkins, J. T., and Webb, G. N.: Acoustic basis of the chest examination. Am. Rev. Tuberc., *72:* 12, 1955.
42. Miller, A., and White, P. D.: Crystal microphone for pulse wave recording. Am. Heart J., *21:* 504, 1941.
43. Mounsey, J. P. D.: The impulse cardiogram and the phonocardiogram. Cardiologia, *48:* 203, 1966.
44. Oreshkov, V.: Indirect measurement of isovolumetric contraction time on the basis of polygraphic tracing (apexcardiogram, carotid tracing, and phonocardiogram). Cardiologia, *47:* 315, 1965.
45. Polis, O., Cleempoel, H., Hanson, J., and VanThiel, E.: Phonocardiographic effect of the Valsalva maneuver. Acta Cardiol., *15:* 441, 1960.
46. Potter, R. K.: Introduction to technical discussions of sound portrayal. J. Acoust. Soc. Am., *18:* 1, 1946.
47. Rappaport, M. B., and Sprague, H. B.: Physiologic and physical laws which govern auscultation and their clinical application; the acoustic stethoscope and the electrical amplifying stethoscope and stethograph. Am. Heart J., *21:* 257, 1941.
48. Richards, J. D. Jr.: Frequency spectra of some normal heart sounds. Am. Heart J., *53:* 183, 1957.
49. Robard, S., Rubinstein, H. M., and Rosenblum, S.: Arrival time and calibrated contour of the pulse wave, determined indirectly from recordings of arterial compression sounds. Am. Heart J., *53:* 205, 1957.
50. Rushmer, R. F.: *Cardiac Diagnosis: A Physiologic Approach.* W. B. Saunders Co., Philadelphia, 1955.
51. Savart, F.: Note sur la communication des mouvements vibratories par les liquids. Ann. Chimie Physique, *31:* 283: 1826.
52. Smith, J. R., Edwards, J. C., and Kountz, W. B.: The use of the cathode ray for recording heart sounds and vibrations; III. Total cardiac vibrations in one hundred normal subjects. Am. Heart J., *21:* 228, 1941.
53. Smith, J. R., and Kountz, W. B.: Total cardiac vibrations in aged hearts and coronary disease. Proc. Soc. Exp. BIOL. Med., *47:* 353, 1941.
54. Tavel, M. E.: *Clinical Phonocardiography and External Pulse Recording,* p. 56. Year Book Medical Publishers, Chicago, 1967.
55. Webb, G. N., and McKusick, V. A.: Analysis of heart sounds. *Proceedings of 1957 National Conference of Instrumental Methods of Analysis.* Instrument Society of America, Pittsburgh, 1957.
56. Wiggers, C. J., and Dean, A. L. Jr.: The nature and time relations of the fundamental heart sounds. Am. J. Physiol., *42:* 476, 1917.
57. Winer, D. E., Perry, L. W., and Caceres, C. A.: Heart sound analysis; a three-dimensional approach. Am. J. Cardiol., *16:* 547, 1965.

chapter 2

Ultrasound

Ultrasound is defined as *sound* with a frequency greater than 20,000 cycles per second. In echocardiography we utilize frequencies in the range of millions of cycles per second (megaHertz). Ultrasound travels in straight lines unless it is reflected or refracted by an interface, or junction, between two different structures or tissues. The more perpendicular the beam to the interface, the more sound will be reflected back. This principle is important when trying to get a good recording of the interventricular septum. The ultrasonic beam must be perpendicular to the plane of the septum before a good recording can be obtained. Certain tissues transmit or conduct ultrasound better than others. Muscle, blood and fat conduct ultrasound very well, whereas bone and air conduct very poorly. Therefore, if the beam is passed through the sternum, ribs or lungs, it will be difficult or almost impossible to obtain a good echocardiographic recording of the cardiac structures.

Assuming that one avoids the bones and lungs, it is possible to differentiate the various cardiac structures because they have different densities; any difference in density is seen as a junction or interface, and they will reflect an echo. The clarity or *resolution* to define structures precisely will depend upon the ability to detect very small interfaces. In order for this to be accomplished, the width of the interface must be greater than 25% of the ultrasound wavelength; thus, the shorter the wavelength of the ultrasound transducer, the greater the resolution power. Unfortunately, because more sound is reflected back from these small interfaces, we have to sacrifice depth of penetration in order to achieve better resolution (figs. 2.1 and 2.2). Recordings in infants and children do not require too much penetration and a high frequency transducer, i.e., 7.5 mHz, which has a small wavelength, is used. For most adults deeper penetration is achieved by using a lower frequency transducer (2.25 mHz). Still deeper penetration can be achieved in obese or barrel-chested individuals by using a wider transducer head such as a 1-inch head as opposed to the usual ½ inch.

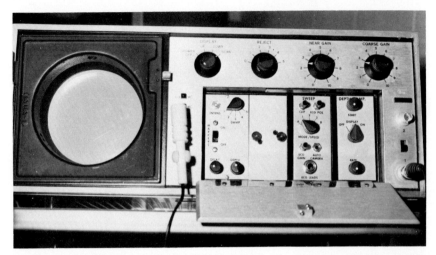

Fig. 2.1. Control panel of the Smith-Kline Ekoline 20, one of several commercially available echocardiographic units showing the various controls used to record echocardiograms (see text).

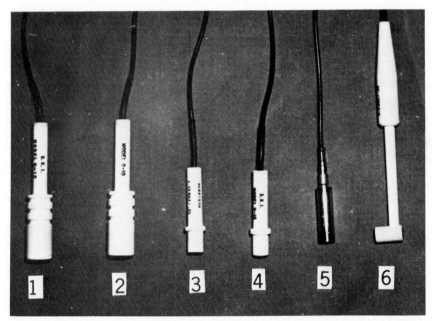

Fig. 2.2. Various types of echocardiographic transducers used during echocardiographic examinations. *Numbers 1* and *2* are most commonly used in adults, *numbers 3, 4* and *5* are used for pediatric echocardiography, and *number 6* is primarily used for the suprasternal approach.

The echocardiographic transducer has a "piezoelectric crystal" which changes shape with changes in electrical fields. Rapid alternation of the electrical field around the crystal causes it to vibrate and produce the ultrasonic beam. The available echocardiographic units emit ultrasonic beams in very short bursts to reduce the total exposure to the ultrasound; the transducer used in these units acts as a receiver 99.9% of the time and as an emitter only 0.1% of the time. This pulsed ultrasound has proved to be practically free of damaging power to the body tissues.

As the ultrasound beam leaves the transducer, it remains parallel for a given distance before it begins to diverge. Objects recorded in a widely divergent beam will appear fainter and may appear to lie on top of each other when they are actually lying side by side. To minimize this effect it is advantageous to use a transducer with a concave focusing lens. As the transducer senses the returning echoes, it generates electrical impulses which correspond in timing to a particular depth from the chest wall. These signals are then amplified and displayed as spikes on the oscilloscope of the unit. This type of display is called the "A-mode," and it does not indicate the motion of the moving object. The "M-mode" or "motion-mode," displays the object moving toward and away from the transducer. The "M-mode" is the most valuable in echocardiography because the various structures can be identified by their characteristic motions.

Recording devices vary from unit to unit. Permanent copies can be made with either Polaroid cameras, strip chart recorders, or various hard copiers. Polaroid copies are limited, in that only a few beats may be seen at a time, whereas strip chart recordings allow a long number of uninterrupted beats, enabling one to establish the interrelationships of the intracardiac structures when scanning from one area of the heart to another. Most medical centers are currently using the Electronics for Medicine or the Honeywell fiberoptic recorder. A further advantage of strip chart recorders is that they may be equipped with amplifiers which allow the simultaneous recording of the echocardiogram with electrocardiogram, carotid pulse tracing, jugular venous pulse tracing or the apexcardiogram. Portability of the echocardiographic unit is of importance, since many pediatric or adult patients may be too ill to be moved to the ultrasonic laboratory. Thus, it is desirable to have a unit which can be moved to a patient's room to obtain the proper recordings.

ECHOCARDIOGRAPHIC CONTROLS

The basic controls of the echocardiograph are usually identical in most ultrasound units. At our institution we use the "Smith-Kline Ekoline 20" unit (fig. 2.1) with the Electronics for Medicine DR8 recorder. The coarse gain knob controls the overall amplitude of all echoes. Increasing

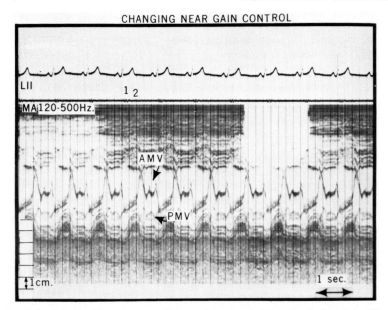

Fig. 2.3. Echocardiogram recorded at the mitral valve level showing effect of changing the near gain control (see text). **AMV** = anterior mitral valve, **PMV** = posterior mitral valve.

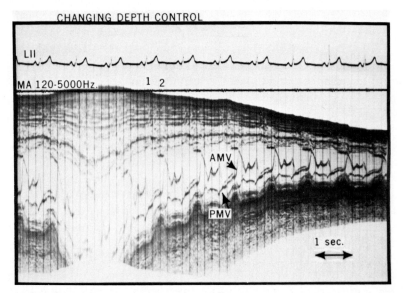

Fig. 2.4. Echocardiogram showing the effect of depth control on the features of motion of the anterior and posterior mitral valve (see text). **AMV** = anterior mitral valve, **PMV** = posterior mitral valve.

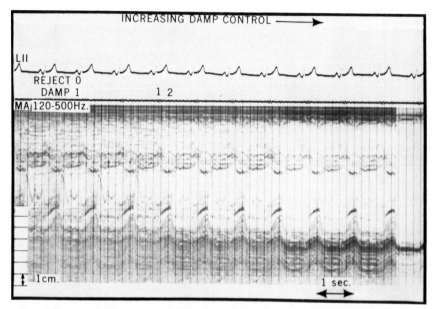

Fig. 2.5. Echocardiogram recorded at the mitral valve level showing the effect of increasing damping control. The reject control was set at 0 position (see text).

or decreasing this setting will affect all echoes to the same degree. The near gain control sets the gain or brightness of the echoes seen in the near field only. In the center portion of figure 2.3, the near gain is too high, and on the right side it is too low.

In figure 2.1, the control panel of the echocardiographic recorder shows the location of the *depth, delay, ramp rate* and *depth compensation* switches. The depth compensation (also called time gain compensation or electronic distance compensation) is an electronic circuit for suppressing near field echoes and enhancing the weaker far field echoes (fig. 2.4). This device is represented on the "A-mode" as a ramp on the depth scale with variable slope. All echoes to the left of the ramp are suppressed in relation to echoes on the right of the ramp. The ramp itself represents increasing depth compensation. In addition, all echoes to the left of the ramp fall within the control of the near gain, whereas all those to the right of the ramp are outside the control of the near gain switch.

The damping control acts much like the coarse gain. By increasing the damp all echoes are suppressed and only the most dominant echoes will remain. In figure 2.5 the pericardium is the only remaining echo after full damping.

The reject control switch selectively eliminates echoes of low amplitude (fig. 2.6). It does nothing to diminish the stronger signals, unlike

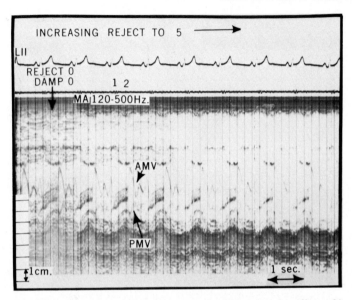

Fig. 2.6. Echocardiogram at the mitral valve level showing the effect of increasing the reject from 0 control to position 5 and maintaining the damping control at 1 position (see text). *AMV* = anterior mitral valve, *PMV* = posterior mitral valve.

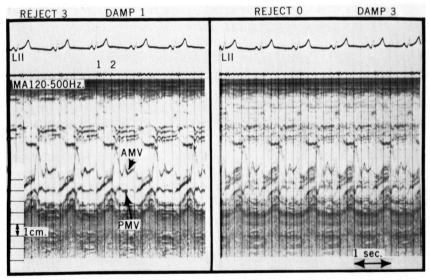

Fig. 2.7. Echocardiogram at the mitral valve level recorded at various reject and damping control settings (see text). *AMV* = anterior mitral valve, *PMV* = posterior mitral valve.

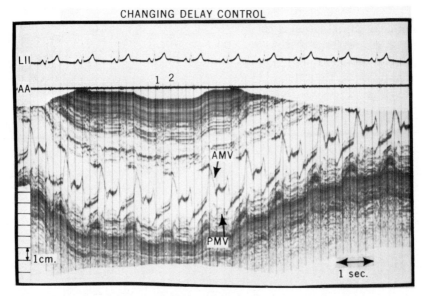

Fig. 2.8. Echocardiogram at the mitral valve level showing the effect of changes in delay control (see text). *AMV* = anterior mitral valve, *PMV* = posterior mitral valve.

coarse gain or damping control. The net effect is to make dominant structures appear as sharper lines by eliminating the smaller echoes. Figure 2.7 illustrates the difference in quality of the echocardiogram when setting up the unit in the two different manners. On the left, the damping control is low and the reject control is high. This combination results in sharp echoes, but does not provide as much detail as when the reject is low as shown on the right panel.

The depth control regulates the depth of the echocardiographic field, as shown in figure 2.4. For most adult echocardiograms, the depth is set at approximately 15 cm or less. Obviously, by setting the depth too shallow, only the anterior cardiac structures will be recognized. On the other hand, by setting the depth too deep, the tracing will be abnormally crowded and the structures will not be easily recognizable.

The delay control is of no importance unless it is incorrectly set. In that event, the anterior structures will be completely cut off (fig. 2.8). When one turns the unit to the "A-mode," the delay should be set so that the transducer artifact can be seen and all echoes will be present on the screen.

RECOGNITION OF NORMAL ECHOCARDIOGRAM

The first step in learning to perform a good echocardiographic study is to learn what a normal echocardiogram is *supposed* to look like. This requires a good knowledge of cardiac anatomy and pathophysiology.

The right side of the heart lies anterior and to the left side. In a horizontal cross section of the heart, the pulmonic valve lies anterior and to the left of the aortic valve, and the mitral valve to the left of the tricuspid valve (fig. 2.9). The interventricular septum is continuous with the anterior aortic wall.

In figure 2.9, cross sectional representations of the heart are seen, showing the echocardiographic transducer placed approximately at the

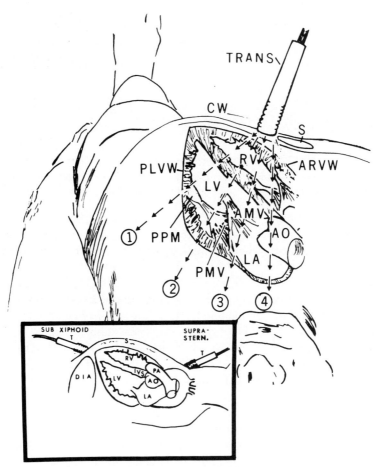

Fig. 2.9. Diagrammatic representation of various positions used during routine recording of conventional echocardiograms. In the *bottom panel*, positioning of the transducer for subxiphoid and suprasternal approaches is shown (see text). TRANS = transducer, *CW* = chest wall, *S* = sternum, *RV* = right ventricle, *LV* = left ventricle, *PLVW* = posterior left ventricular wall, *ARVW* = anterior right ventricular wall, *MV* = mitral valve, *PPM* = posterior papillary muscle, *PMV* = posterior mitral valve, *LA* = left atrium, *PA* = pulmonary artery, IVS = interventricular septum, *DIA* = diaphragm, *AO* = aorta, *1, 2, 3* and *4* = positions 1 through 4, respectively.

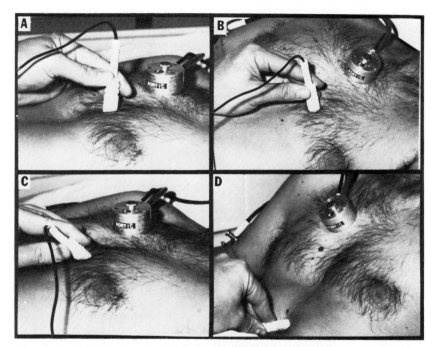

Fig. 2.10. Various positions of the echocardiographic transducer on the chest wall and location of the phonocardiographic microphone. *Panel A* shows the usual approach for right and left ventricular dimensions below the mitral valve apparatus. *Panel B* shows the approach for the mitral valve landmark. *Panel C* shows the typical approach for an aortic valve recording. *Panel D* shows the subxiphoid approach.

fourth intercostal space and to the left of the sternum. The lower part of this diagram is the left saggital cross section of the chest showing the position of the transducer for the suprasternal and subxiphoid approaches. In *position 1*, the ultrasonic beam passes through the chest wall, anterior right ventricular apex and posterior papillary muscle. In *position 2* the ultrasonic beam passes through the anterior right ventricle, right ventricular cavity, interventricular septum, left ventricle, chordae tendinae, and posterior left ventricular wall. In *position 3*, the beam passes through the right ventricular outflow tract, the anterior wall of the aorta, aortic cusps, posterior aortic wall, and the left atrium. Figure 2.10 shows the position of the transducer to record the various cardiac structures described above. Figure 2.11 is an echocardiogram obtained from position 2. The structures seen are as follows: anterior chest wall, right ventricular septum, the M-shaped anterior mitral leaflet, the posterior mitral leaflet, posterior left ventricular wall, pericardium and, finally, the lung and posterior mediastinal structures behind the heart. Examination of mitral valve motion shows that, with

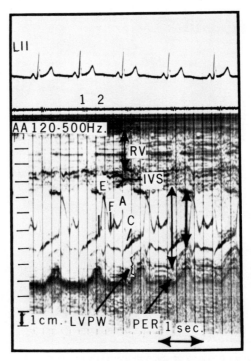

Fig. 2.11. Echocardiogram at the mitral valve in a 21-year-old normal subject showing normal mitral valve motion. This echocardiogram illustrates how various measurements can be made, such as internal right ventricular diameter, thickening of the interventricular septum (*IVS*) and left ventricular internal diameter during systole and diastole. *RV* = right ventricle, *LVPW* = left ventricular posterior wall, *PER* = pericardium.

rapid ventricular filling, the mitral leaflets open maximally and in opposite directions. The time of mitral valve opening is called the E point. The leaflets then drift together to a semiclosed position, called the F point and there is frequently a second, low frequency vibration just after the F point which is seen in longer diastolic intervals. Subsequently, with atrial contraction, the valve reopens and this is called the A point or A wave. With the onset of ventricular systole the mitral valve closes at point C. The closed valve echoes should form an anteriorly directed line during ventricular systole. Figure 2.12 shows the influence of inspiration on the echocardiogram. During that phase of respiration the expansion of the lungs introduces artifacts which obscure the proper recording of the motion of the mitral valve. Figure 2.13 is a scan from the aorta to the left ventricular apex in a normal subject showing the normal motion of the various cardiac structures. During ventricular systole the septum moves posteriorly as the left ventricular posterior wall moves

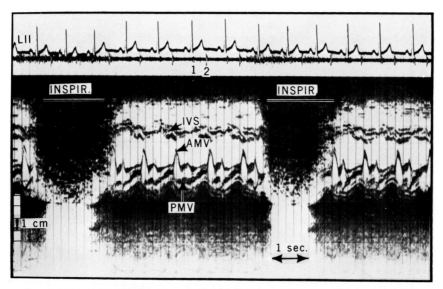

Fig. 2.12. Echocardiogram recorded at the mitral valve of a 29-year-old normal subject showing mitral valve motion. During inspiration the tracing becomes very dark and obscures visualization of mitral valve motion (see text). *INSPIR* = inspiration, *PMV* = posterior mitral valve.

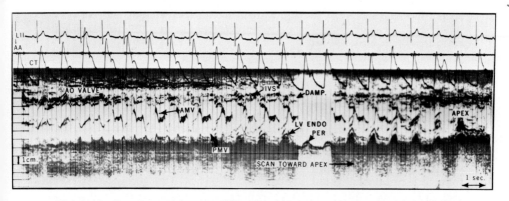

Fig. 2.13. Simultaneously recorded echocardiogram, carotid pulse tracing (*CT*), aortic (*AA*) area phonocardiogram and lead II (*LII*) of the electrocardiogram in a 22-year-old normal subject. The echocardiogram shows an M-scan from the aortic valve to the apex of the left ventricle. There is continuity of the anterior wall of the aorta with the interventricular septum (*IVS*) and of the posterior aortic root with the anterior mitral valve (*AMV*). This tracing indicates the influence of damping on visualization of cardiac structures. By increasing the damping the pericardium (*PER*) is well seen on the right side of the illustration (see text). *PMV* = posterior mitral valve, *LV ENDO* = left ventricular endocardium.

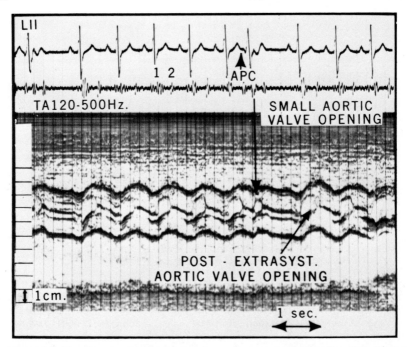

Fig. 2.14. Simultaneously recorded echocardiogram at the aortic valve, tricuspid (*TA*) area phonocardiogram and lead II (*LII*) of the electrocardiogram in a 72-year-old normal subject. Two atrial premature contractions (*APC*) were recorded quite early in the diastolic phase of the cardiac cycle. They result in a very small opening of the aortic valve as compared with the preceding sinus beats. Note the normal, boxlike structure of the aortic valve. There is a slight increase in the aortic valve size in the postextrasystolic beat (see text).

anteriorly. This simply means that the walls of the left ventricle contract toward each other with each heart beat. The normal interventricular septal thickness should not exceed 1.1 cm in the supine position and, normally, it moves slightly less than the posterior left ventricular wall. The normal range of septal motion measured from the standard position through the lower portion of the mitral valve is 0.3–0.8 cm. The amplitude of motion of the left ventricular posterior wall through this same area should be 0.9–1.4 cm. It is important to measure these structures from the standard location, because the interventricular septal motion is usually paradoxical as one angles the echocardiographic transducer too far superiorly. This is due to the fact that the septum follows the normal motion of the aortic root in this area. The normal values for the various measurements made in the echocardiogram are shown in the appendix.

The best recording of the aortic valve should be taken from position 4 and this can be accomplished by angling the transducer medially and toward the right shoulder. In this position the ultrasonic beam passes first through the right ventricular outflow tract, the anterior wall of the aorta, and the aortic cusps. These cusps form a box-shaped structure during systole and a single line during diastole (fig. 2.14). Behind the aortic valve is the posterior wall of the aorta. Note that the normal aortic echoes are thin and occupy the major portion of the aortic root during systole.

The standard left atrial measurement should be taken at the end of systole, at the time of aortic valve closure, from the posterior aortic wall and the left atrial wall. In general, the aortic root and the left atrial dimension should be equal.

An example of the "M-scan" or motion-scan is shown in figure 2.13. The transducer is aimed initially at the aortic area, then angled laterally and inferiorly through the mitral valve and, finally, down through the left ventricle toward the apex of the heart. In this manner the continuity between the anterior aorta and interventricular septum can be appreciated and the anatomic continuity between the posterior aortic wall and the anterior leaflet of the mitral valve can be seen. The shape and size of the ventricle can also be appreciated.

A recording of a tricuspid valve is shown in figures 2.15 and 2.16. Tricuspid valve motion is found by angling the transducer medially from the mitral valve. The tricuspid valve will appear on top of the aortic valve echoes. The echocardiographic features are essentially identical to the mitral valve echoes.

A recording of the pulmonic valve echoes is shown in figure 2.17. The pulmonic valve, like the aortic valve, opens during systole and closes during diastole. Usually, only the posterior leaflet of the pulmonic valve is recordable. The complete box-shaped valve, similar to the motion of the aortic valve, is rarely recorded in normal subjects. The initial downward deflection of the pulmonic valve recording is caused by right atrial contraction and is called the A wave. As the pulmonic valve opens, it forms the box-shaped structure.

After emphasizing the technical aspects and the normal motion of the cardiac structures as seen with sonic echocardiography, it is important to briefly mention other conventional concepts which are currently under investigation by others. These modalities include the two dimensional sector scan concept and the linear array multielement transducer technique. Both of these methods produce two dimensional images of the heart in real time. Current investigational studies have indicated that these methods may have certain advantages over the single element unidimensional technique. These studies have suggested the improvement in visualizing structural cardiac abnormalities in patients with congenital heart disease, a more qualitative analysis of valve motion in

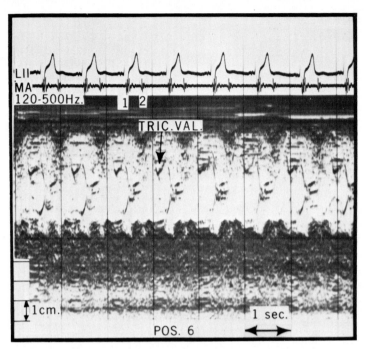

Fig. 2.15. Simultaneously recorded echocardiogram of a normal tricuspid valve, mitral (*MA*) area phonocardiogram and lead II (*LII*) of the electrocardiogram. The contour of the tricuspid valve is similar to the contour of a mitral valve.

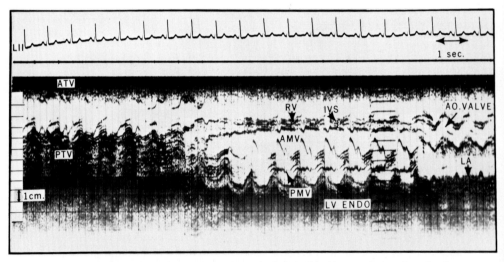

Fig. 2.16. Echocardiographic scan from the tricuspid valve to the aortic valve in a 31-year-old normal subject. Note normal motion of the anterior (*ATV*) and posterior (*PTV*) tricuspid valve (see text). *AMV* = anterior mitral valve, *PMV* = posterior mitral valve, *IVS* = interventricular septum, *LV ENDO* = left ventricular endocardium, *AO VALVE* aortic valve, *LA* = left atrium.

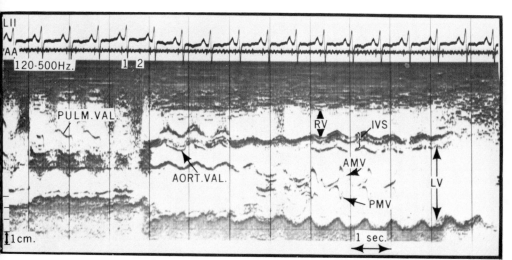

Fig. 2.17. Simultaneously recorded echocardiogram, aortic (*AA*) area phonocardi-ogram and lead II (*LII*) of the electrocardiogram in a 48-year-old woman showing a scan from a normal pulmonic valve (*PULM, VAL*) to the left ventricle (*LV*) (see text). *AORT. VAL* = *aortic valve, RV* = right ventricle, *AMV* = anterior mitral valve, *PMV* = posterior mitral valve, *IVS* = interventricular septum.

patients with valvular heart disease, and the ability to recognize left ventricular wall motion more accurately as well as better accuracy in determining the mitral valve orifice area.

These new concepts are still investigational, and many technical problems in precise resolution of cardiac structures and photographic recording and display features must be resolved before this non-invasive technique can be added to the diagnostic armamentarium.

DOPPLER FLOWMETER TECHNIQUE

Arterial or venous flow velocities have been measured using the trans-cutaneous, and implanted technique or with the use of an intracardiac catheter placed in the various intracardiac chambers or circulatory beds in man. The Doppler ultrasonic flowmeter telemetry system used in our studies was developed by Franklin and has been previously described in detail. The technique, briefly, utilizes the Doppler shift principle. A high frequency sound (7 to 10 mega-Hertz) is coupled to the skin or to the blood vessel wall by means of a piezoelectric crystal. Part of the emitted sound is backscattered and detected by a receiving crystal (figs. 2.18–2.20). The reflected signal differs in frequency from the incident signal by a quantity which is proportional to the velocity of the target, i.e., blood cells. Thus the shift in frequency is proportional to blood

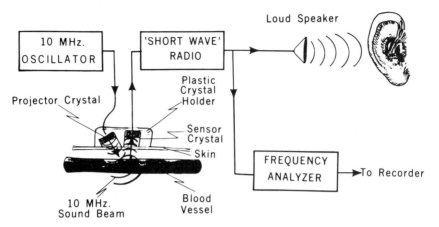

Fig. 2.18. Schematic representation of the Franklin ultrasonic Doppler flowmeter (see text).

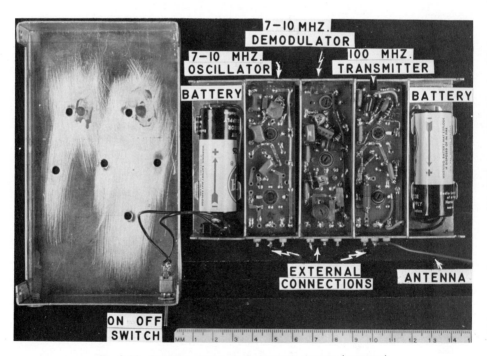

Fig. 2.19. Doppler ultrasonic flowmeter system (see text).

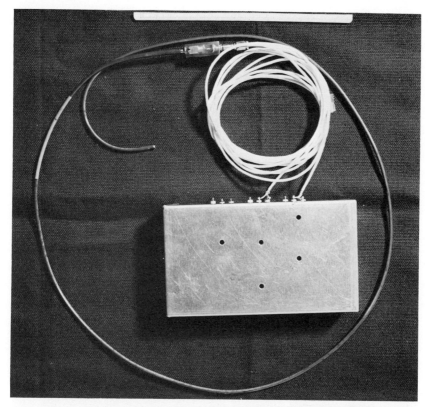

Fig. 2.20. Connection of the intracardiac flowmeter catheter with the Franklin Doppler ultrasonic flowmeter as used to record phasic blood velocities in the various circulatory beds during cardiac catheterization (see text).

velocity. The equipment used in this study consists of a basic flowmeter unit built at Franklin's laboratory. The flowmeter signal is received by any high quality FM tuner amplifier through a standard FM dipole antenna. The demodulated signal is in the audio range and is fed through the "tape" out jack simultaneously to any high quality loudspeaker and a Krohn-Hite band pass filter Model 310C. For analog readout the filtered output is fed to a Vidar frequency to voltage converter Model 320 where the signal is converted to a DC voltage proportional to the frequency of the received signal. An additional filter is necessary at the output of the Vidar unit to smooth out the DC wave form. A 35K ohm resistor across two grounded 1.0 microfarad capacitors accomplishes this final filtering. The output of the frequency to voltage converter can be fed to an oscilloscope or any recorder for analog readout. Calibration is achieved

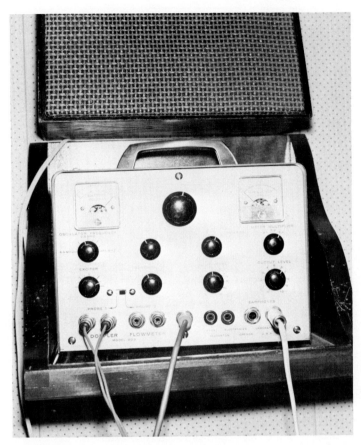

Fig. 2.21. Doppler flowmeter used for transcutaneous measurements of arterial and venous blood velocities (see text).

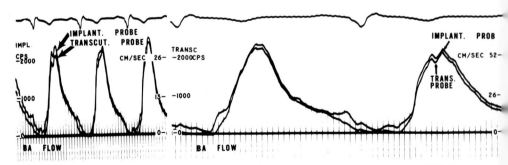

Fig. 2.22. Simultaneous recording of the phasic brachial artery (*BA FLOW*) flow velocity with the probe implant around the brachial artery and a second probe placed transcutaneously over the vessel. Note the similarity of the wave form on these two tracings (see text).

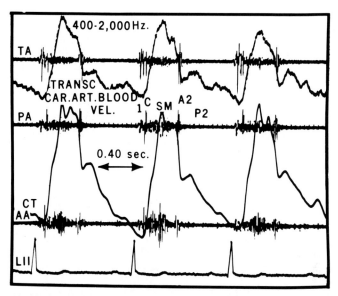

Fig. 2.23. Simultaneously recorded phonocardiogram at the tricuspid (TA), pulmonic (PA) and aortic (AA) areas, carotid pulse tracing (CT), lead II (LII) of the electrocardiogram and transcutaneous carotid artery blood velocity in a 31-year-old patient with aortic valvular stenosis. Note the typical auscultatory findings for patients with aortic valvular stenosis which include the presence of a systolic ejection click followed by a high frequency, high amplitude systolic ejection murmur (SM) recorded in all precordial areas. The carotid pulse tracing shows decreased upstroke time, increased ejection time and a carotid shudder. The transcutaneous carotid artery blood velocity tracing shows decreased upstroke time and prolonged ejection time (see text).

by taking a known frequency from a signal generator (Hewlett-Packard Model 651A) and feeding it to the input of the frequency to voltage converter and adjusting the gain of the DC amplifier channel of the recorder (Electronics for Medicine) to give the oscilloscope a deflection for any given input frequency. The velocity of blood flow can be computed by means of the Doppler shift formula:

$$\Delta f = \frac{2\,ft \cdot v\,\cos x}{c}$$

Δf = frequency shift expressed in cycles per second, ft = twice the transmitted frequency, v = velocity of blood, x = range between the transmitted frequency and the axis of blood, and c = constant speed of ultrasound in a given medium. In this case, soft tissue being 1.5×10^5 cm per second. The calibration figures can be expressed as a frequency shift

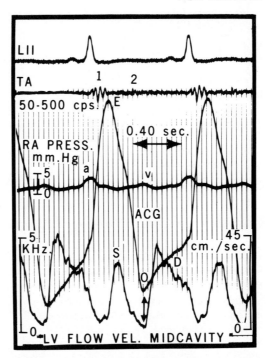

Fig. 2.24. Simultaneously recorded phonocardiogram at the tricuspid (TA) area, right atrial pressure (RA), apexcardiogram (ACG) lead II (LII) of the electrocardiogram and left ventricular flow velocity measured with an intracardiac catheter flowmeter placed near the tricuspid valve in a 44-year-old patient with coronary artery disease. The O point of the apexcardiogram coincides with the beginning of the upstroke of the diastolic wave in the left ventricular flow velocity tracing at the time of mitral valve opening (see text).

(CPS = cycles per second or Hertz) or calculated blood flow velocity (cm per second).

Zero flow is obtained by either occluding the vessel with outside pressure or by briefly disconnecting the input signal to the frequency meter.

For transcutaneous measurements, the transducer containing the transmitting and receiving crystals is placed over the skin at the area of the elbow overlaying the right brachial artery (figs. 2.21–2.24). The probe is positioned so as to obtain a maximally audible audio signal as heard by a loudspeaker or an earphone. When a stable signal is obtained, the transducer is secured in place by means of adhesive tape or rubber strap. For direct measurement of flow the inserted probe is placed around the exposed blood vessel. Several probes of different sizes measuring from 4 to 22 mm in diameter are used according to the outside diameter of the

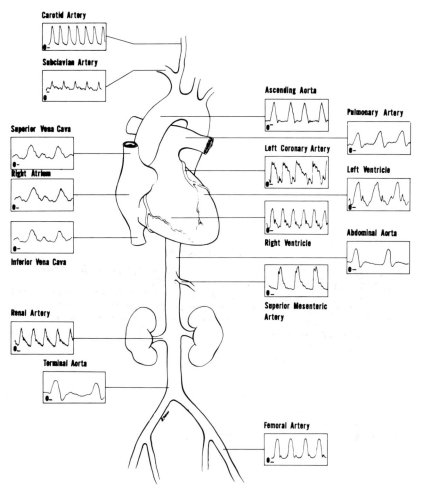

Fig. 2.25. Schematic representation of the phasic blood velocities in the various circulatory beds and intracardiac chambers in man using the Doppler ultrasonic flowmeter system (see text).

vessel. For human studies the probe size most commonly used is 4 or 5 mm in diameter for the brachial artery and 8 mm for the femoral artery.

In some cases the flowmeter curves are recorded during cardiac catheterization simultaneously with intracardiac pressures during right and left heart catheterization (fig. 2.25). As a routine, one or more intracardiac pressures are obtained simultaneously in a multichannel Sanborn tape recorder Model 3900 for storage of data. The original flowmeter audio signal is also recorded on tape. The tracings are monitored and recorded in a DR-12 Electronics for Medicine oscilloscopic photographic recorder at various paper speeds and time lines.

Clinical application of the transcutaneous Doppler flowmeter system at this time is not well recognized. Perhaps it will take several years before this new modality of the use of ultrasound becomes popular in the diagnosis of cardiovascular diseases. Presently, this technique is of value in the study of venous circulation such as deep thrombophlebitis of the lower extremities, peripheral arterial occlusive disease, abnormalities of wave form in carotid artery blood velocity such as those that occur in aortic stenosis, idiopathic hypertrophic subaortic stenosis, and in the examination of jugular venous blood velocity pattern. The transcutaneous recording is relatively easy to obtain and can be done by a skilled technician after proper training.

REFERENCES

1. Abelson, S.: Reciprocal movement of the right and left heart, demonstrated by directional Doppler ultrasound. Am. Heart J., *86:* 651, 1973.
2. Benchimol, A.: Arterial flow in health and diseased states. Proceedings of the 20th Annual Conference on Engineering in Medicine and Biology, *27:* 6, 1967.
3. Benchimol, A.: Blood flow velocity during ventricular fibrillation in man measured with the Doppler flowmeter technique. Chest, *60:* 265, 1971.
4. Benchimol, A., and Desser, K. B.: Clinical application of the Doppler ultrasonic flowmeter. Am. J. Cardiol., *29:* 540, 1972.
5. Benchimol, A., Ellis, J. G., Dimond, E. G., and Wu, T. L.: Hemodynamic consequences of atrial and ventricular arrhythmias in man. Am. Heart J. *70:* 775, 1965.
6. Benchimol, A., and Liggett, M. S.: Cardiac hemodynamics during stimulation of the right atrium, right ventricle and left ventricle in normal and abnormal hearts. Circulation, *33:* 933, 1966.
7. Benchimol, A., Lowe, H. M., and Akre, P. R.: Cardiovascular response to exercise during atrial fibrillation and after conversion to sinus rhythm. Am. J. Cardiol., *17:* 31, 1965.
8. Benchimol, A., Maia, I. G., Gartlan, J. L., Jr., and Franklin, D.: Telemetry of arterial flow in man with a Doppler ultrasonic flowmeter. Am. J. Cardiol., *22:* 75, 1968.
9. Benchimol, A., Pedraza, A., Brener, L., Buxbaum, A., Goldstein, M. R., and Gartlan, J.: Transcutaneous measurement of arterial flow velocity with a Doppler flowmeter in normal subjects and in patients with cardiac dysfunction. Chest, *57:* 69, 1970.
10. Benchimol, A., Stegall, H. F. and Gartlan, J. L.: New method to measure phasic coronary blood flow velocity in man. Am. Heart J., *81:* 93, 1971.
11. Bom, N., Lancee, C. T. Jr., vanZwieten, G., Kloster, F. E., and Roelandt, J.: Multiscan echocardiography; I. Technical description. Circulation, *48:* 1066, 1973.
12. Burggraf, G. W.: Left ventricular volume changes after amyl nitrite and nitroglycerin in man as meaured by ultrasound. Circulation. *49:* 136, 1974.
13. Edler, I.: Atrioventricular valve motility in the living human heart recorded by ultrasound. Acta Med. Scand., *370* (Suppl.): 83, 1961.
14. Edler, I.: Diagnostic use of ultrasound in heart disease. Acta. Med. Scand., *308:* 32, 1955.
15. Feigenbaum, H.: Ultrasonic cardiology. Dis. Chest, *55:* 59, 1969.
16. Feigenbaum, H.: Ultrasound as a clinical tool in valvular heart disease. Cardiovasc. Clin., *5:* 219, 1973.
17. Feigenbaum, H., Popp, R. L., Chip, J. N., and Haine, C. L.: Left ventricular wall thickness measured by ultrasound. Arch. Intern. Med., *1:* 391, 1968.
18. Feigenbaum, H., Popp, R. L., Wolfe, S. B., Troy, B. L., Pombo, J. F., Haine, C. L., and

Dodge, H. T.: Ultrasound measurements of the left ventricle; a correlative study with angiocardiography. Arch. Intern. Med., *129:* 461, 1972.

19. Fortuin, N. J., Hood, W. P. Jr., Sherman, M. E., and Craige, E.: Determination of left ventricular volumes by ultrasound. Circulation, *44:* 575, 1971.

20. Franklin, D. L.: Technique for measurement of blood flow through intact vessels. Med. Electron. Biol. Eng., *3:* 27, 1965.

20. Franklin, D. L., Schlegel, W., and Rushmer, R. F.: Blood flow measured by Doppler frequency shift of backscattered ultrasound. Science, *134:* 564, 1961.

21. Franklin, D. L., Schlegel, W., and Rushmer, R. F.: Ultrasonic Doppler shift blood flowmeter; circuitry and practical application. Proc. I.S.A. Biomed. Sci. Instrum. Symp., *1:* 309, 1963.

22. Franklin, D. L., Watson, N. W., VanCitters, R. L., and Smith, O. A.: Blood telemetered from dogs and baboons. Fed. Proc., *23:* 3030, 1964.

23. Goldberg, B. B.: Suprasternal ultrasonography. J.A.M.A., *215:* 245, 1971.

24. Gramiak, R., and Shah, P. M.: Detection of intracardiac blood flow by pulsed echo-ranging ultrasound. Radiology, *100:* 415: 1971.

25. Gramiak, R., Shah, P. M., and Kramer, D. H.: Ultrasound cardiography; contrast studies in anatomy and function. Radiology, *92:* 939, 1969.

26. Griffith, J. M., and Henry, W. L.: A sector scanner for real time two dimensional echocardiography. Circulation, *49:* 1147, 1974.

27. Hirata, T., Wolfe, S. B., Popp, R. L., Helmen, C. H., and Feigenbaum, H.: Estimation of left atrial size using ultrasound. Am. Heart J., *78:* 43, 1969.

28. Joyner, C. R., and Reid, J. M.: Application of ultrasound in cardiology and cardiovascular physiology. Prog. Cardiovasc. Dis., *5:* 482, 1963.

29. King, D. L.: Real-time cross-sectional ultrasonic imaging of the heart using a linear array multi-element transducer. J. Clin. Ultrasound, *1:* 196, 1973.

30. Kloster, F. E., Roelandt, J., tenCate, F. J., Bom, N., and Hugenholtz, P. G.: Multiscan echocardiography; II. Technique and initial clinical results. Circulation, *48:* 1075, 1973.

31. Kraunz, R. F., and Kennedy, J. W.: Ultrasonic determination of left ventricular wall motion in normal man. Am. Heart J., *79:* 36, 1970.

32. Kraunz, R. F., and Ryan, T. J.: Ultrasound measurements of ventricular wall motion following administration of vasoactive drugs. Am. J. Cardiol., *27:* 464, 1971.

33. Kremkau, F. W., Gramiak, R., Carstensen, E. L., Shah, P. M., and Kramer, D. H.: Ultrasonic detection of cavitation at catheter tips. Am. J. Roentgenol. Radium Ther. Nucl. Med., *110:* 177, 1970.

34. Lundstrom, N. R.: Clinical applications of echocardiography in infants and children; I. Investigations of infants and children without heart disease. Acta Paediat. Scand. *63:* 23, 1974.

35. Lundstrom, N. R.: Clinical applications of echocardiography in infants and children. II. Estimation of aortic root diameter and left atrial size: a comparison between echocardiography and angiocardiography. Acta. Paediatr. Scand., *63:* 33, 1974.

36. Lundstrom, N., and Edler, I.: Ultrasound in infants and children. Acta. Paediatr. Scand., *60:* 116, 1971.

37. Maroon, J. C., Campbell, R. L., and Dyken, M. L.: Internal carotid artery occlusion diagnosed by Doppler ultrasound. Stroke, *1:* 122, 1970.

38. Morris, J. J., Entman, M., North, W. C., Kong, V., and McIntosh, H.: Changes in cardiac output with reversion of atrial fibrillation to sinus rhythm. Circulation, *31:* 670, 1965.

39. Pombo, J., Russell, R. O. Jr., Rackley, C. B., and Foster, G. L.: Comparison of stroke volume and cardiac output determination by ultrasound and dye dilution in acute myocardial infarction. Am. J. Cardiol., *27:* 630, 1971.

40. Roelandt, J., Kloster, F. E., tenCate, F. J., vanDorp, W. G., Honkoop, J., Bom, N., and Hugenholtz, P. G.: Multidimensional echocardiography. An appraisal of its clinical usefulness. Br. Heart J., *36:* 29, 1974.

41. Roper, P. A., Desser, K. B., and Benchimol, A.: Clinical application of echocardiography. Ariz. Med., *32:* 265, 1975.

42. Samet, P., Bernstein, W. H., Medow, A., and Nathan, D. A.: Effect of alterations in ventricular rate upon cardiac output in complete heart block. Am. J. Cardiol., *14:* 477, 1964.

43. Saunders, D. E., and Ord, J. W.: The hemodynamic effects of paroxsymal supraventricular tachycardia in patients with Wolff-Parkinson-White syndrome. Am. J. Cardiol., *9:* 223, 1962.

44. Sjogren, A. L., Hytonen, I., and Frick, M. H.: Ultrasonic measurements of left ventricular wall thickness. Chest, *58:* 37, 1970.

45. Stegall, H. F., Rushmer, R. F., and Baker, D. W.: A transcutaneous ultrasonic blood velocity meter. J. Appl. Physiol., *21:* 707, 1966.

46. Strandness, D. E., McCutchen, E. P., and Rushmer, R. F.: Application of a transcutaneous Doppler flowmeter in evaluation of occlusive arterial disease. Surg. Gynecol. Obstet., *122:* 1039, 1966.

47. Strandness, D. E., and Sumner, D. S.: Application of the ultrasonic flow detector to the study of arterial and venous disease. Proceedings of the 20th Annual Conference on Engineering in Medicine and Biology, *27:* 5, 1967.

48. Tanaka, M.: Ultrasonic evaluation of anatomical abnormalities of the heart in congenital and acquired heart dieases. Br. Heart J., *33:* 686, 1971.

49. VanCitters, R. L., and Franklin, D. L.: The Doppler ultrasonic telemetry flowmeter; application in animal experiments. Proceedings of the 20th Annual Conference on Engineering in Medicine and and Biology, *27:* 7, 1967.

50. Waltenath, C. L.: Assessment of cardiovascular function during operation using Doppler technic. Am. Surg., *38:* 352, 1972.

chapter 3

Normal Heart Sounds, Pulse Waves

CARDIAC CYCLE

The cardiac cycle is primarily divided into systole and diastole. The systolic phase of the cardiac cycle is subdivided into: (1) pre-ejection period, (2) rapid systolic period and (3) slow systolic period.

The pre-ejection period grossly corresponds to isovolumic contraction time, which corresponds to the time when the atrioventricular (mitral and tricuspid) and semilunar (aortic and pulmonic) valves are in closed or semiclosed positions. As soon as the ventricles overcome pulmonic and systemic resistance, the semilunar valves open and the right and left ventricles begin to eject blood into the pulmonary artery and aorta (figs. 3.1 and 3.2). The rapid systolic emptying period corresponds to the first third of ventricular systole at which time the ventricles eject approximately two thirds of the stroke volume into the systemic and pulmonary circulations (figs. 3.2 and 3.3). This phase of the cardiac cycle is represented by a rapid rise on the arterial pulse tracing. A progressive decrease in ventricular emptying then occurs as ventricular volume and systolic pressure progressively decline to the point when ventricular pressure decreases below aortic and pulmonary artery pressures and the semilunar valves close. There is a good correlation between these changes in the aortic pressure and the phasic aortic flow as measured with electromagnetic or Doppler ultrasonic flowmeters. Peak aortic pressure corresponds to peak aortic blood velocity as shown in figure 3.3. As flow velocity and pressure decreases in the latter part of systole, the aortic and pulmonic valves close, producing vibrations corresponding to the second heart sound.

NORMAL HEART SOUNDS

The physiologic factors involved in the production of the first heart sound are still controversial. Most investigators believe that vibrations or

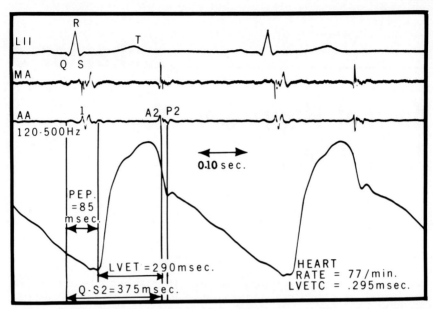

Fig. 3.1. Simultaneously recorded phonocardiogram at the mitral (MA) and aortic (AA) areas, carotid pulse tracing and lead II (LII) of the electrocardiogram in a normal subject demonstrating how measurements of left ventricular ejection time (LVET), pre-ejection period (PEP) and Q-S2 interval are made. The electrical-mechanical systole is measured from the onset of the QRS on the electrocardiogram to the first high frequency vibration of the second heart sound (A2).

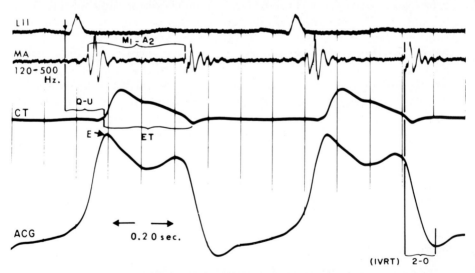

Fig. 3.2. Simultaneously recorded phonocardiogram at the mitral area (MA) at a frequency of 120–500 Hz, carotid pulse tracing (CT), apexcardiogram (ACG) and lead II (LII) of the electrocardiogram demonstrating the measurement of mechanical systole from the first high frequency vibration of the first heart sound to the beginning

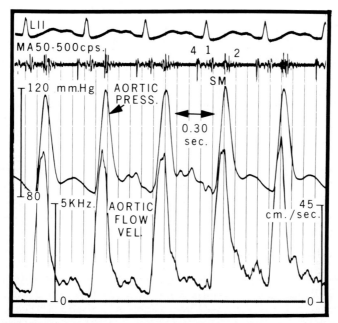

Fig. 3.3. Simultaneously recorded phonocardiogram at the mitral area (MA), lead II (LII) of the electrocardiogram, aortic pressures and aortic flow velocities measured with a catheter tip Doppler flowmeter. Note that the peak aortic velocity occurring in the early part of systole coincides with the maximal rise of aortic pressure.

transients of the first heart sound are due to closure of the mitral and tricuspid valves. Recent investigations have demonstrated that, in addition to the role played by motion of the mitral and tricuspid valves, acceleration and deceleration of the blood into the ventricular cavities as well as the contractile state of the myocardium play a significant role in the production of the first heart sound. The opening of the aortic and pulmonic valves seems to play a relatively small role in the vibration complexes of the first heart sound. The number of vibrations heard and recorded at the time of the first heart sound varies. There are at least three major components of the first heart sound (figs. 3.2 and 3.4). The first component, a low frequency vibration which occurs shortly after the QRS complex of the electrocardiogram, is due to ventricular wall

---

of the high frequency vibration of the second heart sound (M1-A2 interval). The Q-U interval is measured from the onset of the QRS complex on the electrocardiogram to the beginning of the upstroke of the carotid pulse tracing. Ejection time (ET) is measured from the first rapid rise of the ascending limb of the carotid pulse tracing to the dicrotic notch. Isovolumic relaxation time (IVRT) is measured from the aortic valve closure sound to the aortic component of the second heart sound to the O point of the apexcardiogram (2-O interval).

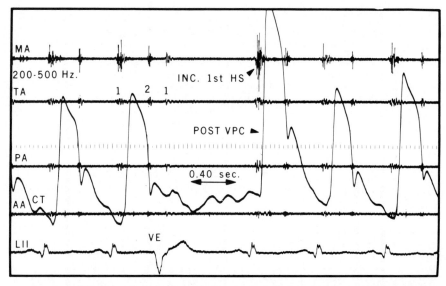

Fig. 3.4. Simultaneously recorded phonocardiogram at the mitral (MA), tricuspid (TA), pulmonic (PA), and aortic (AA) areas, carotid pulse tracing (CT) and lead II (LII) of the electrocardiogram in a 65-year-old patient. The first and second heart sounds are normal. A ventricular extrasystole (VE) was recorded. The post extrasystolic beat is preceded by a compensatory pause resulting in marked increase in the intensity of the first heart sound (HS). Post VPC = postventricular premature contraction.

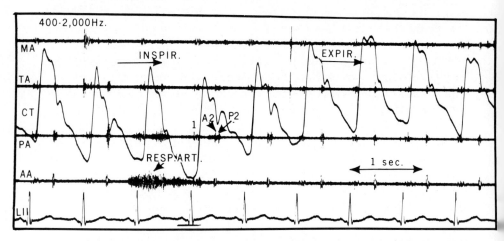

Fig. 3.5. Simultaneously recorded phonocardiogram at the mitral (MA), tricuspid (TA), pulmonic (PA) and aortic (AA) areas, carotid pulse tracing (CT) and lead II (LII) of the electrocardiogram during inspiration and expiration. Note the single second heart sound during expiration and physiologic splitting of the second heart sound during inspiration, best recorded at the pulmonic area. The aortic component of the second sound (A2) precedes the dicrotic notch of the carotid pulse tracing and the pulmonic component follows the dicrotic notch. RESP. ART = respiratory artifacts.

vibration, secondary to atrial contraction. It is called the atrial component of the first heart sound. The other two components have a higher
frequency and most likely are related to mitral and tricuspid valve
closure, respectively. In the absence of any turbulent flow, systole is free
of significant sounds.

SECOND HEART SOUND

The second heart sound corresponds to the time of aortic and pulmonic
valve closure. The aortic valve closes earlier because systemic resistance
is higher than pulmonary resistance. In most adult subjects the second
heart sound is single during both phases of the respiratory cycle. If the
second heart sound is single, the condition of the pulmonary valve and
pulmonary circulation cannot be well defined by the analysis of this
sound because it is probably due to aortic valve closure. Splitting of the
second heart sound may occur during inspiration (figs. 3.5 and 3.6) and is

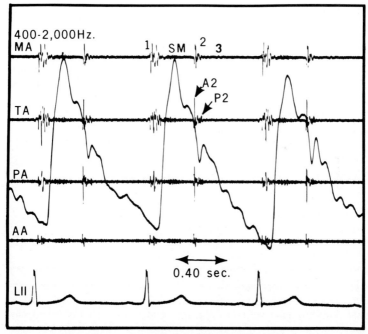

Fig. 3.6. Simultaneously recorded phonocardiogram at the mitral (MA), tricuspid
(TA), pulmonic (PA) and aortic (AA) areas, carotid pulse tracing and lead II (LII) of the
electrocardiogram in a 14-year-old normal subject. The first, second and third heart
sounds are normal. The second heart sound is physiologically split and both
components have normal amplitude. A high frequency, low amplitude systolic
ejection murmur (SM) is best recorded at the tricuspid and pulmonic areas. It has the
features of a functional murmur and the patient did not exhibit any cardiovascular
abnormalities during cardiac catheterization.

related to enhanced venous return and a decrease in pulmonary impedance thus delaying right ventricular systole. This is fairly common in young subjects, but disappears above the age of 30. Recognition of the two components of the second heart sound can be made with accuracy when the phonocardiogram is simultaneously recorded with the transcutaneous carotid pulse. The aortic valve closure sound (A2) precedes the dicrotic notch by 0.02–0.04 sec, and the pulmonary valve closure sound (P2) coincides with or follows the dicrotic notch by 0.01–0.03 sec. Amplitude of the aortic sound is usually twice as large as the amplitude of the pulmonic sound in the phonocardiogram recorded at the pulmonic and tricuspid areas.

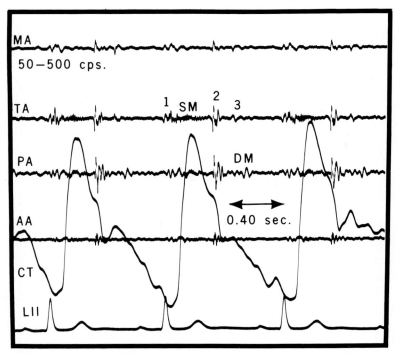

Fig. 3.7. Simultaneously recorded phonocardiogram at the mitral (MA), tricuspid (TA), pulmonic (PA) and aortic (AA) areas, carotid pulse tracing (CT) and lead II (LII) of the electrocardiogram in a 21-year-old patient who was 3 months pregnant. The first and second heart sounds are normal. A prominent third heart sound, recorded best at the tricuspid and pulmonic areas, is followed by a short, low frequency, early mid-diastolic vibration. There is a short, high frequency, low amplitude systolic ejection murmur (SM) recorded best at the tricuspid and pulmonic areas. This type of tracing is not unusual in pregnant women. The systolic murmur probably represents increased flow due to increased blood volume during pregnancy. The short mid-diastolic murmur (DM) may represent turbulent flow across either the mitral or tricuspid valve. The carotid pulse tracing is normal.

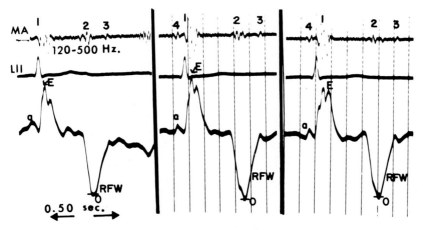

Fig. 3.8. Simultaneously recorded phonocardiogram at the mitral area (MA), lead II (LII) of the electrocardiogram and apexcardiogram in a normal subject. The first and second heart sounds are normal. The third heart sound coincides with the peak of the rapid filling wave (RFW) on the apexcardiogram. In the *left panel*, the apexcardiogram recorded at rest shows a normal A wave, sharp E point and normal systolic retraction. In the *middle panel* recorded 1 minute after a double Masters two-step exercise test the fourth heart sound becomes prominent. The post-exercise tracing coincides with the small A wave on the apexcardiogram. Four minutes after exercise (*right panel*) there is a third and fourth heart sound on the phonocardiogram which coincide with the peak of the A and rapid filling waves of the apexcardiogram.

THIRD HEART SOUND

The third heart sound is a normal physiologic finding in patients until about age 30 (figs. 3.7 and 3.8). Above that age, the third heart sound usually has a pathologic significance. This sound corresponds to the end of rapid filling of the ventricles, and coincides with the peak of the rapid filling wave of the apexcardiogram.

FOURTH HEART SOUND

Following the rapid filling phase of diastole, a progressive slowing of ventricular filling occurs until the atria contract. Atrial contraction causes an increase in flow velocity across the mitral and tricuspid valves resulting in larger ventricular volume. This rapid impact of blood against the ventricular walls creates the fourth heart sound. The mechanism for production of this sound and its clinical significance are still controversial. It has been shown that the fourth heart sound can be heard and recorded in a large number of normal individuals above age 40 (figs. 3.9–3.11). The fourth heart sound is best heard and recorded at the mitral area, but it is well transmitted to the aortic area (fig. 3.11). The fourth heart sound in older subjects seems to be the physiologic

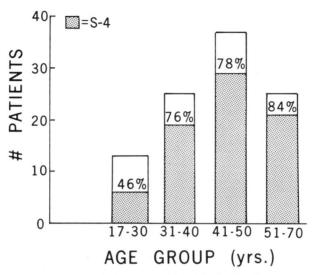

Fig. 3.9. Incidence of the fourth heart sound in a normal population proven by cardiac catheterization and coronary arteriograms. Note the high incidence of the fourth heart sound in the age group from 41 to 50 years of age.

counterpart of the third heart sound heard in the younger age group. The apexcardiogram is the best non-invasive technique to identify these diastolic sounds (figs. 3.12 and 3.13). The third heart sound corresponds to the peak of the rapid filling wave and the fourth heart sound to the atrial wave of the apexcardiogram.

NORMAL CAROTID PULSE

A normal carotid pulse is shown in figure 3.14. The carotid tracing follows the pattern of phasic aortic and carotid artery pressures and flow velocity curves. During early ventricular systole the left ventricle ejects most of its volume into the aorta, thus creating a rapid rise in the carotid pulse (fig. 3.14). The tracing reaches its maximal peak in early systole. The time interval from the beginning of the rise of the carotid tracing to its peak upstroke ranges from 0.04 to 0.10 sec. A progressive downward slope which follows the peak of the tracing is called systolic retraction. It corresponds to progressive decrease in the rate of flow across the aortic valve. The timing of aortic valve closure is represented by a sharp notch known as the dicrotic notch or incisura. The aortic component of the second heart sound precedes the dicrotic notch by 0.02–0.04 sec. This is a consequence of: (1) the delay in transmission of the pulse wave from the aorta to the carotid arteries and (2) delay in the propagated wave through the recording apparatus. The pulmonic component of the second heart sound coincides with or follows the dicrotic notch by 0.01–0.03 sec.

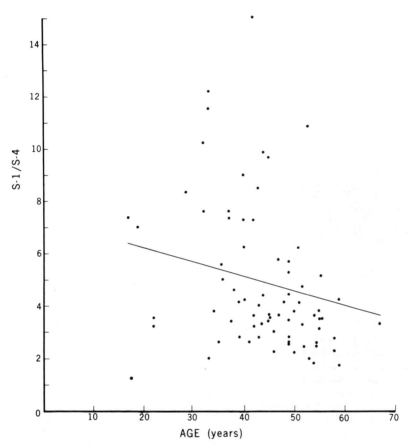

Fig. 3.10. First (S1) and fourth (S4) heart sound ratio in various age groups. There is no correlation of the ratio to age groups.

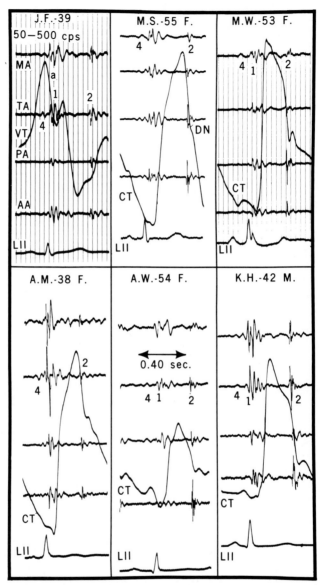

Fig. 3.11. Phonocardiograms at the mitral (MA), tricuspid (TA), pulmonic (PA) and aortic (AA) areas, carotid pulse tracing (CT) and lead II (LII) of the electrocardiogram in six adult subjects who had normal cardiovascular functions proven by right and left heart catheterization, and normal coronary arteriograms. Note the presence of a fourth heart sound in most of the recordings. The carotid pulse tracings are normal. There are no murmurs on the phonocardiograms. VT = venous pulse tracing.

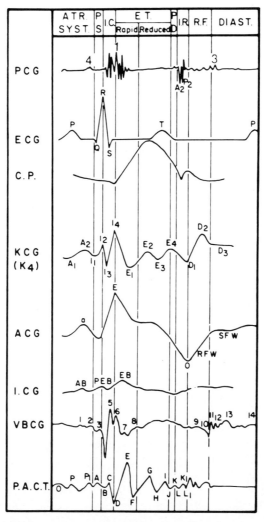

Fig. 3.12. Multiple recordings of the phonocardiogram (PCG) with the electrocardiogram (ECG), carotid pulse tracing (CP), kinetocardiogram (KCG), apexcardiogram (ACG), vibrocardiogram (VBCG), and impulse cardiogram (ICG) showing correlation of the various events of the cardiac cycle with wave forms of these tracings. ATR. SYST. = atrial systole, DIAST. = diastole, PS = pre-systole, IC = isovolumic contraction, ET = ejection time, PD = pre-diastole, IR = isovolumic relaxation, RF = rapid filling period, PACT = precordial acceleration cardiogram tracing (see text).

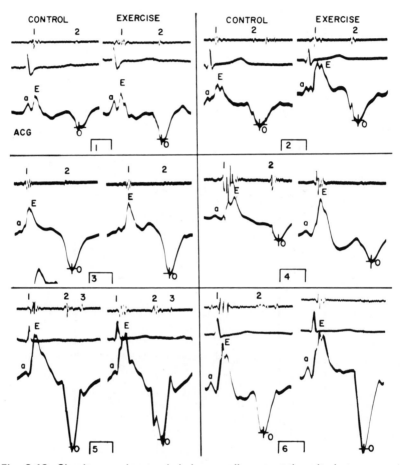

Fig. 3.13. Simultaneously recorded phonocardiogram at the mitral area, apexcardiogram (ACG) and electrocardiogram in six normal subjects. The tracings were recorded before and after double Masters two-step exercise tests. There is a small A wave on the apexcardiogram in the rest and post-exercise tracings. There is no significant increase in amplitude of the A wave on the apexcardiogram after exercise.

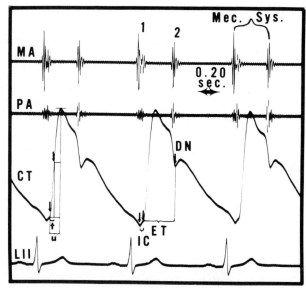

Fig. 3.14. Simultaneously recorded phonocardiogram at the mitral (MA) and pulmonic (PA) areas, carotid pulse tracing (CT) and lead II (LII) of the electrocardiogram showing how various measurements are made on the carotid pulse and phonocardiogram. Mechanical systole (Mec. Sys.) is measured from the first high frequency vibration of the first heart sound to the peak of the high frequency vibration of the aortic component of the second heart sound. Ejection time is measured from the beginning of the rapid rise on the carotid pulse to the dicrotic notch (DN). Isovolumic contraction time (IC) is grossly measured on the carotid pulse from the beginning of the rise of the baseline to the beginning of the upstroke. U time is measured from the beginning of the rise on the carotid pulse to the peak of this tracing. T time is measured from the beginning of the upstroke to the peak of the carotid pulse tracing.

The understanding of this time relationship is important in distinguishing normal physiologic splitting of the second heart sound (A 2 precedes the dicrotic notch and P2 follows the dicrotic notch) from reverse or paradoxical splitting of the second heart sound. In this condition, both components of the second heart sound precede the dicrotic notch. Abnormalities of the wave form of the carotid pulse in various disease states will be described in subsequent chapters. The wave form of the carotid tracing is essentially identical to the carotid artery pressure curve (fig. 3.15).

NORMAL JUGULAR VENOUS TRACING

The jugular venous tracing reflects the events occurring in the right atrium and right ventricle. The phasic wave form of the transcutaneous jugular venous pulse is identical to the pressure wave form of the jugular

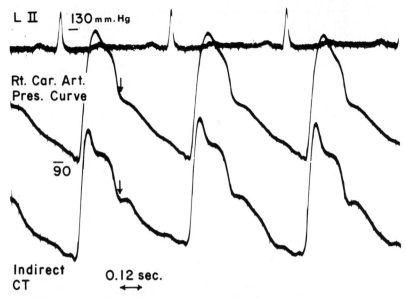

Fig. 3.15. Simultaneously recorded lead II (LII) of the electrocardiogram, right carotid artery pressure curve and indirect transcutaneous carotid pulse tracing (CT) in a normal subject. Note the essentially identical configuration of both wave forms. *Arrows* indicate the time of the dictrotic notch, representing aortic valve closure.

vein, superior vena cava and right atrium. The normal venous tracing shows two major waves, A and V, two descents, X and Y (fig. 3.16). The A wave corresponds to atrial contraction and is of value in identifying the fourth heart sound which occurs approximately at the peak of this wave. Following the A wave, there is a downward deflection called X1 descent, which is inscribed shortly after the first heart sound. In many patients, a small forward deflection is seen, called the C wave. The mechanisms for production of the C wave are not well understood. It is believed to be a "contaminated" wave from the transmitted carotid artery pulsations (fig. 3.17). However, at times this wave can be seen in records obtained from intracavitary right atrial pressures which raises the possibility that this wave may indeed correspond to intracardiac events. If a C wave is present, there is a secondary systolic retraction called X2 descent. The X2 descent continues throughout systole and terminates prior to the inscription of the second heart sound. At this point, there is a continuous upward deflection in the tracing corresponding to progressive increase in atrial pressure. The V wave is then inscribed and closely corresponds to the time of tricuspid valve opening. The peak of the V wave follows the second heart sound by 0.04–0.08 sec. Following the peak of the V wave, there is a progressive downward slope (Y descent) representing

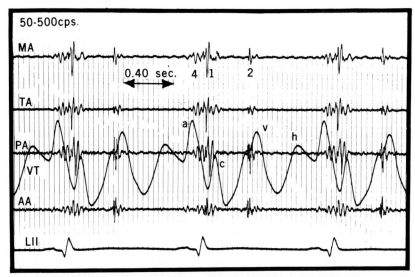

Fig. 3.16. Simultaneously recorded phonocardiogram at the mitral (MA), tricuspid (TA) pulmonic (PA) and aortic (AA) areas, lead II (LII) of the electrocardiogram and jugular venous pulse tracing (VT) in a 46-year-old male with coronary artery disease. The first and second heart sounds are normal. There are no murmurs. A fourth heart sound is recorded in all precordial areas, including the aortic area. The jugular venous tracing shows a normal amplitude relationship of the A and V waves, and normal X and Y descent. Note the presence of an H wave which precedes the A wave. The peak of the A wave coincides with the fourth heart sound.

rapid right atrial emptying. If a right ventricular third heart sound is present, the end of the Y descent nearly corresponds to the time of inscription of this sound. The Y descent of the jugular venous pulse is the physiologic counterpart of the rapid filling wave of the apexcardiogram. Following the Y descent, there is a progressive upward slope corsponding to slow right ventricular filling which terminates with the A wave or occasionally the H wave. The origin and mechanism of the H wave is not well understood. This wave is only seen when there is a long diastolic cycle length. It assumes clinical importance in patients with restrictive myocardial disease and other pathologic states that will be described in subsequent chapters.

APEXCARDIOGRAM

A normal apexcardiogram is shown in figure 3.18. The apexcardiogram is a low frequency recording of the vibrations overlying the apex beat (range 0.1–50 CPS).

The E point corresponds to the time of aortic valve opening and the

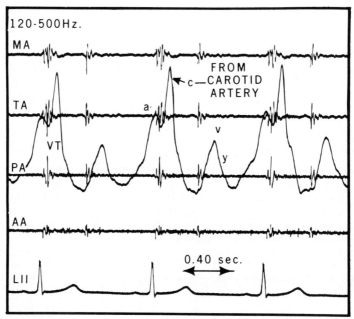

Fig. 3.17. Simultaneously recorded phonocardiogram at the mitral (MA), tri-cuspid (TA), pulmonic (PA) and aortic (AA) areas, jugular venous tracing (VT) and lead II (LII) of the electrocardiogram in a 14-year-old patient. This tracing demonstrates the importance of proper recording technique for the jugular venous pulse. When too much pressure is applied with the transducer over the jugular vein, one might record a prominent systolic wave, representing contamination of the tracing, from the carotid artery pulsations (c). The A and V waves on the venous tracing are normal.

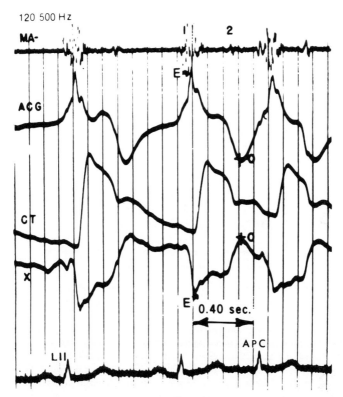

Fig. 3.18. Simultaneously recorded phonocardiogram at the mitral (MA) area, apexcardiogram (ACG), carotid pulse tracing (CT) and lead II (LII) of the electrocardiogram. The first and second heart sounds are normal. There are no murmurs. The tracing recorded with a transducer placed near the apex (X) demonstrates the importance of transducer placement to obtain high quality apexcardiograms. If the transducer is not placed exactly at the point of maximal impulse a mirror image of the apexcardiogram is obtained (X). The E point of the apexcardiogram coincides with the first heart sound. It is followed by a normal systolic retraction. The O point follows the second heart sound. The third beat on this tracing is an atrial premature contraction (APC).

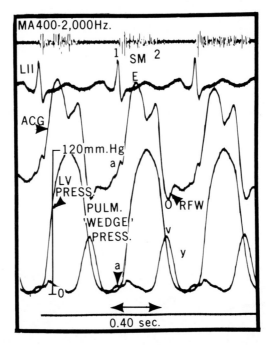

Fig. 3.19. Simultaneously recorded phonocardiogram at the mitral (MA) area, lead II (LII) of the electrocardiogram, apexcardiogram (ACG) left ventricular pressure (LV PRESS) and pulmonary "wedge" pressure in a 52-year-old patient with mitral insufficiency. The slightly diminished first heart sound is followed by a high frequency, high amplitude systolic regurgitant murmur (SM). The second heart sound is normal. There are no extra sounds on the phonocardiogram. The O point of the apexcardiogram coincides with a prominent V wave in the pulmonary "wedge" tracing. The A wave on the apexcardiogram and pulmonary "wedge" pressure tracing have normal amplitude. RFW = rapid filling wave.

beginning of ventricular contraction (fig. 3.19). This point has been well documented by simultaneous measurement of this tracing with intracardiac pressures, phasic aortic measurements and left ventricular blood velocity curves. After the aortic valve opens and ejection begins, the left ventricle decreases in volume, retracts, and moves away from the chest wall. In the apexcardiogram this is called systolic retraction, mid- or late systolic plateau. This retraction continues up to the point when the mitral valve opens. The O point (O = opening) is of value in identifying the opening snap of the mitral valve in patients with mitral stenosis. The validity of the O point corresponding to the time of the opening of the mitral valve has been questioned by some investigators. However, recent observations made with simultaneous measurements of the apexcardiogram and echocardiogram, as well as measurements of phasic left ventricular blood velocity at the mitral valve level, have shown that the O point very nearly corresponds to the time of the opening of the mitral valve or when left ventricular filling begins. This is shown in figure 3.20. Rapid left ventricular filling occurs in the first half of diastole. This phase of the cardiac cycle is represented in the apexcardiogram by the rapid filling wave (RFW) (fig. 3.19). The duration of the rapid filling wave measured from the O point to the peak of this wave is in the range of 0.06 to 0.14 sec. Following the rapid filling wave, there is a second wave in diastole, called the slow filling wave; this wave terminates with atrial contraction. The atrial contraction wave (A) corresponds to active atrial systole and is only present in patients with sinus rhythm (fig. 3.21). The total amplitude of the apexcardiogram follows the changes of left ventricular pressure and left ventricular flow velocity as shown in figures 3.22 and 3.23. Figure 3.24 shows how the apexcardiogram and phonocardiogram can be derived from a vibrocardiogram.

The A wave of the apexcardiogram has gained attention as a diagnostic tool in patients with coronary artery disease, congestive heart failure and any condition associated with diminished left ventricular compliance. Abnormalities of the wave on the apexcardiogram in various disease states will be discussed in subsequent chapters.

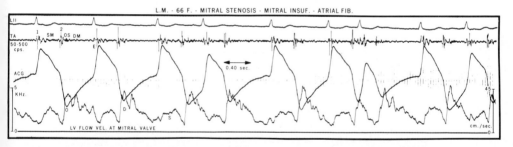

Fig. 3.20. Simultaneously recorded lead II (LII) of the electrocardiogram, tricuspid (TA) area phonocardiogram, apexcardiogram (ACG) and phasic left ventricular flow velocity recorded with a Doppler catheter flowmeter placed near the mitral valve in a 66-year-old patient with mitral stenosis and insufficiency and atrial fibrillation. The sharp E point on the apexcardiogram coincides with the first heart sound. The O point follows the aortic component of the second heart sound and coincides with the opening snap of the mitral valve. The rapid filling wave is absent due to mitral stenosis (see Chapter 4). Note that the O point of the apexcardiogram coincides with the beginning of flow across the mitral valve. In the recording of phasic left ventricular flow velocity, following the maximal diastolic rise in blood velocity across the mitral valve, the tracing gradually returns to near baseline. Systolic components of the flow velocity curves probably represent blood velocities being recorded by the catheter from the mid-cavity and outflow tract of the left ventricle (LV), or they may be due to regurgitant flow across the insufficient mitral valve. SM = systolic murmur, DM = diastolic murmur, OS = opening snap.

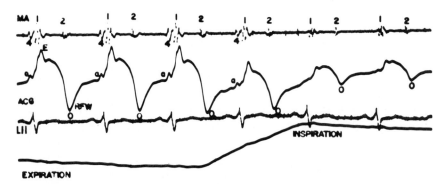

Fig. 3.21. Simultaneously recorded phonocardiogram at the mitral (MA) area, apexcardiogram (ACG) and lead II (LII) of the electrocardiogram during inspiration and expiration. The first and second heart sounds are normal. There is a small fourth heart sound which coincides with the small A wave on the apexcardiogram. During inspiration there is marked reduction in total amplitude of the waves on the apexcardiogram. This tracing illustrates the need for proper recording technique in order to avoid artifacts. In order to obtain a good quality tracing, it should be taken during held expiration. RFW = rapid filling wave.

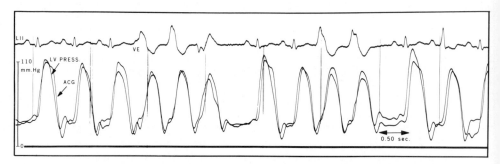

Fig. 3.22. Simultaneously recorded lead II (LII) of the electrocardiogram, apex-cardiogram (ACG) and left ventricular pressure curve in a 40-year-old patient with coronary artery disease during cardiac catheterization. The first three beats are regular sinus beats. Several ventricular extrasystoles (VE) cause a marked decrease in systolic pressures in the left ventricle (LV PRESS.). Note similarity in the wave form of the apexcardiogram and left ventricular pressure during sinus beats and ventricular extrasystoles. As left ventricular pressure falls during the ventricular extrasystole there is a significant decrease in the amplitude of the apexcardiogram.

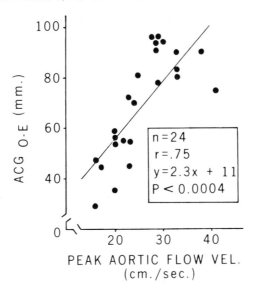

Fig. 3.23. Twenty-four heart beats recorded in a 48-year-old patient with mitral and aortic insufficiencies showing correlation of the total amplitude of the apexcardiogram (ACG) measured from the E to O point in millimeters of deflection. The peak aortic flow velocity curve is measured with a Doppler flowmeter placed at the ascending aorta. The patient had multiple atrial premature contractions (APB) during the recording. With the decrease in amplitude of the apexcardiogram there is a significant decrease in the aortic flow velocity curve (compare with fig. 3.22).

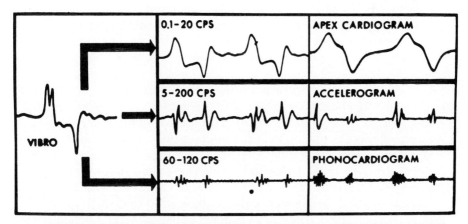

Fig. 3.24. Diagrammatic representation showing how various low and high frequency recordings can be obtained on a vibrocardiogram (VIBRO) using a variable band pass filter. (Courtesy of C. M. Agress, et al.: The common origin of precordial vibrations, American Journal of Cardiology, *13:* 226, 1964.)

HEART MURMURS

Heart murmurs are due to turbulent flow across the cardiac valves or blood vessels as discussed in Chapter 1.

Systolic Murmurs

There are two types of systolic murmurs: (1) the ejection murmur which starts shortly after the period of isovolumic contraction and (2) the regurgitant murmur which starts during the period of isovolumic contraction (figs. 3.25–3.27). The ejection murmur is due to stenosis of the semilunar aortic or pulmonic valves or due to increased flow across these normal valves as seen in patients with intracardiac shunts. Systolic regurgitant murmurs are due to insufficiency of the atrioventricular valves or can be seen with defects in the interventricular septum. These murmurs are described in detail for varying disease states in subsequent chapters.

Diastolic Murmurs

Diastolic murmurs are of two varieties (figs. 3.27 and 3.28): (1) arterial diastolic murmurs, which start during the period of isovolumic relaxation and coincide with the second heart sound. These murmurs are seen in patients with aortic or pulmonic insufficiency; and (2) atrioventricular murmurs, which start after the period of isovolumic relaxation, as seen in patients with mitral and tricuspid stenosis.

Atrial Systolic Murmur

This murmur is due to active atrial contraction. It is frequently present in patients with mitral and/or tricuspid stenosis and in some patients with congestive failure from any cause.

A diagrammatic representation of this murmur is shown in figures 3.27 and 3.28.

In the description of any murmur it is important to recognize its magnitude, location, transmission or radiation, and the frequency characteristics. The combination of all of these findings determines the best probability for the origin of the murmur. For example, murmurs of aortic stenosis may be best heard at the mitral area, but its ejection and musical qualities indicate that the murmur originates in the aortic valve and not at the mitral valve. Transmission of the murmur to the blood vessels in the neck is not necessarily an indication that the patient has aortic stenosis. The murmur of pulmonary valvular stenosis may also be transmitted to the carotid arteries. One must also be aware of the fact that the classical auscultative location of mitral, tricuspid, aortic and pulmonic valves does not reflect the anatomical position of those valves as determined by angiography.

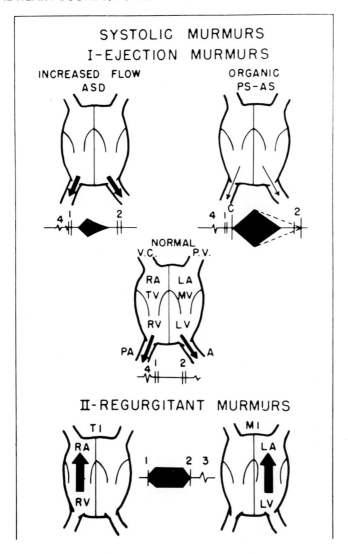

Fig. 3.25. Diagrammatic representation of the configuration of ejection and regurgitant systolic murmurs. Systolic ejection murmurs begin after isovolumic contraction time and there is usually a silent interval between the first sound and the beginning of the murmur. This murmur can be due to increased flow across the valve such as in atrial septal defects (ASD) or organic stenosis of the pulmonic (PS) and aortic (AS) valves. It is frequently preceded by a systolic ejection click (C). Regurgitant systolic murmurs begin with isovolumic contraction time and therefore, with the first heart sound, reaching a plateau in mid-systole and terminating with the second heart sound. They are frequently associated with a third heart sound. The murmur is due to regurgitant flow across the mitral and tricuspid valves as seen in patients with tricuspid (TI) or mitral (MI) insufficiency (compare with fig. 3.26).

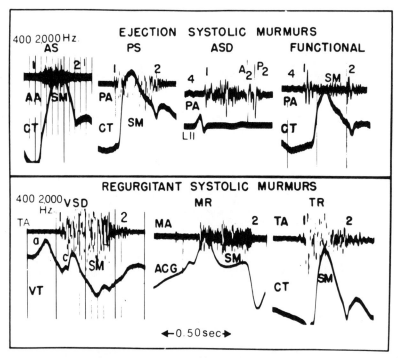

Fig. 3.26. Examples of typical ejection systolic murmurs seen in patients with aortic (AS) and pulmonic (PS) stenosis, atrial septal defect (ASD) and functional murmurs, and of regurgitant systolic murmurs seen in patients with ventricular septal defect (VSD), mitral (MR) and tricuspid (TR) regurgitation. AA = aortic area, CT = carotid pulse tracing, VT = venous pulse tracing, TA = tricuspid area, ACG = apexcardiogram, SM = systolic murmur, LII = lead II.

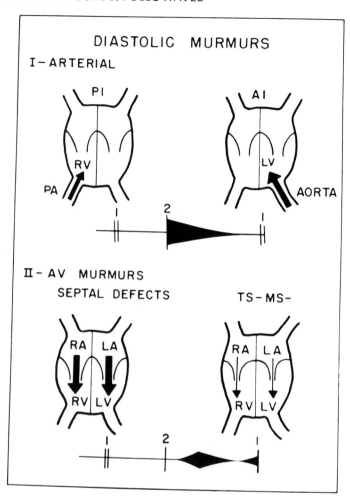

Fig. 3.27. Diagrammatic representation of diastolic murmurs. Arterial diastolic murmurs seen in pulmonic (PI) and aortic (AI) insufficiency start during the period of isovolumic relaxation, therefore, with the second heart sound. They have maximal intensity at this time of the cardiac cycle, progressively decrease in amplitude during mid-diastole, and terminate prior to atrial contraction. Atrioventricular diastolic murmurs (AV) seen in patients with left-to-right shunts are due to increased flow across the tricuspid valve secondary to the shunt. These murmurs start after the period of isovolumic relaxation, shortly after the second heart sound, at the time the mitral and tricuspid valves open. These murmurs have a maximal peak in mid-diastole and terminate prior to atrial contraction. Atriosystolic murmurs, due to active atrial contraction, are seen in patients with mitral (MS) and tricuspid (TS) stenosis. They begin with the P wave of the electrocardiogram and have maximal amplitude at the time of the first heart sound.

DIASTOLIC   MURMURS

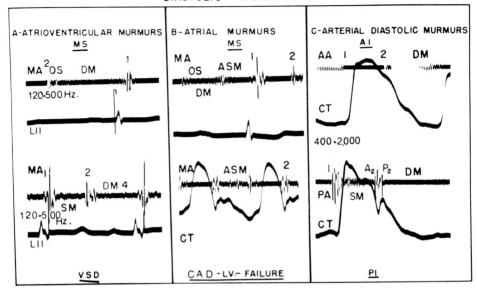

Fig. 3.28. Phonocardiograms demonstrating the various types of diastolic murmurs. Atrioventricular diastolic murmurs (DM) seen in patients with mitral stenosis (MS) are shown in *panel A*. This murmur starts with the opening snap of the mitral valve and terminates prior to atrial contraction. Atriosystolic murmurs, due to active atrial contraction (ASM) are shown in *panel B*. This patient also has first degree atrioventricular block, in which case the typical characteristics of atriosystolic murmurs are clearly seen. At the bottom of *panel B* an example of an atriosystolic murmur is shown. It was recorded with the carotid pulse tracing (CT) in a patient with left ventricular failure. *Panel C* shows arterial diastolic murmurs seen in patients with aortic (AI) and pulmonic (PI) insufficiencies. MA = mitral and AA = aortic areas, SM = systolic murmur, PA = pulmonic area.

References

1. Aygen, M. M., and Braunwald, E.: The splitting of the second heart sound in normal subjects and in patients with congenital heart disease. Circulation, *25:* 328, 1962.
2. Barlow, J., Pocock, W. A., Marshand, P., and Denny, M.: The significance of late systolic murmur. Am. Heart J., *66:* 443, 1963.
3. Benchimol, A., and Dimond, E. G.: The apexcardiogram in normal older subjects and in patients with arteriosclerotic heart disease; effect of exercise on the "A" wave. Am. Heart J., *65:* 789, 1963.
4. Benchimol, A., and Dimond, E. G.: The normal and abnormal apexcardiogram. Am. J. Cardiol., *12:* 368, 1963.
5. Benchimol, A., Fishenfeld, J., and Desser, K. B.: The atrial contribution to the left ventricular apexcardiogram. Chest, *62:* 322, 1972.
6. Benchimol, A., and Maroko, P.: The apex cardiogram. The value of the apex cardiogram in coronary artery disease. Dis. Chest, *54:* 378, 1968.
7. Brough, R. D., and Talley, R. C.: Temporal relation of the second heart sound to aortic flow in various conditions. Am. J. Cardiol., *30:* 237, 1972.

8. Bruns, D. L.: A general theory of causes of murmurs in the cardiovascular system. Am. J. Med., *27:* 360, 1959.

9. Coulshed, N., and Epstein, E. J.: The apexcardiogram: Its normal features explained by those found in heart disease. Br. Heart J., *25:* 697, 1963.

10. Craige, E.: Clinical value of apex cardiography. Am. J. Cardiol., *28:* 118, 1971.

11. Dalla-Volta, S., Vattaglagia, G., and Vincenzi, M.: Paradoxical splitting of the first heart sound. Cardiologia, *40:* 33, 1962.

12. Dickerson, R. D., and Nelson, W. B.: Paradoxical splitting of the second heart sound; an informative clinical notation. Am. Heart J., *67:* 410, 1964.

13. Dimond, E. G., Duenas, A., and Benchimol, A.: Apex cardiography. Am. Heart J., *72:* 124, 1965.

14. Faber, J. J., and Burton, A. C.: Spread of heart sounds over chest wall. Circ. Res., *11:* 96, 1962.

15. Ginn, W. M., Ross, R. S., and Baker, B. M.: Reproducibility of pre and postexercise electrocardiograms and apex cardiograms in subjects with and without coronary heart disease. Clin. Res., *10:* 390, 1962.

16. Gray, I. R.: Paradoxical splitting of the second heart sound. Br. Heart J., *18:* 21, 1956.

17. Grayzel, J.: Gallop rhythm of the heart. Circulation, *20:* 1053, 1959.

18. Kestleloot, H., and Willems, J.: Relationship between the right apexcardiogram and the right ventricular dynamics. Acta Cardiol., *22:* 64, 1967.

19. Kincaid-Smith, P., and Barlow, J.: The atrial sound and the atrial component of the first heart sound. Br. Heart J., *21:* 470, 1959.

20. Leatham, A.: A classification of systolic murmurs. Br. Heart J., *17:* 574, 1955.

21. Leatham, A.: Splitting of the first and second heart sounds. Lancet, *2:* 607, 1954.

22. Legler, J. F., Benchimol, A., and Dimond, E. G.: The apex cardiogram in the study of the 2-OS interval. Br. Heart J., *25:* 246, 1963.

23. Levy, A. M.: Innocent murmurs. Cardiovasc. Clin., *4:* 17, 1973.

24. Luisada, A. A., Szatkowski, J., Testelli, M. R., and Prieto, J. B.: Apical diastolic and presystolic murmurs of proved functional nature. Am. J. Cardiol., *4:* 501, 1959.

25. McKusick, V. A.: *Cardiovascular Sound in Health and Disease.* Williams & Wilkins Co., Baltimore, 1958.

26. McKusick, V. A., Webb, G. N., Humphries, J. O., and Reid, J. A.: On cardiovascular sound. Further observations by means of spectral phonocardiography. Circulation, *11:* 849, 1955.

27. Minhas, K., and Gasul, B. J.: Systolic clicks; a clinical, phonocardiographic and hemodynamic evaluation. Am. Heart J., *57:* 49, 1959.

28. Orias, O., and Braun-Menendez, E.: The heart sounds in normal and pathological conditions. Oxford University Press, New York, 1939.

29. Parisi, A. F.: Relation of mitral valve closure to the first heart sound in man; echocardiographic and phonocardiographic assessment. Am. J. Cardiol., *32:* 779, 1973.

30. Perloff, J. K., and Harvey, W. P.: Mechanisms of splitting of the second heart sound. Circulation, *18:* 998, 1958.

31. Rappaport, M. B., and Sprague, H. B.: The graphic registration of the normal heart sounds. Am. Heart J., *23:* 591, 1942.

32. Reinhold, J., and Rudhe, U.: Relation of the first and second heart sounds to events in the cardiac cycle. Br. Heart J., *19:* 473, 1957.

33. Rich, C. B.: The relation of heart sounds to left atrial pressure. Can. Med. Assoc. J., *81:* 800, 1959.

34. Rios, J. C., and Massumi, R. A.: Correlation between the apexcardiogram and left ventricular pressure. Am. J. Cardiol., *15:* 647, 1965.

35. Roberts, D. V., and Jones, E. S.: A new system for recording the apex beat. Lancet, *1:* 1193, 1963.

36. Robinson, B.: The carotid pulse; II. Relation of external recordings to carotid, aortic, and brachial pulses. Br. Heart J., *25:* 61, 1963.

37. Shafter, H. A.: Splitting of the second heart sound. Am. J. Cardiol., *6:* 1013, 1960.

38. Shah, P. M., Kramer, D. H., and Gramiak, R.: Influence of the timing of atrial systole

on mitral valve closure and on the first heart sound in man. Am. J. Cardiol., *26:* 231, 1970.

39. Shah, P. M., and Slodki, S. J.: The Q-H interval. A study of the second heart sound in normal adults and in systemic hypertension. Circulation, *29:* 551, 1964.
40. Simonyi, J.: The carotid derivative. Am. Heart J., *85:* 842, 1973.
41. Slodki, S. J., Hussain, A. T., and Luisada, A. A.: The Q-II interval; III. Study of the second heart sound in old age. J. Am. Geriatr. Soc., *17:* 673, 1969.
42. Spodick, D. H.: Prevalence of the fourth heart sound by phonocardiography in the absence of cardiac disease. Am. Heart. J., *87:* 11, 1974.
43. Tavel, M. E., Campbell, R. W., Feigenbaum, H., and Steinmetz, E. F.: The apex cardiogram and its relationship to hemodynamic events within the left heart. Br. Heart J., *27:* 829, 1965.
44. Tippit, H., and Benchimol, A.: The apex cardiogram. J.A.M.A., *201:* 549, 1967.
45. Voigt, G. C., and Friesinger, G. C.: The use of apexcardiography in the assessment of left ventricular diastolic pressure. Circulation, *41:* 1015, 1970.
46. Willems, J. L., De Geest, H., and Kestleloot, H.: On the value of apex cardiography for timing intracardiac events. Am. J. Cardiol., *28:* 59, 1971.

chapter 4

Mitral Valve Disease

Rheumatic fever is the most common cause of mitral valve disease. It usually takes several years for patients to become symptomatic. Congenital mitral stenosis and insufficiency are rare as isolated lesions but frequently may be associated with other congenital anomalies (see Chapter 9). Mitral insufficiency may also be seen in patients with coronary artery disease (see Chapter 8).

MITRAL STENOSIS

Auscultation and Phonocardiography

Heart Sounds

The first heart sound is accentuated and is analyzed best at the mitral area. A possible mechanism for accentuation may be that left ventricular contraction starts when left atrial pressure exceeds left ventricular pressure, prolonging closure of the valve. Therefore, the valve is held at its maximal opening position for a longer period, resulting in greater excursion of the valve. Amplitude of the first heart sound is at least twice that of the second sound at the mitral area (figs. 4.1 and 4.2) and is proportional to the length of the P-R interval, i.e., the shorter the P-R interval, the higher the amplitude and vice versa. With a short P-R interval the mitral valve is held wide open at the beginning of ventricular systole and a rapid rate of excursion may be responsible for increased amplitude of the first heart sound.

Calcification and/or thickening of mitral valve leaflets results in a decrease in amplitude of the first heart sound, and is probably due to a diminished rate of excursion of the leaflets (fig. 4.3). The second heart sound is usually split at the pulmonic, tricuspid or mitral areas (fig. 4.3). Amplitude of the pulmonary component of the second heart sound is normal providing that pulmonary artery pressure is normal or only mildly elevated, and the gradient across the mitral valve, at rest, does not exceed 5–8 mm Hg. With the development of pulmonary hyperten-

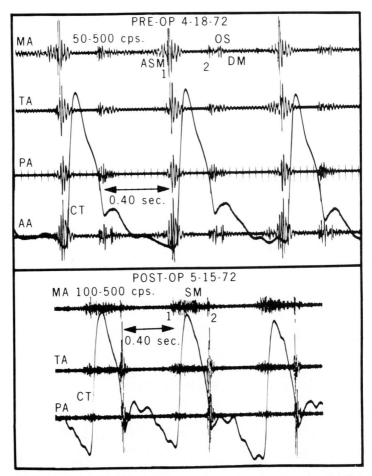

Fig. 4.1. Simultaneously recorded phonocardiogram at the mitral (MA) tricuspid (TA), pulmonic (PA), and aortic (AA) areas and with a carotid pulse tracing (CT) in a 39-year-old patient with severe mitral stenosis and sinus rhythm. Note accentuation of the first (1) heart sound (well seen at the mitral and tricuspid areas), the amplitude of which is at least twice as large as the second heart sound. The opening snap (OS) is present and the 2-OS interval is quite short (0.06 sec) followed by an atrial-ventricular diastolic murmur (DM) which terminates in late diastole. This murmur is then followed by an atrial systolic murmur (ASM) (presystolic accentuation of the diastolic murmur) which terminates with the first heart sound. The opening snap is well transmitted to the aortic area. The post-operative tracing, done on 5/15/72 following mitral valvulotomy, shows a systolic regurgitant murmur of mitral insufficiency. Ejection time measured in the pre-operative carotid pulse tracing recorded on 4/18/72 is slightly decreased.

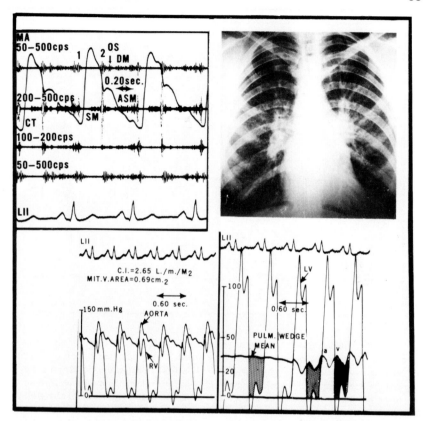

Fig. 4.2. Simultaneously recorded phonocardiogram at the mitral (MA) area with a carotid pulse tracing (CT) and lead II (LII) of the electrocardiogram. The phonocardiogram shown in the top panel was taken with a band pass filter set at 50–500 cycles per second and shows the typical phonocardiographic findings described in figure 4.1. The output gauge of the phonocardiographic amplifier was then connected to 3 other phonocardiographic channels with the band pass filter set at a frequency range of 200–500 cycles per second, 100–200 cycles per second and 50–500 cycles per second. These various recordings demonstrate the frequency characteristics of the diastolic murmur of mitral steonsis. The chest x-ray shows an enlarged left atrial appendage and dilated main pulmonary artery. Recording of the intracardiac pressure shows a marked degree of right ventricular hypertension and severe gradient across the mitral valve. CI = cardiac index, MTV area = mitral valve area.

sion with mean pulmonary artery pressure above 40–60 mm Hg, and a gradient across the mitral valve above 15 mm Hg, the second heart sound becomes single and accentuated. If the sound is split, the pulmonic component will be accentuated due to shortening of right ventricular systole, secondary to increased pulmonary vascular compliance which

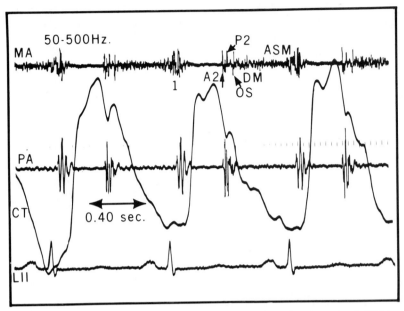

Fig. 4.3. Simultaneously recorded phonocardiogram at the mitral (MA) and pulmonic (PA) areas, carotid pulse tracing (CT) and lead II (LII) of the electrocardiogram in a 37-year-old patient with severe mitral stenosis, calcification of the mitral valve and severe pulmonary hypertension. The first heart sound is diminished. The typical atrioventricular disastolic murmur (DM) of mitral stenosis with an atriosystolic murmur (ASM) is recorded at the mitral area. Note transmission of the pulmonic component of the second heart sound to the mitral area, usually seen in patients with pulmonary hypertension and dilatation of the right ventricle (see text).

forces early closure of the pulmonic valve. When the second heart sound is split and there is moderate or severe pulmonary hypertension and right ventricular enlargement, the pulmonary component can usually be heard and recorded at the mitral and/or aortic areas (fig. 4.3). This may be due to abnormal anterior and rightward displacement of the right ventricle facilitating transmission of the sound to these areas. In these patients the "apex" of the heart represents precordial motion caused by right ventricular contraction.

In most patients with mitral stenosis, a high frequency vibration called an "opening snap" is recorded 0.04–0.12 sec after the aortic valve closure sound (figs. 4.1–4.6). The second sound-opening snap (2-OS) interval is grossly proportional to the degree of pulmonary and left atrial hypertension, and the gradient across the mitral valve. A very short 2-OS interval (0.03-0.05 sec) is usually indicative of severe mitral stenosis with gradients above 15 mm Hg (figs. 4.3-4.5) This can be confused with splitting of the second heart sound. A differential diagnosis can be obtained through simultaneous recording of the phonocardiogram and apexcardiogram (figs. 4.7 and 4.8). If the vibration represents P2 it should precede the O point on the apex tracing. If it represents the opening snap it should coincide with the O point. Following mitral valvulotomy with relief of stenosis the opening snap may disappear, or decrease in amplitude and the 2-OS interval prolongs (fig. 4.6). In the presence of a heavily calcified mitral valve associated with subvalvular stenosis, the amplitude of the opening snap diminishes (fig. 4.7) or may be absent. The opening snap closely coincides with the E point on the echocardiogram. Systolic ejection clicks are seen only when there is pulmonary hypertension with mean pressures exceeding 50 mm Hg. This high frequency sound has been attributed to rapid deceleration of blood during early right ventricular systole against a dilated main pulmonary artery or due to premature opening of the pulmonic valve. A third heart sound is not present in mitral stenosis unless there is significant

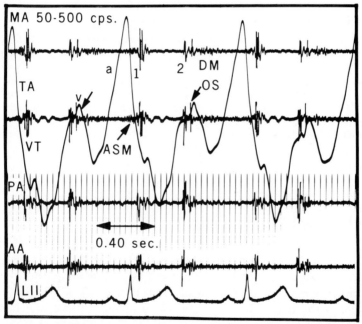

Fig. 4.4. Simultaneously recorded phonocardiogram at the mitral (MA), tricuspid (TA), pulmonic (PA) and aortic (AA) areas with a jugular venous tracing (VT) and lead II (LII) of the electrocardiogram in a 23-year-old patient with mitral stenosis and pulmonary hypertension. Note the typical phonocardiographic features in patients with mitral stenosis. The 2-OS interval is very short (0.05 sec). The jugular venous tracing shows marked increase in the amplitude of the A wave, exceeding the normal ratio of 1.5:1. In addition, the opening snap shortly precedes the peak of the V wave of the jugular venous tracing. DM = diastolic murmur.

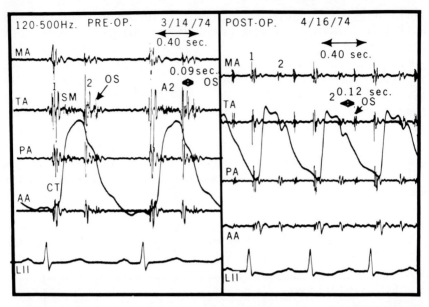

Fig. 4.5. Simultaneously recorded phonocardiogram at the mitral (MA), tricuspid (TA), pulmonic (PA) and aortic (AA) areas with a carotid pulse tracing (CT) and lead II (LII) of the electrocardiogram recorded pre- and post-mitral valvulotomy in a 48-year-old patient with severe mitral stenosis. The diastolic murmurs of mitral stenosis which were difficult to auscultate were not recorded in the phonocardiogram. This is not uncommon in patients with severe mitral stenosis. The pre-operative tracing shows the A2 (2)-opening snap interval of 0.09 sec. After relief of mitral valve obstruction, the second sound opening snap interval increased to 0.12 sec.

pulmonary hypertension and tricuspid insufficiency. In this setting the third heart sound most likely originates in the right ventricle.

Heart Murmurs

The atrioventricular diastolic murmur (diastolic rumble) of mitral stenosis starts with mitral valve opening, after the period of isovolumic relaxation of the left ventricle. This is a low frequency murmur (50–500 Hz) which reaches maximal peak in the first third of diastole. It corresponds to the maximal velocity of flow across the stenotic valve and maximal left ventricular filling (figs. 4.1–4.3). The murmur terminates prior to atrial contraction. In patients with sinus rhythm, a second, late diastolic murmur (atriosystolic murmur) due to active atrial contraction is present. It starts shortly after the P wave of the electrocardiogram and terminates with the high frequency component of the first heart sound (figs. 4.1–4.3). The shape of these murmurs usually follows the gradient across the mitral valve. The atriosystolic murmur, also known as pre-

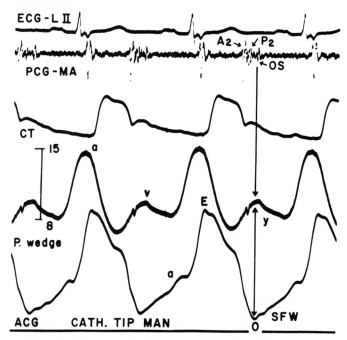

Fig. 4.6. Simultaneously recorded phonocardiogram (PCG) at the mitral area (MA), carotid pulse tracing (CT), pulmonary "wedge" pressure tracing (P. wedge) recorded with a catheter tip manometer (CATH TIP MAN), apexcardiogram (ACG) and lead II (LII) of the electrocardiogram in a patient with mitral stenosis. The opening snap coincides with the peak of the V wave of the pulmonary "wedge" tracing and the O point of the apexcardiogram. Note the marked increase in amplitude of the A wave on the pulmonary "wedge" tracing. On the apexcardiogram the rapid filling wave is absent. SFW = slow filling wave.

systolic accentuation of the diastolic murmur, is absent in patients with atrial fibrillation (fig. 4.7). With first degree atrioventricular block, the atrioventricular diastolic murmur terminates prior to the onset of the first heart sound and has "diamond" shape characteristics. Arterial diastolic murmurs of pulmonary insufficiency are uncommon in patients with mitral stenosis. If present, they occur late in the natural history of the disease. This high frequency diastolic murmur (Graham-Steel murmur) is frequently confused with the murmur of aortic insufficiency (fig. 4.8). Recent data based on pulmonary angiography and aortography have demonstrated that pulmonary insufficiency is uncommon in patients with mitral stenosis. In the majority of cases this arterial diastolic murmur represents regurgitant flow across an insufficient aortic valve. It has a decrescendo characteristic with a maximal peak occurring during the

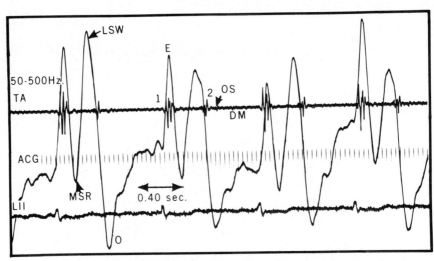

Fig. 4.7. Simultaneously recorded phonocardiogram at the tricuspid (TA) area, apexcardiogram (ACG) and lead II (LII) of the electrocardiogram in a 59-year-old patient with mitral stenosis and left ventricular dyskinesis. The first and second heart sounds are normal in the phonocardiogram. There is a low amplitude opening snap followed by a low frequency, low amplitude mid-diastolic murmur (DM). The apexcardiogram shows a sharp mid-systolic retraction (MSR) followed by a late systolic wave (LSW) as seen in patients with left ventricular disease. The rhythm is atrial fibrillation with a variable ventricular rate.

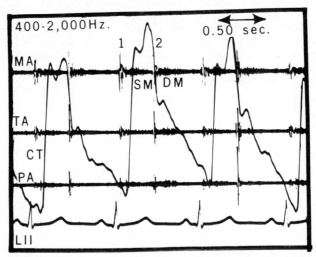

Fig. 4.8. Simultaneously recorded phonocardiogram at the mitral (MA), tricuspid (TA), and pulmonic (PA) areas, carotid pulse tracing (CT) and lead II (LII) of the electrocardiogram in a 29-year-old patient with mitral stenosis and pulmonary insufficiency. Note the accentuation of the second heart sound and the high frequency, high amplitude arterial diastolic murmur (DM) recorded in all areas. This murmur terminates prior to atrial contraction. The carotid pulse is normal. SM = systolic murmur.

period of isovolumic relaxation, i.e., at the time of the second heart sound. It diminishes during mid-diastole and terminates prior to atrial contraction. The murmur is best heard and recorded at the tricuspid and pulmonic areas with the patient in an upright or sitting position during maximal, held expiration. Increase in the amplitude of the murmur during inspiration helps to establish the diagnosis of pulmonic insufficiency.

Carotid Pulse Tracing

Simultaneously recorded carotid pulse tracings and phonocardiograms help to identify the systolic ejection click with occurs during the ascending limb on the carotid pulse. Mitral stenosis does not cause significant abnormalities in the wave form of the carotid tracing except that ejection time may be short (fig. 4.2).

Jugular Venous Pulse Tracing

The jugular venous pulse is normal in mild mitral stenosis and abnormal when the patient develops pulmonary hypertension or tricuspid insufficiency. When pulmonary hypertension is present the venous tracing shows a prominent A wave (arteriovenous ratio greater than normal value of 1.5:1) as shown in figure 4.4. Amplitude of the A wave is grossly proportional to the degree of pulmonary hypertension. Typical abnormalities of the venous pulse in tricuspid insufficiency are described in Chapter 6.

Apexcardiogram

The apexcardiogram is a valuable non-invasive technique for the diagnosis of mitral stenosis. It is important to identify the O point which should coincide with the opening snap of the mitral valve (fig. 4.6). In patients with a heavily calcified mitral valve, the opening snap is absent and the 2-OS interval cannot be measured. However, through simultaneous recording of the apexcardiogram and phonocardiogram it can be obtained by measuring the time interval from aortic valve closure (A2) to the O point of the apexcardiogram (see Chapter 3). This interval grossly represents the period of isovolumic relaxation of the left ventricle. Abnormalities of the systolic wave reflect abnormalities of the left ventricular contraction secondary to rheumatic myocardial disease. The changes noted are a rapid, downward displacement in early systole followed by a late systolic bulge (fig. 4.7). In these patients biplane left ventriculograms show localized areas of left ventricular dyskinesis, probably due to disease of the myocardium secondary to rheumatic process. It is important to obtain a technically adequate apexcardiogram (see Chapter 1) in patients with mitral stenosis and caution should be exercised in interpreting the tracing. Artifacts are recorded if proper recording technique is not used. We are able to record good apexcardiograms in only approximately 75% of our patients with mitral stenosis. A right apexcardiogram may be recorded in patients with mitral stenosis and pulmonary hypertension due to enlargement or dilatation of the right ventricle. If a good right ventricular apex tracing is obtained with the transducer placed at the fourth intercostal space or at the subxyphoid area it may show an exaggerated A wave and a sustained systolic wave.

Systolic Time Intervals

Ejection time is normal in patients with mild mitral stenosis. In the setting of severe stenosis associated with moderate to severe pulmonary hypertension, ejection time is diminished. This is probably due to a decrease in stroke volume and other parameters which determine the status of left ventricular function during the late stage of mitral stenosis. No definite data is available to determine the usefulness of measurement of the pre-ejection period (PEP) or the pre-ejection period/ejection time ratio unless the patient is in heart failure. In this case these indices will be abnormal. They usually will be identical to the findings seen in patients in heart failure of any etiology.

Echocardiography

Echocardiography is important for the evaluation of patients with mitral stenosis. The abnormalities include (1) decreased motion of the anterior leaflet of the mitral valve with a decreased E-F slope (figs. 4.9–4.11), except for patients with atrial fibrillation where the E-F slope varies considerably in relation to cycle length (fig. 4.12). In order to obtain an accurate measurement of the E-F slope at least 7 consecutive cardiac cycles should be recorded. Following mitral valvulotomy the E-F slope changes in proportion to the relief of stenosis (fig. 4.13). (2) The posterior leaflet of the mitral valve has a paradoxical motion, i.e., moving in the same direction as the anterior leaflet (anteriorly) which is the reverse of normal (figs. 4.9–4.11). Calcification or thickening of the mitral valve results in the recording of multiple and disorganized echoes (fig. 4.11). Gross quantitation of the degree of severity of mitral stenosis is possible to obtain by measuring the E-F slope. The E-F slope decreases progressively in proportion to the degree of the stenotic lesion. Measurement of diameters with this technique frequently shows an increase in size of the left atrium (fig. 4.14) and/or right ventricle. In patients with mitral stenosis and severe pulmonary hypertension, the pulmonic valve has an abnormal motion showing a small or absent A wave or "A dip." Caution must be exercised in diagnosing mitral stenosis using only

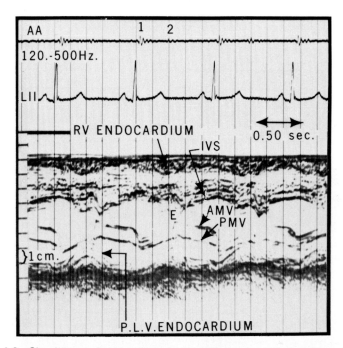

Fig. 4.9. Simultaneously recorded phonocardiogram at the aortic area (AA), echocardiogram of the mitral valve and lead II (LII) of the electrocardiogram in a 44-year-old patient with mitral stenosis. Typical echocardiographic features of patients with mitral stenosis are shown. There is a diminished downslope of the anterior leaflet of the mitral valve. The E point marks the opening of the mitral valve. Note the paradoxical motion of the posterior mitral leaflet which moves in the same direction as the anterior leaflet. This is the reverse of normal. The posterior left ventricular endocardium (PLV endocardium) is indicated. RV = right ventricular endocardium; IVS = interventricular septum; AMV = anterior mitral valve; PMV = posterior mitral valve.

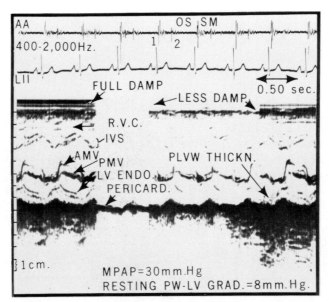

Fig. 4. 10. Simultaneously recorded phonocardiogram at the aortic (AA), area, echocardiogram and lead II (LII) of the electrocardiogram in a 26-year-old patient with non-calcific mitral stenosis and mild degree of mitral insufficiency. The typical echocardiographic features of mitral stenosis are seen. Note that the tracing is recorded at full damping and shows thickening of both the anterior (AMV) and posterior (PMV) mitral valve. With less damping, echoes derived from the mitral valve structure, pericardium and the posterior left ventricular wall (PLVW) are more evident. In this patient, the mean pulmonary artery pressure (MPAP) was 20 mm Hg. The resting pulmonary "wedge"-left ventricular end-diastolic gradient was 8 mm Hg. RVC = right ventricular cavity, IVS = interventricular septum, LV ENDO = left ventricular endocardium, Pericard = pericardium.

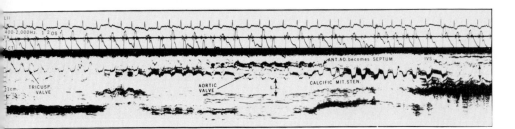

Fig. 4.11. Simultaneously recorded phonocardiogram at the tricuspid (TA) area, echocardiogram and lead II (LII) of the electrocardiogram in a 45-year-old patient with severe mitral stenosis. This is a scan from the aortic valve toward the apex of the left ventricle. The echocardiogram shows typical abnormal motion of the anterior and posterior leaflets of the mitral valve. Note that the anterior aorta becomes the interventricular septum and the posterior aorta becomes the anterior leaflet of the mitral valve. This patient has severe calcification of the mitral valve represented by disorganized multiple echoes derived from this structure. Different degrees of damping were utilized throughout the recording.(Note the good recording of the tricuspid valve shown at the left of the tracing). LA = left atrium, ANT. AO = anterior aorta, IVS = interventricular septum.

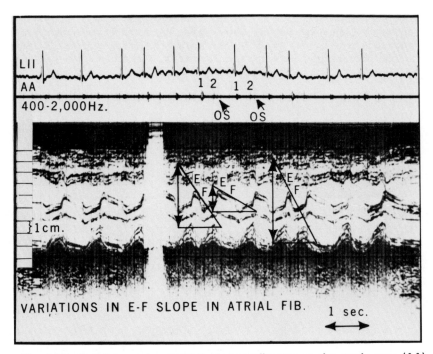

Fig. 4.12. Simultaneously recorded phonocardiogram at the aortic area (AA), echocardiogram and lead II (LII) of the electrocardiogram in a 48-year-old patient with mitral stenosis and atrial fibrillation. Note marked variations in cycle length resulting in marked variations in the E-F slope of the anterior mitral valve. In order to obtain reliable measurements of the E-F slope in patients with atrial fibrillation an average of 6–8 cardiac cycles should be recorded. OS = opening snap.

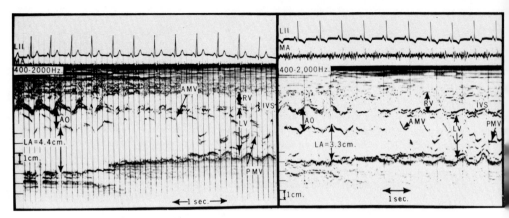

Fig. 4.13. (*Left panel*) Echocardiographic scan from the aorta to the mitral valve
in a 28-year-old patient with moderate mitral stenosis. Note abnormal motion of
the anterior (AMV) and posterior mitral valve (PMV) frequently seen in patients
with mitral stenosis. The left atrial internal diameter is increased to 4.4 cm (*Right
panel*) Echocardiographic scan from the aorta to the mitral valve approximately 2
months after mitral valvulotomy. Note a significant change in the motion of the anterior and posterior mitral valve. The pre-operative E-F slope measured 28 mm/sec
and the post-operative E-F slope was 73 mm/sec. The left atrial internal diameter
has decreased to 3.3 cm which is within the normal range.

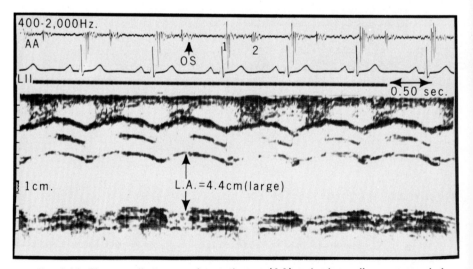

Fig. 4.14. Phonocardiogram at the aortic area (AA) and echocardiogram recorded
at the level of the aortic root in a 26-year-old patient with severe mitral stenosis.
Measurement of left atrial (LA) size is taken from this point and indicates an en-
large left atrium to 4.4 cm (normal range 1.9–4.0 cm with a mean of 2.9 cm). LII
= lead II.

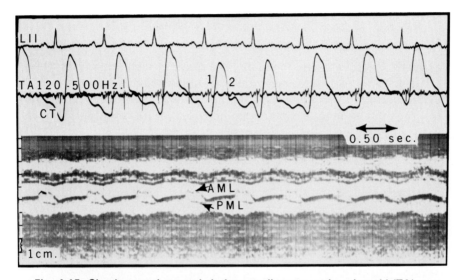

Fig. 4.15. Simultaneously recorded phonocardiogram at the tricuspid (TA) area, carotid pulse tracing (CT), echocardiogram and lead II (LII) of the electrocardiogram in a 63-year-old patient with coronary artery disease. At times in this condition the anterior mitral leaflet may show an abnormal motion with decreased E-F slope. However, the posterior leaflet of the mitral valve moves normally indicating that the patient does not have mitral stenosis. This recording emphasizes the importance of recording the posterior mitral valve motion in order to establish the diagnosis of this condition echocardiographically. Abnormal motion of the anterior mitral valve is frequently seen in patients with decreased cardiac output and stroke volume. AML = anterior mitral leaflet, PML = posterior mitral leaflet.

abnormalities of the anterior mitral valve motion. Good recordings of the posterior mitral leaflet must be obtained because other conditions, such as coronary artery disease or heart failure from any cause, can result in a tracing simulating mitral stenosis (fig. 4.15). Most cardiac arrhythmias will alter the pattern of the mitral valve motion as shown in figures 4.11, 4.12, and 4.16–4.18.

MITRAL INSUFFICIENCY

Auscultation and Phonocardiography

Mitral insufficiency is commonly the result of rheumatic fever. Other etiologic factors include congenital mitral insufficiency due to deformity of the mitral valve, prolapse of the mitral leaflets, mitral insufficiency due to papillary muscle dysfunction in patients with coronary artery disease, rupture of the chordae tendinae during acute myocardial infarction or penetrating injury or trauma to the chest.

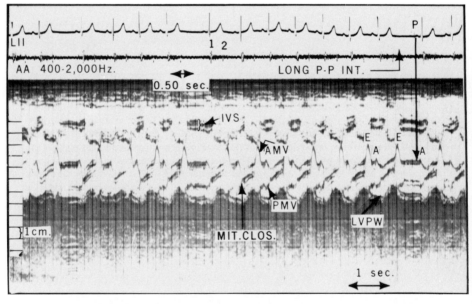

Fig. 4.16. Simultaneously recorded phonocardiogram at the aortic (AA) area, echocardiogram and lead II (LII) of the electrocardiogram in a 7-year-old patient with sinus arrhythmia demonstrating the influence of cycle length on mitral valve motion and the E-F slope. Note the rapid descent of the anterior mitral valve (AMV) with short cycle lengths as compared with a long plateau in the beats preceded by a long diastolic length. IVS = interventricular septum, PMV = posterior mitral valve, LVPW = left ventricular posterior wall. P-P INT. = P-P interval, MIT CLOS. = mitral valve closure.

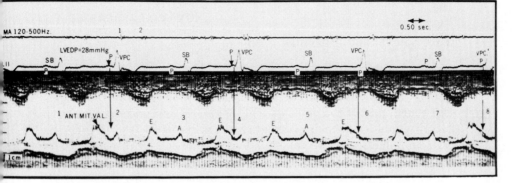

Fig. 4.17. Simultaneously recorded mitral area (MA) phonocardiogram, echocardiogram and lead II (LII) of the electrocardiogram in a 37-year-old patient with aortic insufficiency and elevated left ventricular end-diastolic pressure (LVEDP) to 28 mm Hg. During the recording, the patient had multiple ventricular premature contractions (VPC). Observe the marked variations in the pattern of the anterior mitral valve (ANT. MIT. VAL.) motion during the ventricular premature contractions. In some beats, it resembles the motion seen in patients with mitral stenosis. SB = sinus beats.

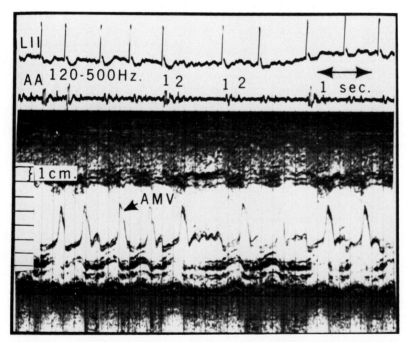

Fig. 4.18. Simultaneously recorded aortic area (AA) phonocardiogram, echocardiogram and lead II (LII) of the electrocardiogram in a 61-year-old patient with atrial fibrillation due to coronary artery disease. Note the coarse fluttering of the mitral valve which is seen in patients with atrial fibrillation. This is best seen in the motion of the anterior mitral valve (AMV).

Heart Sounds and Murmurs

The first heart sound is usually diminished in mitral insufficiency due to decreased excursion of the mitral valve secondary to a dilated mitral annulus (figs. 4.19–4.21). The second heart sound is normal. The third heart sound, part of the phonocardiographic and auscultatory findings in this condition, is due to increased diastolic filling of the left ventricle (fig. 4.19), and should not be taken as evidence of left ventricular failure. Fourth heart sounds are recorded in about 20% of patients with mitral insufficiency and they do not have any major clinical significance. The third heart sound coincides with the peak of the rapid filling wave (fig. 4.19) and the fourth heart sound with the A wave of the apexcardiogram. An opening snap of the mitral valve is present in 8 to 12% of patients with pure mitral insufficiency (fig. 4.20), and the explanation for its presence is unknown. The regurgitant systolic murmur of mitral insufficiency is a high frequency murmur which starts during the period of isovolumic contration, therefore, immediately or shortly after the first heart sound. The best way to recognize the beginning of the systolic murmur is by multiple simultaneous recording of the heart sounds with high frequency

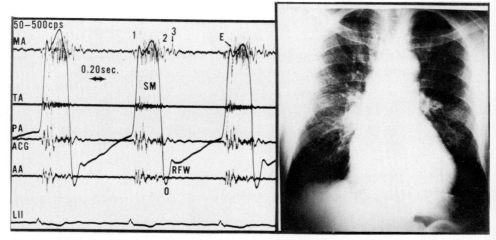

Fig. 4.19. Simultaneously recorded phonocardiogram at the mitral (MA), tricuspid (TA), pulmonic (PA) and aortic (AA) areas, apexcardiogram (ACG) and lead II (LII) of the electrocardiogram in a 68-year-old patient with severe mitral insufficiency. The first (1) heart sound is diminished. The second (2) heart sound is normal. There is a prominent third heart sound (3) which coincides with the peak of a prominent rapid filling wave (RFW) in the apexcardiogram. The high amplitude, high frequency systolic regurgitant murmur begins with the first heart sound and ends with the second heart sound. The patient's rhythm is atrial fibrillation. The apexcardiogram shows a prominent systolic wave. The chest x-ray shows an enlarged cardiac silhouette with left ventricular and left atrial enlargement.

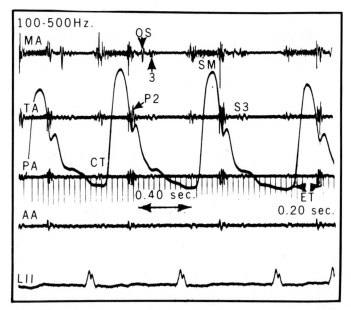

Fig. 4.20. Simultaneously recorded phonocardiogram at the mitral (MA), tricuspid (TA), pulmonic (PA) and aortic areas (AA) with a carotid pulse tracing (CT) and lead II (LII) of the electrocardiogram in a 63-year-old patient with mitral insufficiency. The systolic regurgitant murmur (SM) of mitral insufficiency is shown. The first (1) heart sound is diminished. There is an opening snap (OS) as well as a third heart sound (3). The carotid tracing shows a rapid ascending limb with a normal dicrotic notch. The ejection time (ET) is markedly diminished to 0.20 sec which is frequently seen in this condition.

filter setting. With logarithmic or log-log recordings, low frequency vibrations are eliminated and the beginning of the murmur may be easier to identify. This murmur has a continuous plateau during systole and terminates with the second heart sound (figs. 4.19–4.29). The amplitude of this murmur changes slightly during variations in cycle length in patients with atrial fibrillation (fig. 4.21), or during cardiac arrhythmias (fig. 4.22). In acute stages of bacterial endocarditis of the mitral valve, the systolic murmur of mitral insufficiency may be musical and will subsequently change in quality (fig. 4.23). In patients with severe mitral insufficiency the increase in diastolic flow across the mitral valve may cause a soft low amplitude mid-diastolic murmur.

Carotid Pulse Tracing

The carotid pulse is of little diagnostic value in mitral insufficiency. However, in patients with severe mitral insufficiency the carotid tracing

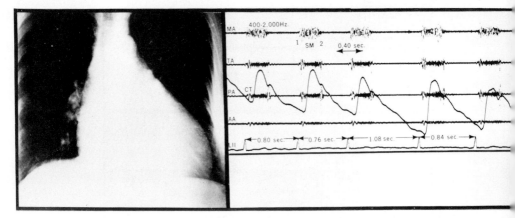

Fig. 4.21. Simultaneously recorded phonocardiogram at the mitral (MA) tricuspid (TA), pulmonic (PA) and aortic (AA) areas, carotid pulse tracing (CT) and lead II (LII) of the electrocardiogram in a 55-year-old patient with mitral insufficiency and atrial fibrillation. The first heart sound (1) is diminished. The second (2) heart sound is normal. There is a high frequency, high amplitude systolic regurgitant murmur (SM) which changes in amplitude in relation to cycle length. Note in the beats which are preceded by a long cycle length that the systolic regurgitant murmur increases slightly in amplitude. Measurements for each cycle length are indicated. The chest x-ray shows marked cardiomegaly with enlargement of the left atrium and the left ventricle.

may show a rapid ascending limb and diminished ejection time (figs. 4.20 and 4.27).

Jugular Venous Pulse Tracing

The jugular venous pulse is usually normal in patients with mitral insufficiency. When there is a significant degree of pulmonary hypertension there is exaggeration of the A wave.

Apexcardiogram

The apexcardiogram is abnormal showing increased amplitude of the rapid filling wave, reflecting large left ventricular diastolic loading (figs. 4.19 and 4.27). The A wave may be prominent in patients with sinus rhythm. Abnormalities of the systolic wave showing systolic retraction followed by a late systolic bulge or sustained and round systolic wave may be seen. They reflect left ventricular dyskinesis or left ventricular hypertrophy. Systolic wave abnormalities can be exaggerated if they follow an atrial or ventricular extrasystole (fig. 4.29). Apexcardiograms showing a sustained systolic wave are usually indicative of severe left ventricular hypertrophy (figs. 4.19 and 4.27).

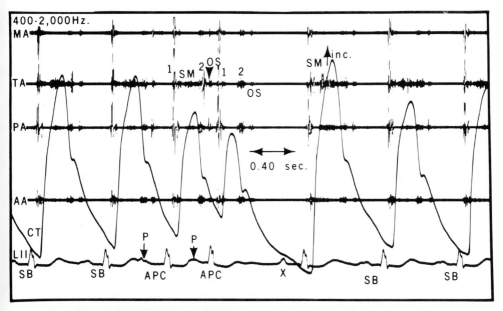

Fig. 4.22. Simultaneously recorded phonocardiogram at the mitral (MA), tricuspid (TA), pulmonic (PA) and aortic (AA) areas, carotid pulse tracing (CT) and lead II (LII) of the electrocardiogram in a 46-year-old patient with mitral insufficiency showing the effects of arrhythmias on the configuration and amplitude of the systolic murmur (SM). During sinus beats (SB) the tracing shows the typical features of mitral insufficiency. Atrial premature contractions (APC) result in a marked decrease in amplitude of the systolic regurgitant murmur. Note in the fourth beat, which is an early atrial premature contraction, that the systolic murmur is practically absent. The post-extrasystolic beat (X) shows a slight increase in amplitude of the systolic regurgitant murmur as compared with pre-extrasystolic sinus beats. At times, this is seen in patients with mitral insufficiency, but most frequently it is characteristic of patients with aortic stenosis.

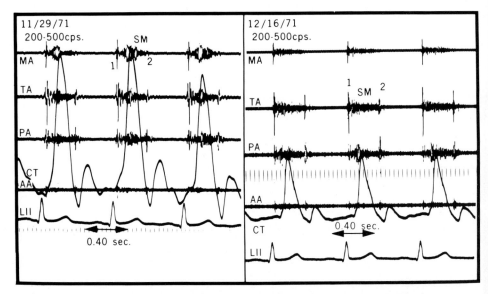

Fig. 4.23. Simultaneously recorded phonocardiogram at the mitral (MA), tricuspid (TA), pulmonic (PA) and aortic (AA) areas, carotid pulse tracing (CT) and lead II (LII) of the electrocardiogram in a 40-year-old patient with mitral insufficiency. The tracing taken on 11/29/71 was obtained during an acute episode of bacterial endocarditis involving the mitral valve. It shows the typical "musical" characteristics with various harmonic components best seen at the mitral area. The tracing taken on 12/16/71, after the clinical condition became stable, shows the usual features of pansystolic regurgitant murmur of mitral insufficiency without "musical" characteristics.

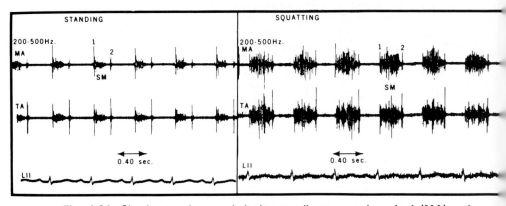

Fig. 4.24. Simultaneously recorded phonocardiogram at the mitral (MA) and tricuspid (TA) areas and lead II (LII) of the electrocardiogram in a 37-year-old patient with mitral insufficiency showing the effect of position on the systolic murmur (SM). While standing, the murmur decreases in amplitude, is early, and terminates prior to the second heart sound. During squatting, there is a marked increase in the amplitude of the systolic regurgitant murmur.

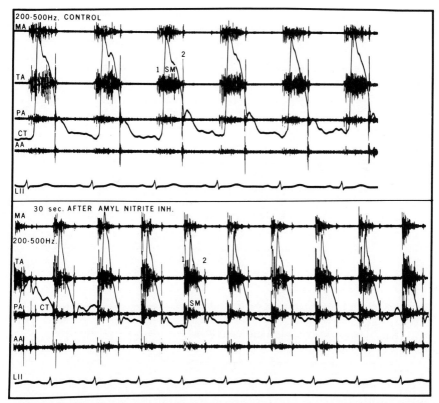

Fig. 4.25. Simultaneously recorded phonocardiogram at the mitral (MA), tricuspid (TA), pulmonic (PA) and aortic (AA) areas, carotid pulse tracing (CT) and lead II (LII) of the electrocardiogram in a 37-year-old patient with mitral insufficiency. In the control tracings the typical systolic regurgitant murmur (SM) of mitral insufficiency is seen. There is a diminished first (*1*) heart sound and the second (*2*) heart sound is normal. The *lower panel* shows the effect of inhalation of amyl nitrite on the systolic murmur. During inhalation of this drug there is marked diminution of the systolic murmur. Observe that the murmur becomes more prominent in the early part of systole and terminates prior to the second heart sound.

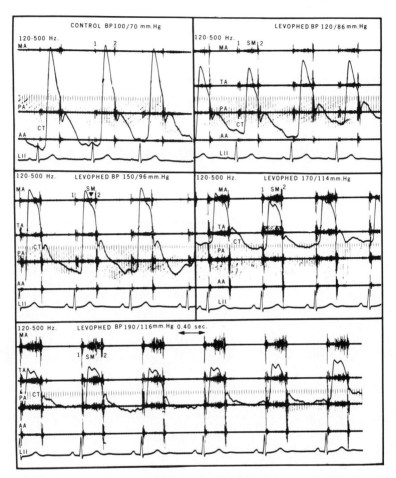

Fig. 4.26. Simultaneously recorded phonocardiogram at the mitral (MA), tricuspid (TA), pulmonic (PA) and aortic (AA) areas, carotid pulse tracing (CT) and lead II (LII) of the electrocardiogram in a 16-year-old patient with rheumatic mitral insufficiency. The control tracing shows a low amplitude, high frequency systolic murmur (SM). Intravenous administration of Levophed results in a significant rise in blood pressure from the control reading of 100/70 mm Hg to 190/116 mm Hg (*bottom panel*). A progressive increase in amplitude of the systolic regurgitant murmur is best seen in the bottom panel.

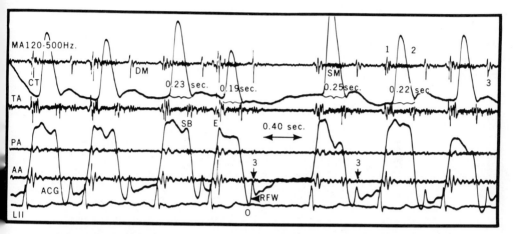

Fig. 4.27. Simultaneously recorded phonocardiogram at the mitral (MA), tricuspid (TA), pulmonic (PA) and aortic (AA) areas with carotid pulse tracing (CT), apexcardiogram (ACG) and lead II (LII) of the electrocardiogram in a 38-year-old patient with mitral insufficiency and atrial fibrillation. The first (1) heart sound is slightly diminished. There is a high frequency, low amplitude systolic regurgitant murmur (SM) which begins with the first heart sound and terminates prior to the second heart sound. There is a low frequency, low amplitude mid-diastolic murmur (DM), probably representing increased flow across the mitral valve. There is a third heart sound which coincides with the peak of the rapid filling wave (RFW) of the apexcardiogram. The carotid pulse tracing shows diminished ejection time and a rapid ascending limb. The apexcardiogram shows an abnormal systolic wave, a late systolic bulge (SB) and a prominent rapid filling wave (RFW).

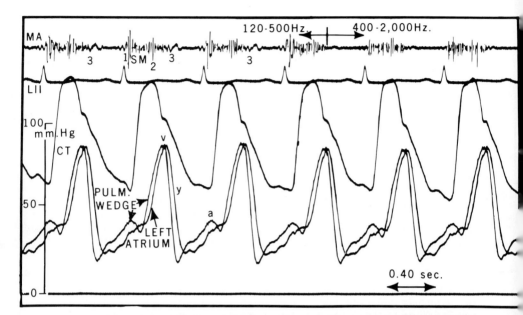

Fig. 4.28. Simultaneously recorded phonocardiogram at the mitral (MA) area, carotid pulse tracing (CT), pulmonary "wedge" pressure curve, left atrial pressure curve and lead II (LII) of the electrocardiogram in a 53-year-old patient with severe mitral insufficiency. The first (1) sound is of normal amplitude. The second heart sound is single and normal. There is a high frequency, low amplitude systolic regurgitant murmur. A prominent third heart sound is present. The patient is in sinus rhythm. The carotid pulse shows a rapid upstroke time and a diminished ejection time. Note that the third heart sound coincides with the downslope of the Y descent in both the pulmonary "wedge" and left atrial pressure curves. Both the pulmonary "wedge" and left atrial pressure curves show a prominent V wave followed by a rapid Y descent though the A wave is of normal amplitude. The peak of the V wave in both intracardiac pressure recordings is approximately 85 mm Hg. The right panel, with the band pass filter set at 400-2000 Hz, shows a decrease in amplitude of the systolic murmur. The third heart sound is not recordable. SM = systolic murmur.

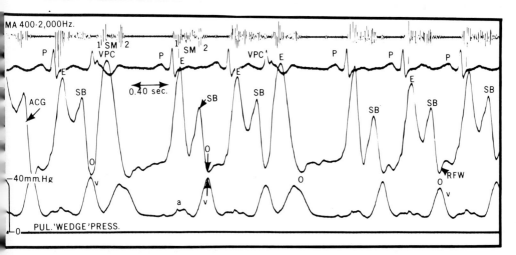

Fig. 4.29. Simultaneously recorded phonocardiogram at the mitral area (MA), apexcardiogram (ACG), pulmonary "wedge" pressure curve and lead II (LII) of the electrocardiogram in a 52-year-old patient with mitral insufficiency. The rhythm is sinus with multiple ventricular premature contractions (VPC). The first (1) and second (2) heart sounds are normal. There is a high frequency, high amplitude systolic regurgitant murmur (SM). In the apexcardiogram the sinus beats show a prominent systolic bulge (SB) and a slightly conspicuous rapid filling wave (RFW). With the ventricular premature contractions, the systolic bulge disappears. In the post-extrasystolic beat (E), the systolic bulge becomes quite prominent, returning to control values in the subsequent sinus beats. The O point of the apexcardiogram coincides with the peak of the V wave in the pulmonary "wedge" pressure curve. There is marked elevation of pulmonary "wedge" pressure.

Maneuvers and Pharmacologic Agents

The influence of supraventricular and ventricular arrhythmias, as well as changes in cycle length, significantly alter the amplitude of the heart sounds and murmurs (figs. 4.21, 4.22, 4.27, and 4.29). Squatting causes a marked increase in the amplitude of the systolic murmur in patients with rheumatic mitral insufficiency (fig. 4.24). Inhalation of a vasodilator such as amyl nitrite causes a decrease and shortening of the systolic murmur (fig. 4.25) and vasopressors, such as intravenous administration of levarterenol, cause an increase in the amplitude of the systolic murmur (fig. 4.26).

Echocardiogram

Mitral insufficiency secondary to rheumatic heart disease is difficult to detect with the echocardiogram. Separation of the mitral leaflets during systole is technically difficult to record and, therefore, the technique is of little diagnostic value.

PROLAPSE OF THE MITRAL VALVE

The syndrome of mid- or late systolic clicks with or without mid- or late systolic murmurs (Barlow syndrome) has been recognized with increasing frequency during the past few years.

Auscultation and Phonocardiography

Heart Sounds

The first and second heart sounds are normal. If mitral insufficiency is severe, the second heart sound is split due to early closure of the aortic valve. Single or multiple early, mid- or late systolic clicks are the characteristic findings (figs. 4.30–4.35). In general, location of the click during systole is related to the degree of mitral insufficiency. The greater the degree of mitral insufficiency, the earlier the onset of the click. The presence of multiple systolic clicks has no relationship to the degree of mitral insufficiency (fig. 4.31). Third heart sounds may be present if mitral insufficiency is hemodynamically significant.

Heart Murmurs

The murmur of prolapse of the mitral valve characteristically starts in mid-systole following the mid-systolic click. It progressively increases in amplitude in late systole and terminates with aortic valve closure (figs. 4.30 and 4.31). This is a high frequency murmur, at times musical, with varying intensity. The murmur usually radiates posteriorly to the axillary line and toward the spine. If the posterior leaflet is involved, the murmur transmits anteriorly toward the sternum. As the degree of mitral insufficiency increases, the murmur and the click move toward the first heart sound. In some patients the systolic click may be inscribed during mid-systole and at times is preceded by a short systolic murmur (fig. 4.33).

Carotid Pulse Tracing

The carotid pulse is of some use in the evaluation of patients with prolapse of the mitral valve. The tracing shows rapid upstroke time and a systolic retraction followed by a late systolic bulge (fig. 4.35). This type of tracing sometimes simulates those seen in idiopathic hypertrophic subaortic stenosis and other hyperdynamic circulatory disease states.

Jugular Venous Tracing

The jugular venous tracing is of no value in this disease state.

Apexcardiogram

The apexcardiogram shows a sharp E point and abnormal systolic

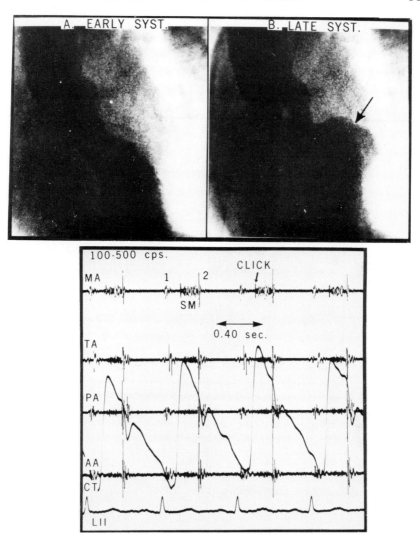

Fig. 4.30. Simultaneously recorded phonocardiogram at the mitral (MA), tricuspid (TA), pulmonic (PA) and aortic (AA) areas, carotid pulse tracing (CT) and lead II (LII) of the electrocardiogram in an 18-year-old patient with mitral insufficiency due to prolapse of the mitral valve. The first (1) and second (2) heart sounds are normal. Observe the presence of a mid-systolic click followed by a late, high frequency systolic murmur (SM) which terminates with the second heart sound. The left ventricular angiogram (top panel), taken during early and late systole, demonstrates prolapse of the mitral valve.

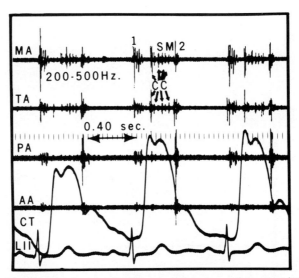

Fig. 4.31. Simultaneously recorded phonocardiogram at the mitral (MA), tricuspid (TA), pulmonic (PA) and aortic areas (AA), carotid pulse tracing (CT) and lead II (LII) of the electrocardiogram in a 45-year-old patient with prolapse of the posterior leaflet of the mitral valve. The first (1) and second (2) heart sounds are normal. Note the presence of multiple clicks (C) during systole with variations in amplitude in the three recorded beats. There is also a late, high frequency, medium amplitude systolic murmur (SM). The carotid tracing has a normal configuration and the pre-ejection period and ejection time are normal.

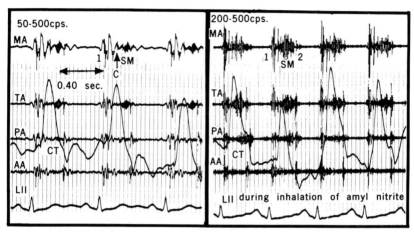

Fig. 4.32. Simultaneously recorded phonocardiogram at the mitral (MA), tricuspid (TA), pulmonic (PA) and aortic (AA) areas, carotid pulse tracing (CT) and lead II (LII) of the electrocardiogram in a 21-year-old patient with mitral insufficiency and prolapse of the mitral valve. In the left panel the first (1) and second (2) heart sounds are normal. There is a mid-systolic click followed by a high frequency, medium amplitude systolic regurgitant murmur (SM) which terminates with the first heart sound. Inhalation of amyl nitrite (*right panel*) results in a marked increase in amplitude of the systolic regurgitant murmur. The first heart sound becomes slightly accentuated. Observe that the maximal peak of the systolic murmur is near the first heart sound.

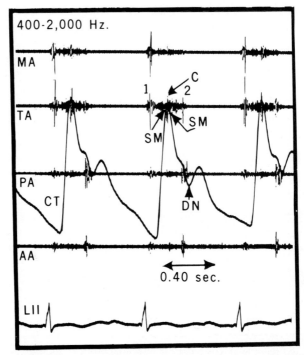

Fig. 4.33. Simultaneously recorded phonocardiogram at the mitral (MA), tricuspid (TA), pulmonic (PA) and aortic (AA) areas, carotid pulse tracing (CT) and lead II (LII) of the electrocardiogram in a 39-year-old patient with prolapse of the mitral valve. The first (*1*) and second (*2*) heart sounds are of normal amplitude. Note the presence of a systolic click (C) which occurs in mid-systole. The systolic murmur (SM) starts with the first heart sound, reaches a maximal peak at the time of the mid-systolic click and terminates with the second heart sound (see text).

retraction which coincides with the onset of the mid-systolic click (fig. 4.34). A late systolic rise follows and is inscribed at the time of the late crescendo systolic murmur. These changes reflect abnormal left ventricular contraction which has been well documented by left ventriculograms (figs. 4.35 and 4.36). The rapid filling wave is exaggerated only if the mitral regurgitant flow is significant and exceeds approximately 25% of the total left ventricular output.

Systolic Time Intervals

Ejection time is normal or shortened slightly in this condition.

Maneuvers and Pharmacologic Agents

Maneuvers such as Valsalva, squatting, exercise and the use of amyl nitrite (fig. 4.32) and vasopressors increase the amount of mitral

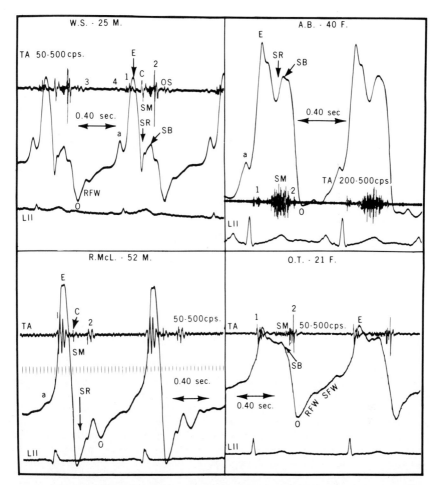

Fig. 4.34. Abnormalities of the apexcardiogram seen in patients with prolapse of the mitral valve. In these four recordings of the apexcardiogram, phonocardiogram and electrocardiogram one can appreciate the presence of a mid-systolic click (C) followed by a late systolic murmur (SM). In the majority of cases of prolapse of the mitral valve, the mid-systolic click coincides with a sharp systolic retraction (SR) in the apexcardiogram followed by a late systolic bulge (SB). These abnormalities in the apexcardiogram are probably related to abnormalities of left ventricular contraction as seen in biplane left ventricular angiograms. TA = tricuspid area, LII = lead II, RSW and SFW, rapid and slow filling wave.

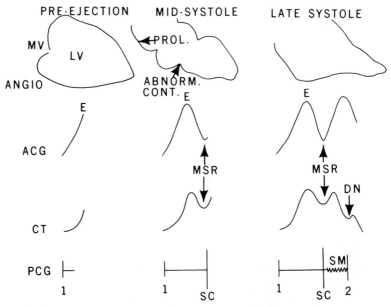

Fig. 4.35. Diagrammatic representation of various abnormalities seen in the apexcardiogram (ACG), carotid pulse tracing (CT) and phonocardiogram (PCG) in patients with prolapse (PROL.) of the mitral valve. The schematic representation of the left ventricular (LV) angiogram (ANGIO) shows constricting rings, indicated by *arrows*, in the inferoposterior aspect of the left ventricle. This is particularly prominent during mid- and late systole. This abnormality seems to be responsible for the mid-systolic retraction (MSR) and late systolic bulge in the apexcardiogram, as well as the systolic retraction seen in the carotid pulse tracing. They occur, as shown in figure 4.34, at the time that the mid-systolic click is inscribed on the phonocardiogram. MV = mitral valve, SM = systolic murmur, DN = dicrotic notch, SC = systolic click.

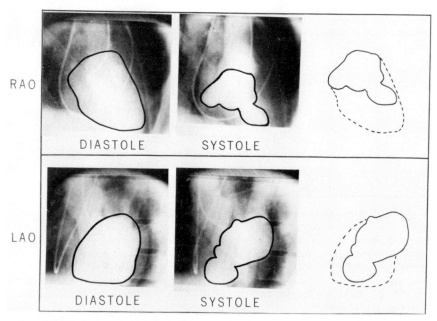

Fig. 4.36. Left ventricular angiogram in a 25-year-old patient with prolapse of the mitral valve, as seen from right (RAO) and left (LAO) anterior oblique projections showing the typical constricting ring during systole.

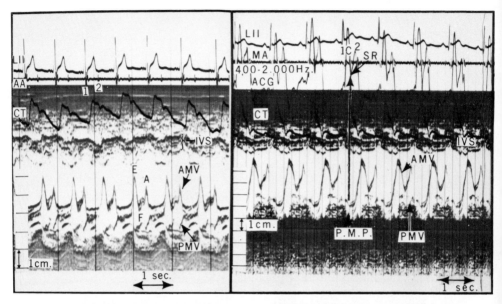

Fig. 4.37. Simultaneously recorded echocardiogram, aortic area (AA) phonocardiogram , carotid pulse tracing (CT) and lead II (LII) of the electrocardiogram (*left panel*)
showing normal mitral valve motion on the echocardiogram. An example of mitral
valve prolapse is shown in the *right panel*. During ventricular systole the posterior
leaflet of the mitral valve prolapses into the left atrial cavity (PMP) at the time of
inscription of the mid-systolic click (C) on the phonocardiogram and the systolic
retraction (SR) on the apexcardiogram (ACG). AMV = anterior mitral valve, PMV =
posterior mitral valve.

insufficiency and cause an early onset of the click-murmurs. Diastolic
murmurs are not present in this condition unless mitral insufficiency is
very severe. In this case, a third heart sound is present, followed by a
mid-low frequency diastolic rumble due to increased diastolic flow across
the mitral valve.

Echocardiogram

The echocardiogram is a very valuable non-invasive technique in the
diagnosis of prolapse of the mitral valve leaflet. Several patterns of the
echocardiogram have been described by investigators. They all reflect
abnormal mitral valve motion with the valve closing early in systole,
opening again in mid- or late systole, and prolapsing into the left atrial
cavity. Various types of abnormalities seen on echocardiograms in this
condition are shown in figures 4.37–4.41.

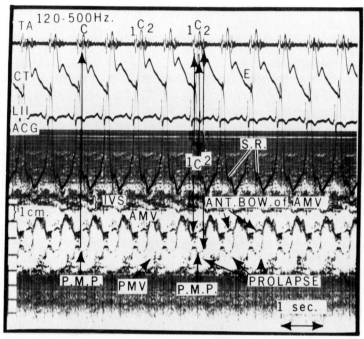

Fig. 4.38. Simultaneously recorded echocardiogram, mitral area (MA) phono-cardiogram, carotid pulse tracing (CT), apexcardiogram (ACG) and lead II (LII) of the electrocardiogram in a 45-year-old patient with prolapse of the mitral valve. The phonocardiogram shows the mid-systolic click (C) and late systolic murmur charac-teristic of this condition. Note the abnormal motion of the mitral valve. There is an-terior bowing of the anterior mitral valve (AMV), and prolapse of the posterior mitral valve (PMP). PMV = posterior mitral valve, IVS = interventricular septum.

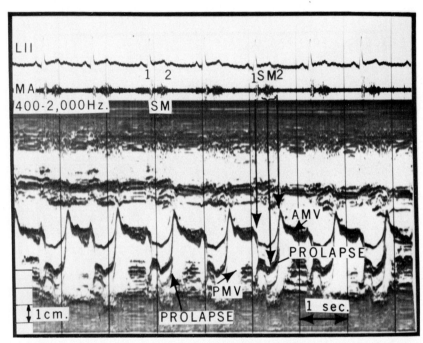

Fig. 4.39. Echocardiogram of a mitral valve recorded simultaneously with a phonocardiogram at the mitral area (MA) and lead II (LII) of the electrocardiogram in a 25-year-old patient with prolapse of the mitral valve. Note the abnormal posterior motion of the posterior mitral valve (PMV) during systole and the typical pansystolic prolapse of the mitral valve. The phonocardiogram shows a high frequency systolic murmur (SM) with a mid-to-late systolic peak. AMV = anterior mitral valve.

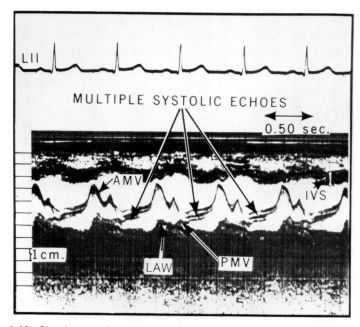

Fig. 4.40. Simultaneously recorded echocardiogram and lead II (LII) of the electrocardiogram in a 13-year-old patient with acute mitral insufficiency showing exaggerated motion of the left atrial wall (LAW) and multiple systolic echoes of the mitral valve. AMV = anterior mitral valve, PMV = posterior mitral valve.

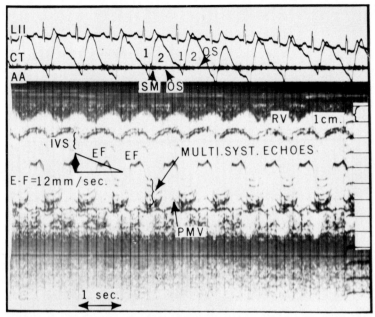

Fig. 4.41. Simultaneously recorded echocardiogram, aortic area (AA) phonocardiogram, lead II (LII) of the electrocardiogram and carotid pulse tracing (CT) in a
47-year-old patient with rheumatic mitral stenosis and insufficiency. Note the decreased E-F slope (12 mm/sec) and the presence of multiple systolic echoes which
are sometimes seen in patients with rheumatic mitral valve disease. IVS = interventricular septum, PMV = posterior mitral valve, RV = right ventricle, SM = systolic murmur and OS = opening snap.

REFERENCES

1. Aronow, W. S., Kaplan, M. A., and Ellestad, M.: Prediction of left ventricular contrac-
   tility in mitral valve disease by EICT and LVET/EICT measurements (abstract).
   Clin. Res., *17:* 226, 1969.
2. Aykent, Y., Thurmann, M., and Bussmann, B. W.: Continuous murmur in mitral
   stenosis. Am. J. Cardiol., *15:* 715, 1965.
3. Barlow, J. B., and Bosman, C. K.: Aneurysmal protrusion of the posterior leaflet of the
   mitral valve. An auscultatory-electrocardiographic syndrome. Am. Heart J., *71:* 166,
   1966.
4. Benchimol, A., Dimond, E. G., Waxman, D., and Shen, Y.: Diastolic movement of the
   procordium in mitral stenosis and regurgitation. Am. Heart J., *60:* 417, 1960.
5. Benchimol, A., Harris, C. L., and Desser, K. B.: Midsystolic carotid pulse wave
   retraction in subjects with prolapsed mitral valve leaflets. Chest, *62:* 614, 1972.
6. Bridgen, W., and Leatham, A.: Mitral insufficiency. Br. Heart J., *15:* 55, 1953.
7. Cheng, T. O.: Loud S_1 with murmur of mitral regurgitation. N. Engl. J. Med., *287:* 988,
   1972.
8. Craige, E.: Phonocardiographic studies in mitral stenosis. N. Engl. J. Med., *257:* 650,
   1957.
9. DeMaria, A. N.: The variable spectrum of echocardiographic manifestations of the
   mitral valve prolapse syndrome. Circulation, *50:* 33, 1974.

10. Dock, W.: Production mode of systolic clicks due to mitral cusp prolapse. Arch. Intern. Med., *132:* 118, 1972.
11. Duchak, J. M., Chang, S. J., and Feigenbaum, H.: The posterior mitral valve echo and the echocardiographic diagnosis of mitral stenosis. Proceedings of the American Institute of Ultrasound Medicine, 1971.
12. Edler, I.: Mitral valve function studied by the ultrasound echo method. In Grossman, C. C., Holmes, J. H., Joyner, C., and Purnell, E. W. (eds.): *Diagnostic Ultrasound. Proceedings of the First International Conference, University of Pittsburgh, 1965,* p. 168. Plenum Press, New York, 1966.
13. Edler, I.: Ultrasound cardiogram in mitral valve disease. Acta Chir. Scand., *111:* 230, 1956.
14. Edler, I., and Gustafson, A.: Ultrasonic cardiogram in mitral stenosis. Acta Med. Scand., *159:* 85, 1957.
15. Effert, S.: Pre- and postoperative evaluation of mitral stenosis by ultrasound. Am. J. Cardiol., *19:* 59, 1967.
16. Fischer, J. C., Chang, S., Konecke, L. L., and Feigenbaum, H.: Echocardiographic determination of mitral valve flow. Am. J. Cardiol., *29:* 262, 1972.
17. Fleming, H. A., and Wood, P.: The myocardial factor in mitral valve disease. Br. Heart J., *21:* 117, 1959.
18. Friedman, N. J.: Echocardiographic studies of mitral valve motion; genesis of opening snap in mitral stenosis. Am. Heart J., *80:* 177, 1970.
19. Gabor, G. E., and Winsberg, F.: Motion of mitral valves in cardiac arrhythmias; ultrasonic cardiographic study. Invest. Radiol., *5:* 355, 1970.
20. Gustafson, A.: Correlation between ultrasoundcardiography, haemodynamics and surgical findings in mitral stenosis. Am. J. Cardiol., *19:* 32, 1967.
21. Hancock, E. W., and Cohn, K.: The syndrome associated with midsystolic click and late systolic murmur. Am. J. Med., *41:* 183, 1966.
22. Hubbard, T. F., Dunn, F. L., and Neis, D. D.: A phonocardiographic study of apical diastolic murmur in pure mitral insufficiency. Am. Heart J., *57:* 223, 1959.
23. Hultgren, H. N., and Leo, T. F.: The tricuspid component of the first heart sound in mitral stenosis. Circulation, *18:* 1012, 1958.
24. Joyner, C. R., Dyrda, I. Barrett, J. S., and Reid, J. M.: Preoperative determination of the functional anatomy of the mitral valve. Circulation, *32:* 110, 1965.
25. Joyner, C. R., Reid, J. M., and Bond, J. P.: Reflected ultrasound in the assessment of mitral valve disease. Circulation, *27:* 506, 1963.
26. Kelly, J. J., Jr.: Diagnostic value of phonocardiography in mitral stenosis. Am. J. Med., *19:* 862, 1955.
27. Leo, T., and Hultgren, H.: Phonocardiographic characteristics of tight mitral stenosis. Medicine, *38:* 85, 1959.
28. McLaurin, L. P.: An appraisal of mitral valve echocardiograms mimicking mitral stenosis in conditions with right ventricular pressure load. Circulation, *48:* 801, 1973.
29. Meadows, W. R., Sharp, J. T., and Zachariudakis, S.: Premature mitral valve closure; a hemodynamic explanation for absence of the first heart sound in aortic insufficiency. Circulation, *28:* 251, 1963.
30. Mercer, J. L.: Presystolic murmur in mitral stenosis. Lancet, *2:* 765, 1972.
31. Mounsey, P., Brigden, W.: The apical systolic murmur in mitral stenosis. Br. Heart J., *16:* 255, 1954.
32. Nixon, P. G. F., and Wooler, G. H.: Phases of diastole in various syndromes of mitral valvular disease. Br. Heart J., *25:* 393, 1963.
33. Nixon, P. G. F., Wooler, G. H., and Radigan, L. R.: The opening snap in mitral incompetence. Br. Heart J. *22:* 395, 1960.
34. Oreshkov, V. I.: Isovolumic contraction time and isovolumic contraction time index in mitral stenosis. Study on basis of polygraphic tracing (apex cardiogram, phonocardiogram, and carotid tracing.) Br. Heart J., *34:* 533, 1972.
35. Popp, R. L.: Echocardiographic abnormalities in the mitral valve prolapse syndrome. Circulation, *49:* 428, 1974.

36. Proctor, M. H., Walker, R. C., Hancock, E. W., and Abelmann, W. H.: The phonocardiogram in mitral valvular disease. Am. J. Med., *24:* 861, 1958.
37. Sasse, L.: Echocardiography of mitral valve prolapse. Circulation, *49:* 595, 1974.
38. Segal, B. L., Likoff, W., and Kingsley, B.: Echocardiography; clinical application in mitral stenosis. J.A.M.A., *193:* 161, 1956.
39. Silver, W., Rodriguez-Torres, R., and Newfeld, E.: The echocardiogram in a case of mitral stenosis before and after surgery. Am. Heart J., *78:* 811, 1969.
40. Sutton, G. C., and Craige, E.: Clinical signs of severe acute mitral regurgitation. Am. J. Cardiol., *20:* 141, 1967.
41. Tatemichi, K.: The ultrasono-cardiographic criterion for the operative procedures of mitral valvular disease. Jap. Circ. J., *37:* 473, 1973.
42. Tavel, M. E.: The "closing snap" in mitral stenosis. Am. Heart J., *84:* 282, 1972.
43. Weissler, A. M., Leonard, J. J., and Warren, J. V.: Observations in delayed first heart sound in mitral stenosis and hypertension. Circulation, *18:* 165, 1958.
44. Wells, B. G.: The assessment of mitral stenosis by phonocardiography. Br. Heart J., *16:* 261, 1954.
45. Wharton, C. F. P., Bescos, L. L.: Mitral valve movement; a study using an ultrasound technique. Br. Heart J., *16:* 261, 1954.
46. Wood, P.: An appreciation of mitral stenosis. Br. Med. J., *1:* 1051, 1954.
47. Zaky, A., Nasser, W. K., and Feigenbaum. H.: A study of mitral valve action recorded by reflected ultrasound and its application in the diagnosis of mitral stenosis. Circulation, *37:* 789, 1968.

chapter 5

Aortic Valvular Disease

Aortic valvular disease is usually due to rheumatic heart disease, or calcification of the aortic valve in older subjects with diffuse atherosclerosis. It can also result from a congenital bicuspid aortic valve which calcifies later in life. Aortic valve disease is also seen with conditions such as Paget's disease, Marfan's syndrome, rheumatoid arthritis and others. In this chapter non-invasive diagnosis of aortic valvular and idiopathic hypertrophic subaortic stenosis will be discussed, as well as subvalvular and supravalvular disease.

AUSCULTATION AND PHONOCARDIOGRAPHY

Heart Sounds and Murmurs

The first heart sound is normal in patients with aortic valvular disease (fig. 5.1). The second heart sound may be normal providing that the gradient between the left ventricle and aorta is not above 30 mm Hg (fig. 5.1). If the gradient is above this level and there is decreased mobility of the aortic cusps due to sclerosis or calcification, the aortic component of the second heart sound decreases in amplitude (figs. 5.2 and 5.3). When a stenotic lesion at the valvular or subvalvular level is severe, and the left ventricular aortic pressure gradient exceeds 50 mm Hg, the second sound exhibits paradoxical or reverse splitting (pulmonary valve closure sound precedes the aortic closure sound) secondary to increased duration of left ventricular systole (fig. 5.2). If the second heart sound is paradoxically split both components are well heard during expiration and become single, or the A2-P2 interval shortens considerably during inspiration. This finding is best recognized through simultaneous recording of the phonocardiogram and carotid pulse tracing. Both components of the second heart sound should precede the dicrotic notch (fig. 5.2). A systolic ejection click, common in young patients with valvular or subvalvular aortic stenosis and dilatation of the ascending aorta (fig. 5.1), is probably a consequence of the rapid impact of high velocity jets from the left ventricle into a dilated aorta. A third heart sound auscultated in young

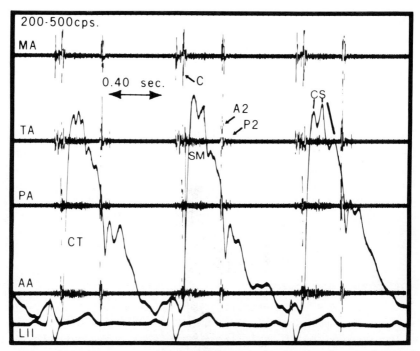

Fig. 5.1. Simultaneously recorded phonocardiogram at the mitral (MA), tricuspid (TA), pulmonic (PA) and aortic areas (AA), carotid pulse tracing (CT) and lead II (LII) of the electrocardiogram in a 15-year-old patient with congenital aortic valvular stenosis. A systolic ejection click (C) follows the first heart sound. The click is inscribed during the first 40 msec of the ascending limb of the carotid pulse tracing. In this patient with discrete aortic valvular stenosis the aortic component of the second heart sound and the dicrotic notch of the carotid pulse tracing are normal. There is a high frequency, low amplitude systolic ejection murmur (SM). Observe the normal, rapid rise in the carotid pulse tracing and the presence of carotid shudder (CS). The gradient across the aortic valve was 18 mm Hg.

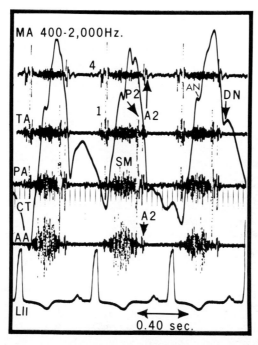

Fig. 5.2. Simultaneously recorded phonocardiogram at the mitral (MA), tricuspid (TA), pulmonic (PA) and aortic (AA) areas, carotid pulse tracing (CT) and lead II (LII) of the electrocardiogram in a 12-year-old patient with severe aortic valvular stenosis. The first heart sound is normal. There is a low amplitude fourth heart sound recorded best at the mitral area. The second heart sound shows a paradoxical splitting and both components (P2-A2) precede the dicrotic notch (DN) of the carotid pulse tracing. This recording was taken during inspiration. Amplitude of the aortic component of the second heart sound is diminished. There is a high frequency, high amplitude aortic systolic ejection murmur (SM) which has mid-to-late systolic accentuation. The carotid pulse tracing shows an anacrotic notch (AN), carotid shudder, dicrotic notch and prolonged ejection time.

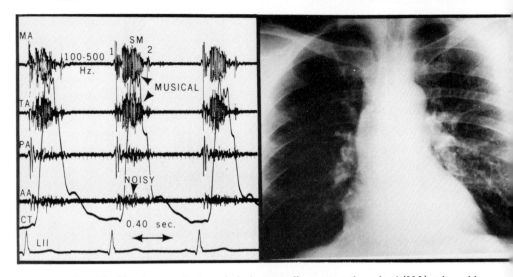

Fig. 5.3. Simultaneously recorded phonocardiogram at the mitral (MA), tricuspid (TA), pulmonic (PA), and aortic (AA) areas, carotid pulse tracing (CT) and lead II (LII) of the electrocardiogram in a 40-year-old patient with calcific aortic valvular stenosis. The musical characteristic of the systolic murmur (SM) is best recorded at the mitral and tricuspid areas. The noisy characteristic of the murmur, consisting of "disorganized" vibrations of varying frequencies and amplitudes are best recorded at the aortic area. The varying characteristics of the murmur recorded at different precordial areas is called the Gallavardin phenomenon. The noisy murmur is probably the result of turbulence around the central velocity jet across the diseased aortic valve, while the musical component recorded at the mitral and tricuspid areas represents regular harmonic vibrations from the stenotic valve lesion. In the *right panel* a chest x-ray shows overall cardiac enlargement, particularly of the left ventricle, and moderate post-stenotic dilatation of the ascending aorta.

patients with congenital aortic stenosis is not of diagnostic value unless it is associated with other signs of congestive heart failure. However, the third heart sound assumes clinical importance in subjects over age 30 to 40 where it is usually indicative of impaired left ventricular function.

The fourth heart sound is part of the auscultatory and phonocardiographic features of adult patients with aortic valvular disease. It does not necessarily indicate severe aortic stenosis or heart failure (fig. 5.2). If one or both of these conditions are noted, the fourth heart sound is always present if the patient is in sinus rhythm. This sound may be due to sudden deceleration of blood into the left ventricular cavity due to forceful atrial contraction against a hypertrophic left ventricle which has slightly elevated end-diastolic pressure and decreased compliance. The systolic murmurs of rheumatic aortic valvular stenosis, congenital bicuspid aortic stenosis or membranous aortic stenosis are similar. These high frequency ejection murmurs have a diamond shape and begin with a systolic ejection click, or shortly after the first heart sound (fig. 5.2). The maximum peak, reached in the first half of systole, corresponds to the period of maximum rapid left ventricular ejection (figs. 5.1–5.10). It decreases in amplitude during late systole, terminating at, or shortly before, the second heart sound. It is heard best at the mitral, tricuspid and aortic areas. In many subjects with aortic stenosis, the murmur is recorded best at the mitral area and may, therefore, be confused with the murmur of mitral insufficiency. The characteristic ejection and noisy qualities of the murmur of aortic stenosis are helpful in differential diagnosis, as are abnormalities of the carotid pulse tracing. At times, this murmur may have musical characteristics (fig. 5.3) and in adults it usually is associated with calcification of the aortic valve (fig. 5.3). The shape of the murmur is similar to the shape of the pressure gradient

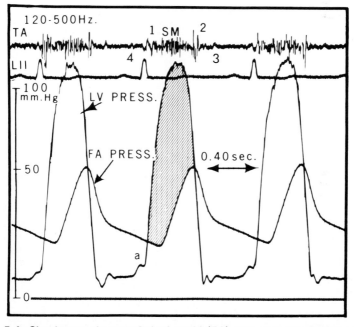

Fig. 5.4. Simultaneously recorded tricuspid (TA) area phonocardiogram at filter gain setting of 120–500 Hz, lead II (LII) of the electrocardiogram, left ventricular (LV PRESS) and femoral (FA PRESS) artery pressures in a 53-year-old patient with severe aortic valvular stenosis. The *shaded area* indicates systolic pressure gradient between the left ventricle and femoral artery. The configuration of the systolic ejection murmur (SM) follows the gradient between the left ventricle and the femoral artery pressure with peak amplitude of the high frequency systolic ejection murmur corresponding to peak left ventricular systolic pressure. Note the presence of high frequency vibrations at the peak of left ventricular pressure.

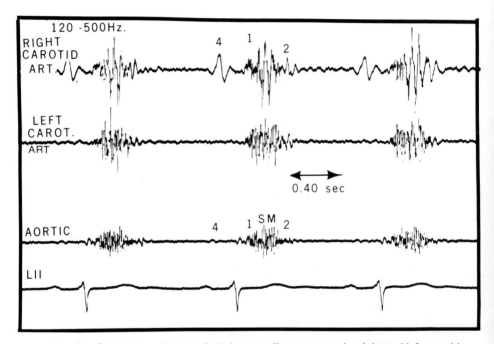

Fig. 5.5. Simultaneously recorded phonocardiogram over the right and left carotid arteries, aortic area and lead II (LII) of the electrocardiogram in a 65-year-old patient with aortic stenosis. The first heart sound is normal. The second heart sound is single with diminished amplitude. A prominent fourth heart sound is recorded best over the right carotid artery and at the aortic area. A high frequency, high amplitude systolic ejection murmur (SM) is recorded in all areas. At times in patients with aortic valvular stenosis the fourth heart sound can be heard and recorded best over the right carotid artery as shown in this illustration.

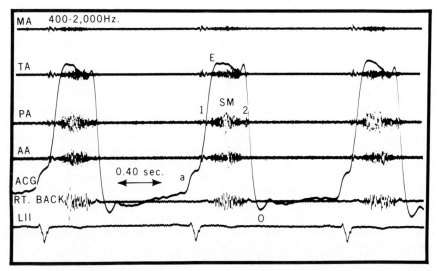

Fig. 5.6. Simultaneously recorded phonocardiogram at the mitral (MA), tricuspid (TA), pulmonic (PA), and aortic (AA) areas with a microphone placed at the fifth intercostal space near the lumbar spine, apexcardiogram (ACG) and lead II (LII) of the electrocardiogram, in a 68-year-old patient with severe aortic valvular stenosis. Note transmission of the systolic ejection murmur (SM) toward the right back (RT BACK). The second heart sound is single and markedly diminished. The apexcardiogram shows a conspicuous A wave and sustained systolic wave usually seen in patients with aortic valvular stenosis and severe left ventricular hypertrophy.

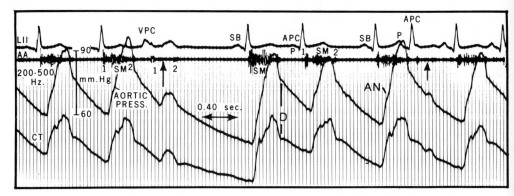

Fig. 5.7. Simultaneously recorded aortic (AA) area phonocardiogram, aortic pressure curve (AORTIC PRESS) and carotid pulse tracing (CT) obtained during cardiac catheterization in a 40-year-old patient with severe aortic valvular stenosis. Note the presence of ventricular (VPC) and atrial (APC) premature contractions on the electrocardiogram. In patients with aortic valvular stenosis, the systolic murmur (SM) decreases in amplitude during premature contractions because of a small stroke volume. However, because of the long compensatory pause which follows the ventricular premature contraction, the amplitude of the systolic ejection murmur increases in the post-extrasystolic beat as compared with the pre-extrasystolic beat. In the sinus beats (SB) following the ventricular premature contraction, there is an increase in aortic pressure and in the amplitude of the carotid pulse tracing. The increase in amplitude of the systolic ejection murmur following atrial premature contraction is not as noticeable as the increase after the post-extrasystolic ventricular premature contraction. Abnormalities of the carotid pulse tracing include a slow upstroke time, a low placed anacrotic notch (AN), inconspicuous dicrotic notch (D) and prolonged ejection time. These abnormalities are similar to those observed in the aortic pressure curve.

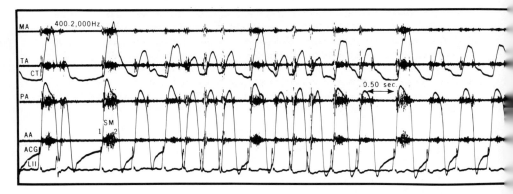

Fig. 5.8. Simultaneously recorded phonocardiogram at the mitral (MA), tricuspid (TA), pulmonic (PA) and aortic (AA) areas, carotid pulse tracing (CT), apexcardiogram (ACG), and lead II (LII) of the electrocardiogram in a 66-year-old patient with aortic valvular stenosis and atrial fibrillation with rapid ventricular rate. In beats with short cycle length, amplitude of the systolic murmur (SM) decreases. In beats preceded by a long cycle length, the murmur becomes quite prominent. The typical abnormalities of the carotid pulse tracing described previously are seen (compare with fig. 5.7).

116

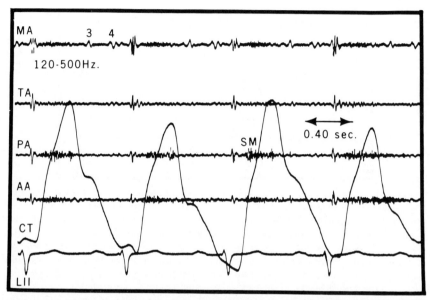

Fig. 5.9. Simultaneously recorded phonocardiogram at the mitral (MA), tricuspid (TA), pulmonic (PA) and aortic areas (AA), carotid pulse tracing (CT) and lead II (LII) of the electrocardiogram in a 58-year-old patient with severe aortic valvular stenosis and left heart failure. The tracing, recorded during expiration, shows typical alteration of the carotid pulse tracing. Strong left ventricular contractions are associated with high amplitude carotid pulse waves and the weaker ventricular contractions with lower amplitude. This phenomenon is usually indicative of severe left ventricular failure and a marked decrease in left ventricular stroke volume. Note alternation of the systolic ejection murmur (SM) recorded at several precordial areas but observed best at the pulmonic area. Murmurs with high amplitude characteristics are associated with stronger left ventricular contractions. There are prominent third and fourth heart sounds at the mitral area.

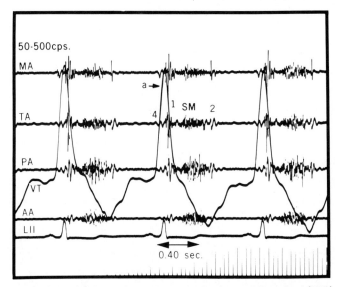

Fig. 5.10. Simultaneously recorded phonocardiogram at the mitral (MA), tricuspid (TA), pulmonic (PA) and aortic (AA) areas, jugular venous tracing (VT) and lead II (LII) of the electrocardiogram in a 68-year-old patient with severe aortic stenosis and heart failure. The gradient across the aortic valve was 90 mm Hg and left ventricular end-diastolic pressure was elevated to 18 mm Hg. There was also marked elevation of pulmonary artery pressure with a mean of 62 mm Hg. Right atrial mean pressure was 12 mm Hg. The phonocardiogram shows the typical characteristics of a systolic ejection murmur (SM) as described previously. There is a fourth (4) heart sound which coincides with the peak of a markedly exaggerated A wave on the jugular venous tracing.

across the aortic valve as shown in figure 5.4. The murmur radiates to both carotid arteries (fig. 5.5) but is transmitted best to the right carotid artery. It can also be radiated to the back at the level of the fourth and fifth intercostal spaces near the spine (fig. 5.6). Amplitude varies with cycle length during cardiac arrhythmias as shown in figures 5.7 and 5.8.

The time interval between the onset of the QRS on the electrocardiogram and the peak of the systolic murmur has some correlation with the systolic gradient across the aortic valve. The longer this time interval, the higher the gradient across the stenotic aortic valve.

Maneuvers and Pharmacologic Agents

An increase in the murmur of aortic valvular stenosis during exercise is probably related to increased heart rate, stroke volume and the resultant increase in the gradient across the aortic valve. Inhalation of vasodilators such as amyl nitrite results in a significant increase in amplitude of the ejection murmur, probably as a result of a decrease in systemic resistance and an increased gradient across the aortic valve (fig. 5.11). Administration of vasopressor agents results in a decrease in the amplitude of the ejection murmur because of an increase in the after load.

Carotid Pulse Tracing

Abnormalities of the carotid pulse tracing have diagnostic value in the assessment of aortic valvular disease. Typical features of the arterial pulse wave form in this condition are a slow rise in upstroke time (U time measured from its beginning until the tracing reaches its peak), prominent anacrotic notch, inconspicuous dicrotic notch, carotid shudder and prolonged ejection time (figs. 5.1–5.3 and 5.7–5.9). This type of pulse is called pulsus tardus. The probable mechanism for the configuration of this pulse wave seems to be due to prolongation of left ventricular ejection time and to the Venturi effect in the aorta. The late systolic peak and low amplitude of the arterial pulse are due to relative decrease in lateral pressure of the aortic walls.

A similar situation occurs when aortic stenosis and aortic insufficiency coexist. The aortic pulse pressure may be normal or increased but the upstroke limb of the arterial pulse wave form is interrupted by a notch (anacrotic notch) which is most prominent at the time of maximal left

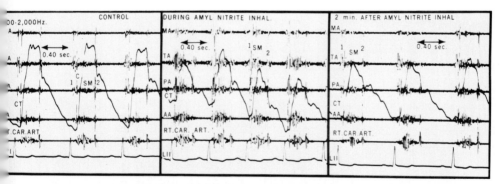

Fig 5.11. Simultaneously recorded phonocardiogram at the mitral (MA), tricuspid (TA), pulmonic (PA), aortic (AA) and right carotid artery (RT. CAR. ART.) areas, carotid pulse tracing (CT) and lead II (LII) of the electrocardiogram in a 31-year-old patient with severe aortic valvular stenosis. The tracings were taken at control, during, and 2 minutes after inhalation of amyl nitrite. The control tracing shows the typical phonocardiographic features described previously. The carotid pulse tracing shows an anacrotic notch, carotid shudder and prolonged ejection time. During inhalation of amyl nitrite, there is marked accentuation of the systolic ejection murmur (SM) in all areas. The peak of the systolic ejection murmur occurs in early systole as compared with mid-systolic accentuation seen in the control tracing.

Table 5.1. Ejection Time in Aortic Stenosis and Mitral Stenosis*

Group and No. of Subjects	Total Ejection Time		U Time		T Time		Ejection Angle (degrees)	
	Range	Average	Range	Average	Range	Average	Range	Average
	sec	*sec*	*sec*	*sec*	*sec*	*sec*		
Control, 30	0.28–0.34	0.302 ± 0.017	0.06–0.11	0.008 ± 0.013	0.02–0.04	0.033 ± 0.007	4.6–10.3	6.86 ± 1.51
Mitral stenosis, 40	0.23–0.32	0.274 ± 0.024	0.04–0.13	0.075 ± 0.057	0.01–0.04	0.031 ± 0.013	4.9–11.9	7.91 ± 1.92
Aortic stenosis, 25	0.31–0.41	0.364 ± 0.031	0.08–0.29	0.179 ± 0.071	0.02–0.10	0.059 ± 0.021	4.8–2.73	14.29 ± 5.75

* Ejection time in patients with aortic valvular stenosis was compared with normal subjects and patients with mitral stenosis. The diagnosis of patients with mitral and aortic valvular stenosis was documented by right and left heart catheterization and cineangiography. Note the increase in ejection time in patients with aortic stenosis as compared with the control group. Patients with mitral stenosis have a slightly decreased ejection time. The figure preceded by the ± symbol in the "Average" columns is the standard deviation. Values for total left ventricular ejection time were corrected for heart rate by dividing observed ejection time by the square root of the cycle length. Values for U time and ejection angle are given.

ventricular ejection. The time of inscription of the anacrotic notch is grossly proportional to the gradient across the aortic valve. The higher the gradient, the lower the inscription of the anacrotic notch. If heart failure is present, ejection time tends to normalize, representing a decrease in stroke volume (Table 5.1). In addition, pulsus alternans may be observed on the carotid pulse tracing (fig. 5.9).

Jugular Venous Pulse Tracing

The jugular venous pulse tracing is not useful in the diagnosis of aortic valvular stenosis unless the patient has pulmonary hypertension second-ary to left ventricular failure, at which time the A wave becomes quite prominent (fig. 5.10).

Apexcardiogram

The apexcardiogram is very useful in evaluating patients with aortic valvular stenosis. Amplitude of the A wave, representing forceful left atrial contraction against a non-distensible left ventricle, is increased above 15% of the total amplitude of the apexcardiogram (fig. 5.6). The E point, which coincides with the opening of the aortic valve, at times is difficult to identify due to the presence of left ventricular hypertrophy. In this condition, the E point is in direct continuation with the round and sustained systolic wave (figs. 5.6, 5.8 and 5.12). The O point is normal and is followed by a small rapid filling wave. If a third heart sound is present in patients with heart failure, the rapid filling wave becomes prominent and its peak coincides with the time of inscription of the third heart sound (fig. 5.12).

Systolic Time Intervals

As stated earlier, left ventricular ejection time is prolonged in patients with aortic stenosis without heart failure (fig. 5.13). Total left ventricular systole (M1-A2) is also prolonged (fig. 5.14). Prolongation of left ventricular ejection time (Table 5.1) is basically proportional to the severity of aortic valvular stenosis and correlates with the pressure gradient across the aortic valve. The pre-ejection period is slightly decreased in subjects with aortic valvular stenosis. This probably is a result of an increase in the rate of rising of left ventricular pressure during the period of isovolumic contraction. The combination of pro-longed left ventricular ejection time and pre-ejection period results in a pre-ejection period to left ventricular ejection time ratio lower than normal.

When patients with aortic stenosis develop left ventricular failure, ejection time decreases and the pre-ejection period increases above the normal range. These patients usually present a prominent third heart

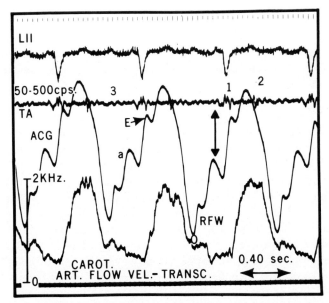

Fig. 5.12. Simultaneously recorded tricuspid (TA) area phonocardiogram, apexcardiogram (ACG), transcutaneous carotid artery flow velocity curve and lead II (LII) of
the electrocardiogram in a 70-year-old patient with severe aortic valvular stenosis
and heart failure. Note the marked increase in the A wave of the apexcardiogram. A
late systolic bulge reaches its peak near the second heart sound. The peak of the
prominent rapid filling wave (RFW) coincides with the third heart sound on the
phonocardiogram. The wave form of the transcutaneous flow velocity curve is similar
to that described for the carotid pulse tracing in patients with this condition. It shows
a slowly ascending limb, high frequency vibrations during systole (carotid shudder)
and an inconspicuous dicrotic notch.

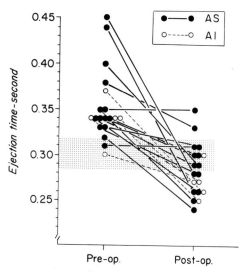

Fig. 5.13. Corrected ejection time measured on the carotid pulse tracing in patients with aortic stenosis (AS) and aortic insufficiency (AI) before and after aortic valve replacement with a ball valve prosthesis. The *shaded bar* on this graph indicates the normal range. Note significant increase in the ejection time in pre-operative tracings and a decrease in ejection time following aortic valve replacement.

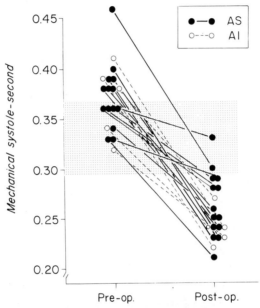

Fig. 5.14. Mechanical systole (M1-A2 interval) in patients with aortic valvular stenosis (AS) and in patients with aortic insufficiency (AI) before and after aortic valve replacement with a ball valve prosthesis. Note prolongation of ejection time in most of the pre-operative tracings and a decrease in ejection time following aortic valve replacement.

sound (figs. 5.9 and 5.12). This is associated with a decrease in the amplitude of the systolic ejection murmur (fig. 5.12). A shortening of the systolic left ventricular ejection time, mechanical systole and pre-ejection time is usually seen in patients subjected to successful aortic valvulotomy or aortic valve replacement as shown in figures 5.13 and 5.14 (Table 5.1).

Echocardiogram

Echocardiography is a useful technique for evaluating patients with aortic valvular disease. Angling the transducer to position 4 (pointing toward the base of the heart) usually produces good aortic valve echoes particularly in patients with aortic valvular stenosis. It is important to obtain multiple cardiac cycles and a scan from the base of the heart to the apex for proper identification of the cardiac structures. Simultaneous recording of the phonocardiogram and/or carotid pulse tracing is helpful to identify the beginning and end of ventricular systole. The normal range of aortic valve opening is 1.6 – 2.6 cm with an average of 1.9 cm. Normally, echoes from the aortic valve seem to represent motion of the right and non-coronary cusps. However, this is controversial and it appears that it is better to refer to anterior and posterior aortic cusp motion. Aortic valvular lesions can be detected by a decrease in the size of the aortic valve opening, and this measurement should be compared with the size of the aortic root which is frequently dilated, especially in patients with severe aortic stenosis. Echocardiograms of a normal aortic valve and in a patient with aortic valvular stenosis are shown in figure 5.15. A decrease in size of the aortic valve opening may be seen in other cardiac diseases associated with low blood flow across a normal aortic valve (fig. 5.16); therefore, this may not necessarily indicate the presence of an obstructed aortic valve. Calcification or thickening can be recognized by the presence of multiple and disorganized echoes originating from the aortic valve structure during systole and diastole (fig. 5.15). Echocardiography is also useful for measurements of left atrial and left ventricular internal diameters. These measurments are above normal limits in patients with moderate-to-severe aortic stenosis with or without heart failure (fig. 5.17). If a technically satisfactory recording of the aortic valve cannot be obtained, a good recording of the interventricular septum and the posterior wall of the left ventricle will help to determine the degree of left ventricular involvement. An increase in thickness of the interventricular septum and of the posterior wall of the left ventricle is usually associated with hemodynamically significant aortic valvular stenosis (concentric left ventricular hypertrophy). Caution must be exercised in the interpretation of echocardiograms in patients with aortic

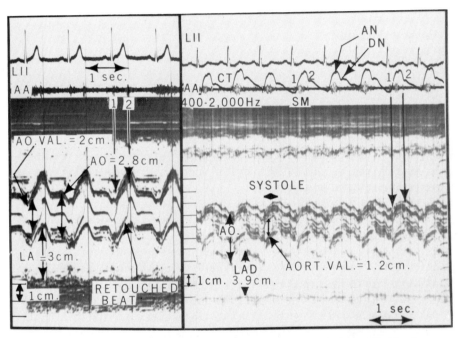

Fig. 5.15. Echocardiogram showing a normal aortic valve (*left panel*). Simultaneously recorded lead II (LII) of the electrocardiogram, carotid pulse tracing (CT), aortic
area (AA) phonocardiogram and echocardiogram of a 69-year-old patient with aortic
stenosis (*right panel*). The carotid pulse tracing is abnormal and shows an anacrotic
notch (AN), dicrotic notch (DN) and carotid shudder. A systolic ejection murmur(SM)
was recorded on the phonocardiogram. The echocardiogram reveals a reduced
systolic opening of the aortic valve (1.2 cm) and multiple diastolic echoes emanating
from the valvular apparatus. These findings are typical for patients with calcific aortic
valvular stenosis.

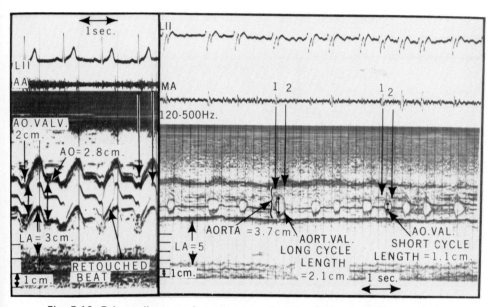

Fig. 5.16. Echocardiogram of a normal aortic valve (*left panel*). The aortic root (AO) measures 2.8 cm and the left atrium (LA) measures 3 cm. Echodardiogram of the aortic valve in a patient with atrial fibrillation without aortic stenosis and with decreased cardiac output (*right panel*). Time of inscription of the first and second heart sounds is indicated. Note the variation in excursion of the aortic value related to cycle length. In beats preceded by a long cycle length the aortic valve opening is approximately 2.1 cm and in beats preceded by a short cycle length it is 1.1 cm. This change is related to variations in stroke volume. The aortic root measures 3.7 cm and left atrial (LA) internal diameter is increased to 5 cm. LII = lead II, **AA** = aortic and **MA** = mitral areas.

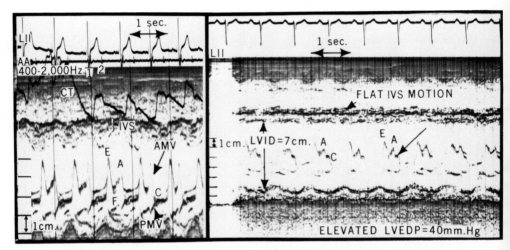

Fig. 5.17. Echocardiogram on a normal subject (*left panel*) and a patient with severe calcific aortic stenosis and left ventricular failure (*right panel*). In the normal subject, note the normal posterior motion of the interventricular septum (IVS) during systole. In the patient with severe calcific aortic stenosis and left ventricular failure, the left ventricular end-diastolic pressure was elevated to 40 mm Hg. Note the flat interventricular septal motion. The left ventricular internal diameter (LVID) was markedly increased to 7 cm. Note the abnormal motion of the anterior mitral valve (AMV) with prolonged A-C interval usually seen in patients with elevated end-diastolic pressures.

stenosis because normal echocardiograms have been recorded in a few patients with proven, severe aortic valvular stenosis.

AORTIC SUBVALVULAR STENOSIS—MEMBRANOUS TYPE

The auscultatory, phonocardiographic, pulse wave and systolic time interval abnormalities in this condition do not differ significantly from those of patients with aortic valvular stenosis. The echocardiogram in patients with membranous aortic stenosis usually shows an early, partial closure of the aortic valve during the first third of systole followed by a secondary opening during the remaining phase of systole as shown in figure 5.18.

SUPRAVALVULAR AORTIC STENOSIS

In patients with congenital supravalvular stenosis, the findings are nearly identical to those described for aortic valvular stenosis. The

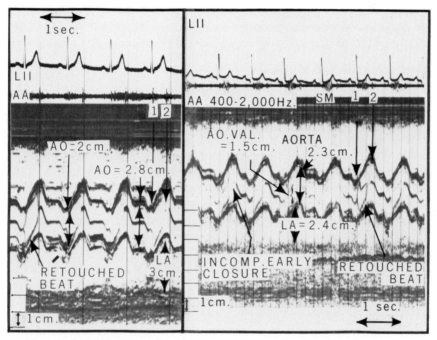

Fig. 5.18. Echocardiogram of a normal aortic valve (*left panel*). Simultaneously recorded lead II (LII) of the electrocardiogram, aortic area (AA) phonocardiogram and echocardiogram in a patient with subaortic stenosis (*right panel*). The echocardiogram shows incomplete, early closure of the aortic valve which is in an eccentric position. Left atrial (LA) internal diameter, 2.4 cm, is within normal limits. A high frequency, high amplitude systolic ejection murmur (SM) was recorded on the phonocardiogram. Time of inscription of the first and second heart sounds is indicated.

systolic ejection click is usually absent. A systolic ejection murmur is more frequently radiated to the left carotid artery with poor transmission to the right carotid artery. The right carotid pulse may show normal features while the left carotid pulse tracing will show the characteristic findings described for aortic valvular stenosis.

AORTIC INSUFFICIENCY

The most common type of aortic insufficiency or regurgitation is due to rheumatic heart disease. Other pathologic states associated with aortic insufficiency are dissecting aortic aneurysm, spondylitis, rheumatoid arthritis, Marfan's syndrome, idiopathic cystic medial necrosis of the aorta, systemic hypertension, atherosclerosis, congenital bicuspid valve, penetrating trauma to the chest wall, bacterial endocarditis with rupture of the cusps and, in some cases, ventricular septal defect with abnormal position of the aortic cusps. In the majority of cases, the auscultatory, phonocardiographic and pulse wave abnormalities are alike, with few exceptions. The characteristic noisy murmur of aortic insufficiency is seen in most of these conditions. The murmur is musical in patients with rupture of the aortic cusps or in patients with rheumatoid arthritis.

Heart Sounds and Murmurs

The first heart sound is normal or slightly accentuated. A systolic ejection click is present in 30–40% of patients with aortic insufficiency due to dilatation of the ascending aorta (fig. 5.19). The second heart sound is single and accentuated due to increased intensity of the aortic valve closure sound secondary to increased aortic pulse pressure. It is best recorded at the aortic and tricuspid areas (figs. 5.19 and 5.20). A third heart sound, frequently heard or recorded on the phonocardiogram in patients with aortic insufficiency, is usually due to increased diastolic volume of the left ventricle secondary to the regurgitation fraction. A fourth heart sound (atrial gallop) is present but should not be considered a sign of heart failure.

A typical, noisy, high frequency arterial diastolic murmur is heard and best recorded at the tricuspid, aortic and mitral areas, particularly when the patient is sitting or standing. It begins with the aortic valve closure sound during the period of isovolumic relaxation, which is the point of maximum intensity of the murmur. It corresponds to the maximum peak of regurgitant flow from the aorta into the left ventricle. This noisy, high frequency murmur in the range of 500 to 2,000 Hz decreases progressively through mid-diastole, terminating prior to atrial contraction (figs. 5.19–5.21). Musical diastolic murmurs may be found in patients with rupture of the aortic valve. A systolic ejection murmur is heard frequently but does not necessarily indicate the presence of significant aortic valvular stenosis. This murmur is the result of increased stroke

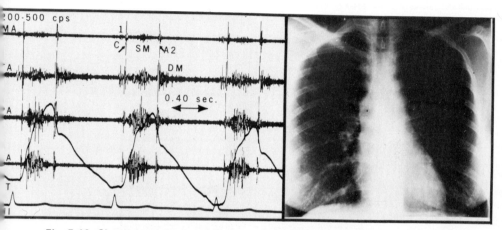

Fig. 5.19. Simultaneously recorded phonocardiogram at the mitral (MA), tricuspid (TA), pulmonic (PA) and aortic areas (AA), carotid pulse tracing (CT) and lead II (LII) of the electrocardiogram in a 28-year-old patient with combined aortic stenosis and insufficiency. The predominant lesion at cardiac catheterization was aortic insufficiency with a small pressure gradient (15 mm Hg) across the aortic valve. The second heart sound is accentuated at the mitral area. It has over twice the amplitude of the first heart sound. A systolic ejection click (C) follows the first heart sound. A high amplitude, high frequency, decrescendo, noisy arterial diastolic murmur (DM) is recorded best at the tricuspid and pulmonic areas. It begins with a second heart sound and terminates prior to atrial contraction. A high frequency, high amplitude, diamond shaped systolic ejection murmur (SM) is recorded in all precordial areas. The carotid pulse tracing shows an anacrotic notch and prolonged ejection time. The chest x-ray shows a dilated ascending aorta and a normal sized heart.

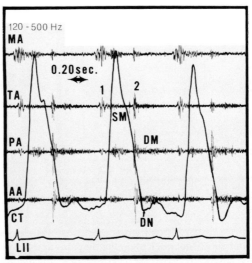

Fig. 5.20. Simultaneously recorded phonocardiogram at the mitral (MA), tricuspid (TA), pulmonic (PA) and aortic (AA) areas, carotid pulse tracing (CT) and lead II (LII) of the electrocardiogram in a 15-year-old patient with severe rheumatic aortic insufficiency. Note the normal first heart sound and accentuation of the second heart sound which is single. There is a high frequency, high amplitude arterial diastolic murmur (DM) with an early diastolic peak terminating at the time of atrial contraction. A high frequency, low amplitude systolic ejection murmur (SM) is recorded in all precordial areas. This murmur has a mid-systolic peak and terminates before the second heart sound. At cardiac catheterization, there was no systolic pressure gradient across the aortic valve. The murmur in this illustration is best recorded at the tricuspid, pulmonic and aortic areas. The carotid pulse tracing shows a rapid upstroke and a dicrotic notch (DN) which is located almost at the baseline level.

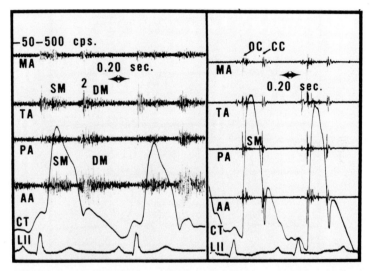

Fig. 5.21. Simultaneously recorded phonocardiogram at the mitral (MA), tricuspid (TA), pulmonic (PA) and aortic areas (AA), carotid pulse tracing (CT) and lead II (LII) of the electrocardiogram before (*left panel*) and after (*right panel*) aortic valve replacement with a Starr-Edwards prosthesis. In the pre-operative tracing note the high frequency, high amplitude arterial diastolic murmur (DM) of aortic insufficiency. The systolic ejection murmur (SM) is probably secondary to increased flow across the aortic valve. Note the opening (OC) and closing clicks (CC) of the prosthetic aortic valve in the post-operative tracing. A short, high frequency, low amplitude systolic ejection murmur is recorded in most precordial areas. The diastolic murmur is absent.

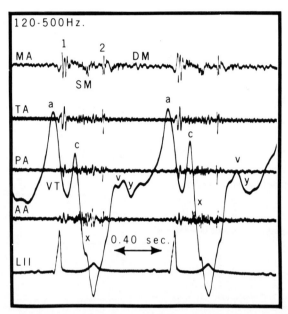

Fig. 5.22. Simultaneously recorded phonocardiogram at the mitral (MA), tricuspid
(TA), pulmonic (PA), and aortic (AA) areas, jugular venous pulse tracing (VT) and lead
II (LII) of the electrocardiogram in a 42-year-old patient with aortic insufficiency and
an Austin Flint murmur. Note the presence of a high frequency, low amplitude systolic ejection murmur (SM) recorded in all precordial areas. The first and second
heart sounds are normal. There is a low frequency, mid-diastolic murmur (DM) best
recorded at the mitral area. There are some low frequency vibrations recorded
following the P wave of the electrocardiogram. The jugular venous tracing is normal.

volume across a non-stenotic aortic valve (figs. 5.20 and 5.21). A short, low frequency, mid-diastolic murmur called the Austin Flint murmur may also be heard in patients with aortic insufficiency and it is recorded best at the mitral area (fig. 5.22). This murmur may be confused with the murmur of mitral stenosis because at times it has a presystolic accentuation. It seems to be related to turbulent, regurgitant aortic flow against the mitral valve.

Carotid Pulse Tracing

Abnormalities on the carotid pulse tracing include the presence of a rapid ascending limb followed by a rapid mid-systolic retraction, a late systolic bulge (pulsus bisferiens) and prolonged ejection time (figs. 5.20–5.28). The dicrotic notch, located near the baseline, is quite conspicuous. The mechanism of the pulsus bisferiens is still not well understood. The probable mechanism seems to be related to a large, rapidly ejected left ventricular stroke volume causing an early, high percussion wave; the mid-systolic retraction may be the result of a rapid decrease in aortic

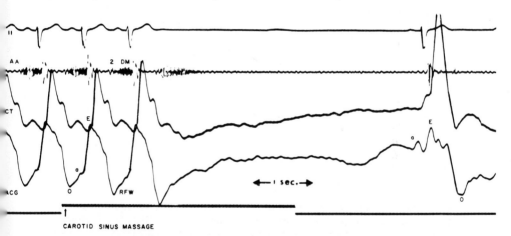

CAROTID SINUS MASSAGE

Fig. 5.23. Simultaneously recorded phonocardiogram at the aortic area (AA), carotid pulse tracing (CT), apexcardiogram (ACG) and lead II (LII) of the electrocardiogram in a patient with aortic insufficiency due to rupture of the aortic cusp secondary to bacterial endocarditis. Note the presence of sinus tachycardia and the musical characteristic of the diastolic murmur (DM) which begins with the second heart sound. During tachycardia (first three beats) the murmur seems to have pre-systolic accentuation. Carotid sinus massage results in a marked decrease in heart rate. The murmur starts with the second heart sound, has a maximal peak during early diastole and terminates in mid-diastole. The remaining part of diastole is clear. Pre-systolic accentuation of the murmur is no longer apparent. The carotid pulse tracing shows a slightly late systolic bulge and a low placed dicrotic notch. The apexcardiogram has a small A wave during sinus tachycardia and a more prominent A wave in the beat preceded by a long cycle length. RFW = rapid filling wave.

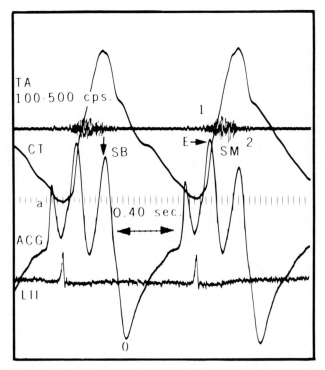

Fig. 5.24. Simultaneously recorded tricuspid (TA) area phonocardiogram, apexcardiogram (ACG), carotid pulse tracing (CT), and lead II (LII) of the electrocardiogram in a 65-year-old patient with aortic stenosis and insufficiency. The diastolic murmur of aortic insufficiency was not well recorded. A systolic ejection murmur (SM) is present. The apexcardiogram shows a triple impulse configuration with a prominent A wave, late systolic bulge (SB) and sharp E point. There is also a mid-systolic retraction. The rapid filling wave is slightly prominent.

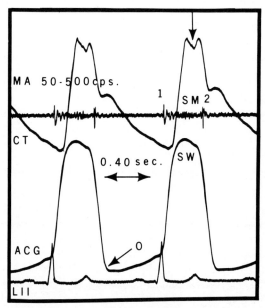

Fig. 5.25. Simultaneously recorded mitral (MA) area phonocardiogram, carotid pulse tracing (CT), apexcardiogram (ACG), and lead II (LII) of the electrocardiogram in a 40-year-old patient with aortic stenosis and predominant aortic insufficiency. The apexcardiogram shows a sustained systolic wave (SW) and the E point cannot be clearly identified. There is a diminutive rapid filling wave following the O point. This type of tracing is seen in patients with severe left ventricular hypertrophy and diminished left ventricular compliance. The carotid pulse tracing shows a rapid ascending limb, mid-systolic retraction (*arrow*) and a normal dicrotic notch. SM = systolic murmur.

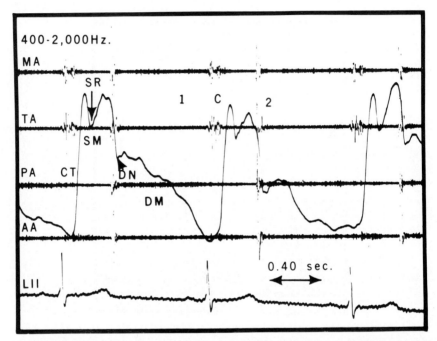

Fig. 5.26. Simultaneously recorded phonocardiogram at the mitral (MA), tricuspid (TA), pulmonic (PA) and aortic areas (AA), carotid pulse tracing (CT) and lead II (LII) of the electrocardiogram in a 63-year-old patient with aortic insufficiency. The first heart sound is normal. There is a systolic ejection click (C) followed by a short, high frequency, low amplitude systolic ejection murmur (SM). The second heart sound is single and markedly accentuated. There is a high frequency, high amplitude arterial diastolic murmur (DM) of aortic insufficiency best recorded at the pulmonic and tricuspid areas. The carotid pulse tracing shows the features of pulsus bisferiens consisting of systolic retraction (SR) and late systolic bulge. DN = dicrotic notch.

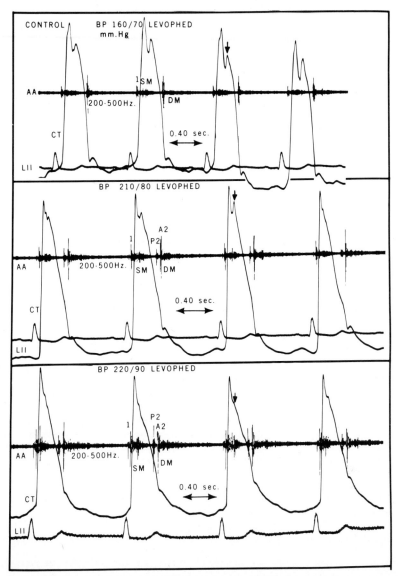

Fig. 5.27. Simultaneously recorded aortic area (AA) phonocardiogram, carotid pulse tracing (CT) and lead II (LII) of the electrocardiogram before and during administration of a vasopressor (Levophed) in a 35-year-old patient with aortic insufficiency. In the control tracing, there is a high frequency, low amplitude systolic ejection murmur (SM) and a high frequency, low amplitude arterial diastolic murmur (DM) of aortic insufficiency. The second heart sound is single. Administration of Levophed with elevation of blood pressure of 210/80 and 220/90 mm Hg results in significant increase in the amplitude of the systolic and arterial diastolic murmur. The second heart sound becomes paradoxically split with the pulmonic component preceding the aortic component and is inscribed before the dicrotic notch in the carotid pulse tracing. Note also that the administration of this agent changes the configuration of the carotid pulse which shows a very rapid rise and rapid fall off.

139

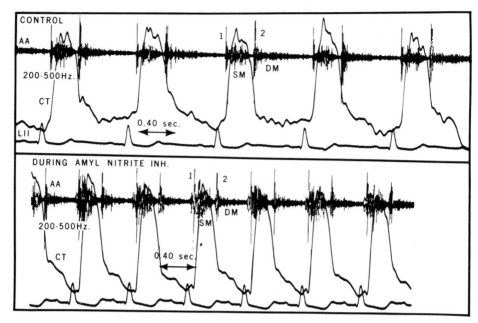

Fig. 5.28. Simultaneously recorded aortic (AA) area phonocardiogram, carotid pulse tracing (CT) and lead II (LII) of the electrocardiogram in a 32-year-old patient with severe aortic insufficiency. The control tracing shows the typical diastolic murmur (DM) of aortic insufficiency as well as a systolic murmur (SM). Inhalation of amyl nitrite results in slightly decreased amplitude of the diastolic murmur and the systolic murmur shows an early systolic peak. Also note that with the tachycardia effect of this drug, the dicrotic notch becomes low placed, close to the baseline, but ejection time is increased to above the normal range.

pulse pressure prior to the inscription of a normally timed tidal or reflected wave.

Systolic Time Intervals

Patients with aortic insufficiency have prolonged left ventricular ejection time due to large total left ventricular stroke volume. The pre-ejection period is reduced probably related to low systemic arterial diastolic pressure and the pre-ejection period to left ventricular ejection time ratio is decreased. As described for patients with aortic valvular stenosis, the presence of congestive heart failure will normalize these systolic time intervals.

Jugular Venous Pulse Tracing

The jugular venous pulse is normal in this condition (fig. 5.22) unless the patient develops heart failure and pulmonary hypertension. In this setting, the A wave is prominent due to right ventricular failure.

Apexcardiogram

The apexcardiogram shows a prominent A wave, a sustained or bifid systolic wave (figs. 5.24 and 5.25) and an accentuated rapid filling wave. In patients with severe left ventricular hypertrophy, the systolic wave is round and the E point is difficult to identify (fig. 5.25).

Maneuvers and Pharmacologic Agents

Cardiac arrhythmias can cause significant changes in the configuration and the maximal time amplitude of the murmur of aortic insufficiency. As shown in figure 5.23, in patients with sinus tachycardia and aortic insufficiency the murmur may simulate the one seen in patients with mitral stenosis because of a short diastolic cycle length. However, if sinus bradycardia can be induced by carotid sinus massage (fig. 5.23), it will help in the differential diagnosis. If the murmur is due to aortic insufficiency, it shows an early diastolic peak terminating in mid-diastole.

Administration of vasopressor agents which result in an increase in systemic resistance and aortic pulse pressure causes an increase in the diastolic regurgitant flow and accentuation of the diastolic murmur of aortic insufficiency (fig. 5.27), and the second heart sound may become paradoxically split. As shown in figure 5.27, the second heart sound is single in the control tracing when the arterial blood pressure is 160/70 mm Hg. Intravenous administration of levarterenol results in progressive increase in blood pressure to 210/80 mm Hg and, at 220/90 mm Hg, the second heart sound becomes split and both the pulmonic and aortic components precede the dicrotic notch of the carotid pulse tracing.

Administration of vasodilators such as inhalation of amyl nitrite causes a decrease in amplitude of the diastolic murmur of aortic insufficiency and a slight increase in amplitude of the systolic ejection murmur as shown in figure 5.28.

Echocardiogram

The echocardiogram is useful in studying patients with aortic insufficiency. The most common finding is the presence of a dilated aortic root with or without thickening or calcification of the aortic valve, multiple diastolic echoes and incomplete closure of the valve during diastole. Increased thickening of the interventricular septum and an increase in left ventricular and left atrial diameters can be seen (figs. 5.29–5.33). Abnormal motion of the aorta and/or leaflets of the mitral valve can be seen, including the presence of "flutter" of the anterior leaflet during diastole. This is a fine fluttering as compared with coarse fluttering as seen in patients with atrial fibrillation or flutter (fig. 5.33) without aortic insufficiency. However, if the patient has associated mitral valve disease

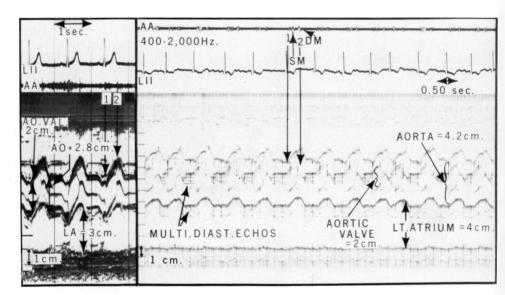

Fig. 5.29. Echocardiogram of a normal aortic valve (**AO VAL.**) (*left panel*). Echocardiogram in a patient with hemodynamically significant aortic valvular insufficiency (*right panel*). Note the presence of multiple diastolic echoes. The aortic root measures 4.2 cm as compared with left atrial internal diameter of 4 cm. The aortic valve opening averages about 2 cm. The rhythm is atrial fibrillation. The phonocardiogram shows an aortic systolic ejection murmur (**SM**) and the arterial diastolic murmur (**DM**) of aortic insufficiency. **LII** = lead II,. **LA** = left atrium, **AA** = aortic area.

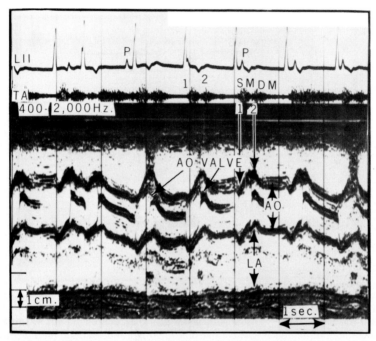

Fig. 5.30. Simultaneously recorded lead II (LII) of the electrocardiogram, tricuspid area (TA) phonocardiogram and echocardiogram in a 16-year-old patient with severe aortic insufficiency and complete heart block. Time of inscription of the first and second heart sounds is indicated. The phonocardiogram shows a typical arterial diastolic murmur (DM) of aortic insufficiency and a prominent systolic ejection murmur (SM) due to increased flow across the aortic valve. Note heavy echoes originating from the aortic valve. The left atrium (LA) measures 3.5 cm, aortic root, 3 cm; and the aortic valve, 2.4 cm. AO = aorta.

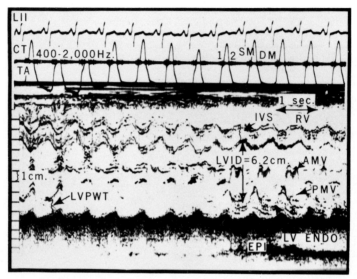

Fig. 5.31. Simultaneously recorded tricuspid area (TA) phonocardiogram, carotid pulse tracing (CT), lead II (LII) of the electrocardiogram and echocardiogram in a 59-year-old patient with aortic insufficiency and dilatation of the left ventricle. The phonocardiogram shows a systolic murmur (SM) and the diastolic murmur (DM) of aortic insufficiency. The echocardiogram shows increased thickness of the interventricular septum (IVS) and posterior wall of the left ventricle (LVPWT) which measures approximately 1.6 cm (concentric hypertrophy). Left ventricular internal diameter (LVID) is increased to 6.2 cm. During cardiac catheterization the patient was found to have marked aortic insufficiency and a markedly enlarged left ventricle. AMV = anterior mitral valve, PMV = posterior mitral valve, LV ENDO = left ventricular endocardium, EP = epicardium, RV = right ventricle.

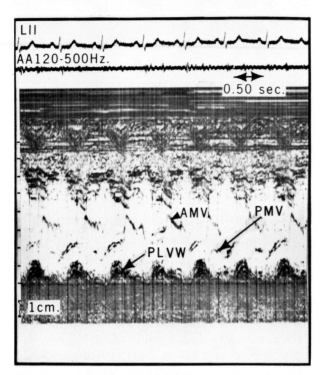

Fig. 5.32. Simultaneously recorded echocardiogram, aortic area (AA), phonocardiogram and lead II (LII) of the electrocardiogram in a 51-year-old patient with
rheumatic aortic insufficiency. Note the fine fluttering of the mitral valve in the
echocardiogram. AMV = anterior mitral valve, PMV = posterior mitral valve, PLVW
= posterior left ventricular wall.

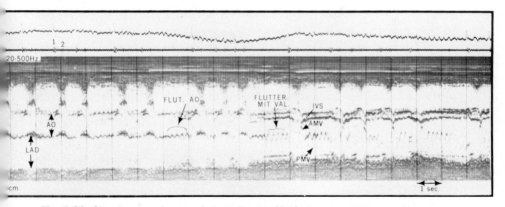

Fig. 5.33. Simultaneously recorded aortic area (AA) phonocardiogram, lead II (LII)
of the electrocardiogram and echocardiographic scan from the aorta (AO) to the
mitral valve in a 70-year-old patient with idiopathic atrial fibrillation and a normal
aortic valve. Note the coarse fluttering waves of the aortic valve and mitral leaflets.
IVS = interventricular septum, LAD = left atrial diameter, AMV = anterior mitral
valve, PMV = posterior mitral valve.

with thickening or calcification of the mitral valve, fluttering may not be detected. Fluttering of the mitral valve in patients with aortic insufficiency seems to explain the Austin Flint murmur seen in this condition. It probably corresponds to regurgitant aortic flow against the mitral valve resulting in a diastolic murmur which simulates mitral stenosis. Additional, important echocardiographic signs in aortic insufficiency are premature closure of the mitral valve, with the C point occurring, at times, even before the QRS complex of the electrocardiogram, and a small E wave in relation to the A wave.

IDIOPATHIC HYPERTROPHIC SUBAORTIC STENOSIS

Idiopathic hypertrophic subaortic stenosis (IHSS) is a disease of unknown etiology in which there is asymmetrical septal hypertrophy (ASH phenomenon), causing obstruction of ventricular ejection.

Heart Sounds and Murmurs

The first heart sound is normal. The second heart sound shows normal amplitude of the aortic valve closure sound which helps in the differentiation from aortic valvular stenosis. Reverse splitting of the second heart sound is frequently seen, particularly in patients with a significant gradient at rest. Systolic ejection clicks are infrequent in this condition and are seen in less than 10% of patients. Prominent fourth heart sounds are quite common (figs. 5.34 and 5.35). Third heart sounds are infrequent unless the patient develops heart failure.

High frequency, high amplitude systolic ejection murmurs are common. They are recorded at the aortic and/or mitral areas and may radiate to both carotid arteries. This murmur probably represents turbulent flow across the mid-cavity obstruction and it usually has noisy characteristics (figs. 5.34–5.43). This murmur will increase in amplitude during maneuvers such as Valsalva (fig. 5.41) and during administration of isoproterenol (fig. 5.40), inhalation of amyl nitrite, squatting and in cardiac cycles following an atrial, junctional or ventricular premature contraction or postural changes (figs. 5.42 and 5.44).

An arterial diastolic murmur of aortic insufficiency has been described in this condition, although it is rare. Its mechanism seems to be due to deformity of the aortic cusps resulting in dilatation of the aortic ring, thus allowing regurgitation to occur. When this murmur is present, it has the same characteristics described in patients with aortic valvular insufficiency. (See "Aortic Insufficiency.")

Carotid Pulse Tracing

The carotid pulse tracing is useful in the diagnosis of idiopathic hypertrophic subaortic stenosis. The usual features include a rapid

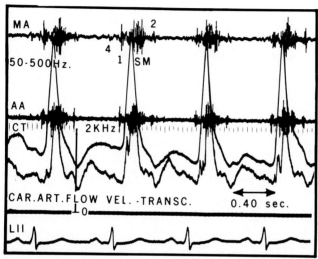

Fig. 5.34. Simultaneously recorded phonocardiogram at the mitral (MA) and aortic areas (AA), carotid pulse tracing (CT), and lead II (LII) of the electrocardiogram and transcutaneous carotid artery flow velocity curves in a 28-year-old patient with idiopathic hypertrophic subaortic stenosis. The phonocardiogram shows normal first and second heart sounds. There is a fourth heart sound at the mitral area. A typical high frequency systolic ejection murmur (SM) is present with a mid-systolic peak, terminating prior to the second heart sound. The carotid pulse tracing shows a rapid rise with rapid fall-off and prolonged ejection time. The wave form of the transcutaneous carotid flow velocity curves is quite similar to the contour of the carotid artery pulse tracing.

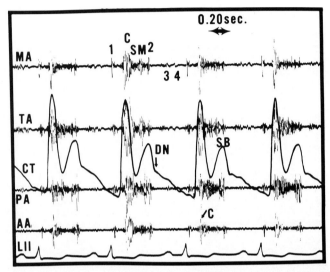

Fig. 5.35. Simultaneously recorded phonocardiogram at the mitral (MA), tricuspid (TA), pulmonic (PA) an aortic (AA) areas, carotid pulse tracing (CT) and lead II (LII) of the electrocardiogram in a 31-year-old patient with idiopathic hypertrophic subaortic stenosis. Note normal first and second heart sounds. A third and fourth heart sound are recorded, as well as a systolic ejection click (C), which is followed by a high frequency systolic ejection murmur (SM). The carotid pulse tracing shows rapid upstroke followed by a prominent, late systolic bulge (SB). The dicrotic notch (DN) is inconspicuous and ejection time is prolonged. At cardiac catheterization, the patient had a gradient of 85 mm Hg across the outflow tract of the left ventricle, and left ventricular end-diastolic pressure was elevated despite the clinical evidence of heart failure.

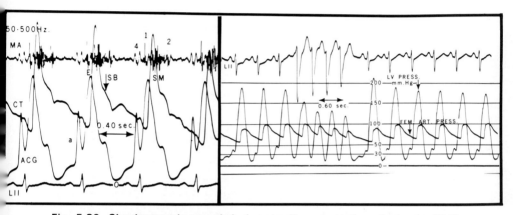

Fig. 5.36. Simultaneously recorded phonocardiogram at the mitral area (MA), carotid pulse tracing (CT), apexcardiogram (ACG) and lead II (LII) of the electrocardiogram (*left panel*) in a 28-year-old patient with idiopathic hypertrophic subaortic stenosis. There are normal first and second heart sounds and a prominent fourth heart sound. A high frequency systolic ejection murmur (SM) terminates prior to the second heart sound. The carotid pulse tracing shows a discrete systolic retraction followed by a small late systolic bulge (SB). The apexcardiogram shows a prominent A wave and a diminished rapid filling wave. The simultaneous recording of left ventricular (LV PRESS.), and femoral artery pressures (FEM ART PRESS.) with lead II of the electrocardiogram (*right panel*) shows a pressure gradient between the left ventricle and femoral artery of 35 mm Hg during sinus rhythm. During ventricular tachycardia the gradient is decreased to 20 mm Hg due primarily to a decrease in left ventricular peak systolic pressure. However, the post ventricular tachycardia gradient increased to approximately 105 mm Hg.

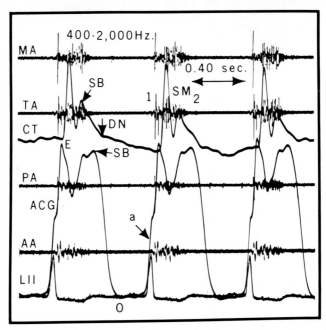

Fig. 5.37. Simultaneously recorded phonocardiogram at the mitral (MA), tricuspid (TA), pulmonic PA) and aortic (AA) areas, carotid pulse tracing (CT), apexcardiogram (ACG) and lead II (LII) of the electrocardiogram in a 39-year-old patient with severe idiopathic hypertrophic subaortic stenosis. Note the typical systolic ejection murmur (SM) which was described earlier. The carotid pulse tracing shows a rapid upstroke time with an early systolic retraction followed by a late systolic bulge (SB). The dicrotic notch (DN) is normal. The apexcardiogram shows a sharp E point with early systolic retraction coinciding with retraction in the carotid pulse tracing. It is followed by a late systolic bulge. The A wave of the apexcardiogram is markedly exaggerated.

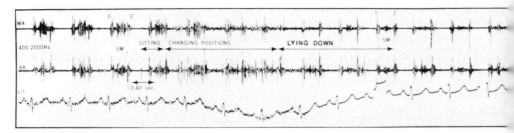

Fig. 5.38. Simultaneously recorded phonocardiogram at the mitral (MA) and aortic areas (AA) and lead II (LII) of the electrocardiogram in a 54-year-old patient with idiopathic hypertrophic subaortic stenosis. On the left side the systolic ejection murmur (SM) is more prominent in the sitting position as compared with the decubitus position shown at the right. The change in position produces changes in left ventricular end-diastolic pressure due to venous return. While the patient is lying down venous return is augmented and left ventricular end-diastolic pressure is increased with a subsequent reduction in the outflow tract gradient.

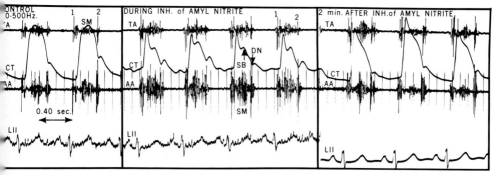

Fig. 5.39. Simultaneously recorded phonocardiogram at the tricuspid (TA) and aortic areas (AA), carotid pulse tracing (CT) and lead II (LII) of the electrocardiogram in a 54-year-old patient with idiopathic hypertrophic subaortic stenosis. The control tracing (*left panel*) shows a systolic ejection murmur (SM) and prolonged ejection time on the carotid pulse tracing. However, contour of the carotid pulse tracing is normal. During inhalation of amyl nitrite (*middle panel*) there is a marked increase in amplitude of the systolic ejection murmur and the contour of the carotid pulse tracing is typical for patients with idiopathic hypertrophic stenosis. Two minutes after inhalation of amyl nitrite (*right panel*) the carotid pulse tracing still shows a rapid rise but the systolic retraction and systolic bulge are much less conspicuous as compared with the middle panel. Again, the effects of alteration in venous return and end-diastolic pressure have produced changing characteristics of the outflow tract gradient as shown in figure 5.38.

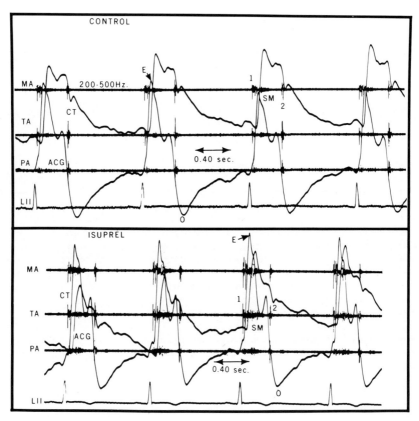

Fig. 5.40. Simultaneously recorded phonocardiogram at the mitral (MA), tricuspid (TA) and pulmonic (PA) areas, apexcardiogram (ACG) carotid pulse tracing (CT) and lead II (LII) of the electrocardiogram in a 17-year-old patient with idiopathic hypertrophic subaortic stenosis. In the control tracing note the normal first and second heart sounds. There is a low frequency, high amplitude systolic ejection murmur (SM) which terminates in mid-systole. Contour of the carotid pulse tracing and apexcardiogram are normal. During intravenous administration of Isuprel there is a significant increase in amplitude of the systolic ejection murmur. The carotid pulse tracing shows a rapid rise followed by a systolic retraction and prolonged ejection time. The apexcardiogram shows an increase in amplitude of the late systolic bulge.

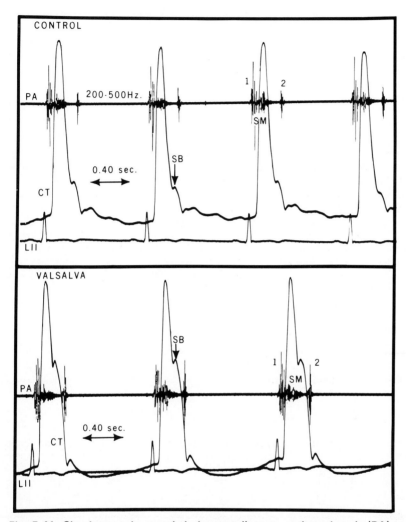

Fig. 5.41. Simultaneously recorded phonocardiogram at the pulmonic (PA) area, carotid pulse tracing (CT), and lead II (LII) of the electrocardiogram in a 17-year-old patient with idiopathic hypertrophic subaortic stenosis before and during Valsalva maneuver. The systolic ejection murmur (SM) is well recorded in the pulmonic area. The carotid pulse tracing shows a rapid upstroke, a small, late systolic bulge (SB) and normal dicrotic notch. The Valsalva maneuver results in a slight increase in amplitude of the systolic murmur with earlier inscription and higher amplitude of the systolic bulge in the carotid pulse tracing.

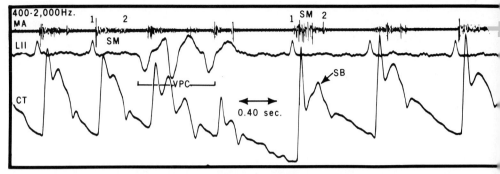

Fig. 5.42. Simultaneously recorded phonocardiogram at the mitral (MA) area, lead II (LII) of the electrocardiogram and carotid pulse tracing (CT) in a 63-year-old patient with idiopathic hypertrophic subaortic stenosis. The first two sinus beats show a high frequency, medium amplitude systolic ejection murmur (SM). The carotid pulse tracing shows a rapid rise followed by a mid-systolic retraction and late systolic bulge (SB). Three recorded ventricular premature contractions (VPC) result in diminution of the systolic murmur and in the amplitude of the carotid pulse tracing. The first sinus beat following the premature contractions shows an increase in amplitude of the systolic murmur and exaggeration of the abnormalities of the carotid pulse tracing.

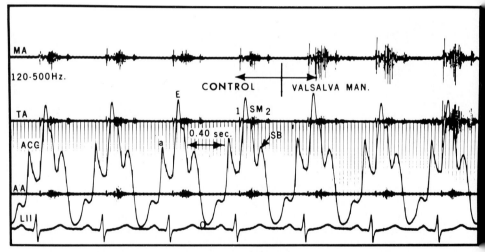

Fig. 5.43. Simultaneously recorded phonocardiogram at the mitral (MA), tricuspid (TA), and aortic (AA) areas, apexcardiogram (ACG) and lead II (LII) of the electrocardiogram in a 28-year-old patient with idiopathic hypertrophic subaortic stenosis before and during Valsalva maneuver. Note the marked increase in amplitude of the systolic ejection murmur (SM) during the Valsalva maneuver. The apexcardiogram shows a prominent A wave, sharp E point and a late systolic bulge (SB).

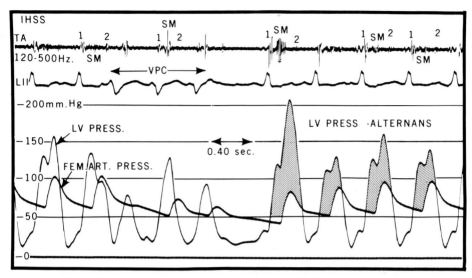

Fig. 5.44. Simultaneously recorded tricuspid area (TA) phonocardiogram, lead II (LII) of the electrocardiogram, left ventricular (LV PRESS.) and femoral artery pressures (FEM. ART. PRESS.) in a patient with idiopathic hypertrophic subaortic stenosis (IHSS). The first two sinus beats are followed by three ventricular premature contractions (VPC). The *shaded area* in the pressure curves indicates the presence of a systolic gradient between the left ventricle and femoral artery. There is a low amplitude, high frequency systolic ejection murmur (SM) in the sinus beats preceding ventricular premature contractions. Following the premature contractions there is a marked increase in amplitude of the systolic ejection murmur and an increase in the gradient between the left ventricle and femoral artery. Sinus beats following the ventricular premature contractions exhibit the appearance of pulsus alternans.

upstroke time due to rapid emptying of blood between the mid-cavity obstruction and the aortic valve causing a sudden distension of the peripheral arteries. This is followed by a rapid systolic retraction and a late systolic bulge which is usually inscribed in the last third of ventricular systole. The dicrotic notch is normal and an anacrotic notch is not present (figs. 5.34–5.37). If the carotid pulse tracing has a normal contour at rest, the pressure gradient across the mid-cavity of the left ventricle is usually small. If the features described above are not present and if this diagnosis is suspected clinically, administration of amyl nitrite (fig. 5.39), isoproterenol (fig. 5.40) and the Valsalva maneuver (fig. 5.41) will usually induce them.

Jugular Venous Pulse Tracing

The jugular venous pulse usually is not helpful in the diagnosis of this disease. At times, one may detect a large A wave which probably represents a marked degree of asymmetrical septal hypertrophy which would impair normal right ventricular contraction. However, it must be emphasized that cases of idiopathic hypertrophy of the outflow tract of the right ventricle have been described simulating the findings seen in idiopathic hypertrophic subaortic stenosis.

Apexcardiogram

The apexcardiogram shows a prominent A wave, probably due to decreased left ventricular compliance causing a forceful left atrial systole against a non-distensible left ventricle (figs. 5.36 and 5.43). The E point is usually sharp and well recognized. Following the E point, there is a mid-systolic retraction; for this retraction to be significant, the maximal downward systolic deflection should reach approximately one-third of the total amplitude of the apexcardiogram as measured from the E to the O point. After the systolic retraction, there is a late systolic bulge which has a maximal peak near the second heart sound (fig. 5.37). Occasionally, a round systolic wave of the type seen in patients with other types of severe left ventricular hypertrophy from any cause is seen. The rapid filling wave is usually small and the transition between this wave and the slow filling wave is inconspicuous. As described for the heart murmurs and carotid pulse tracing, some of these changes, if not present at rest, may be induced by exercise, Valsalva maneuver, administration of drugs, extrasystoles, etc.

Systolic Time Intervals

Corrected ejection time is increased in patients with idiopathic hypertrophic subaortic stenosis who have significant outflow tract obstruction. Valsava maneuver, exercise, post-extrasystolic beats (fig. 5.42), administration of vasopressor agents and inhalation of amyl nitrite will increase the gradient across the outflow tract of the left ventricle, therefore, increasing ejection time.

Echocardiogram

Echocardiography, a very important non-invasive technique in the diagnosis of idiopathic hypertrophic subaortic stenosis (figs. 5.45–5.48) is also useful for follow-up. Several investigators have shown that a very common finding in patients with idiopathic hypertrophic subaortic stenosis with or without gradients at rest is an increase in thickness of the interventricular septum in relation to left ventricular posterior wall thickness. Most patients will have a ratio of interventricular septum to the ventricular posterior wall greater than the normal ratio, 1.3:1 (figs. 5.45 and 5.47). It must be emphasized that the pathophysiology of this disease is still not fully understood. Echocardiographic studies show abnormal systolic anterior motion of the mitral valve which may

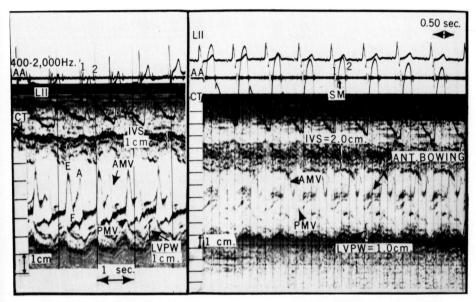

Fig. 5.45. Simultaneously recorded echocardiogram, aortic area (AA) phonocardiogram, lead II (LII) of the electrocardiogram and carotid pulse tracing (CT) in a normal subject (*left panel*) showing normal thickness of the interventricular septum (IVS) and normal motion of the mitral valve. The typical echocardiogram of a patient with idiopathic hypertrophic subaortic stenosis is shown in the right panel. Interventricular septal thickness is increased to 2 cm as compared with left ventricular posterior wall (LVPW) thickness of 1 cm, constituting asymmetrical septal hypertrophy. Note the abnormal, anterior systolic motion of the anterior leaflet of the mitral valve (AMV). PMV = posterior mitral valve, SM = systolic murmur.

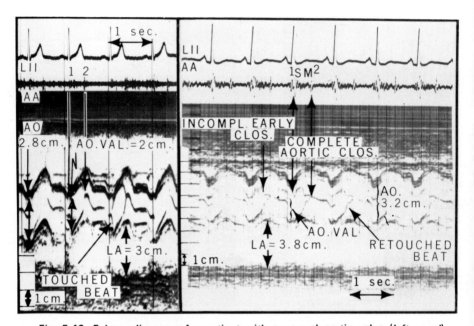

Fig. 5.46. Echocardiogram of a patient with a normal aortic valve (*left panel*). Simultaneously recorded lead II (LII) of the electrocardiogram, aortic area (AA) phonocardiogram and echocardiogram in a patient with idiopathic hypertrophic subaortic stenosis (*right panel*). Note the incomplete, early closure of the aortic valve. The aortic root which measures 3.2 cm and left atrial (LA) internal diameter of 3.8 cm are within normal limits. The phonocardiogram shows normal first and second heart sounds and a high frequency, low amplitude systolic ejection murmur (SM). Time of inscription of the first and second heart sounds is indicated. AO = aorta.

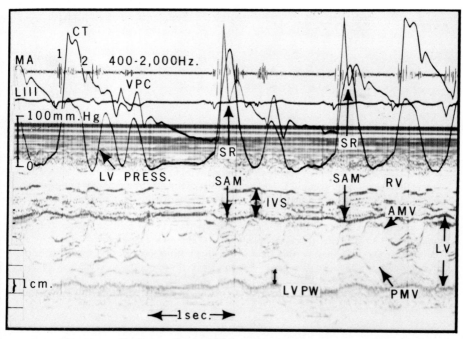

Fig. 5.47. Simultaneously recorded mitral area (MA) phonocardiogram, lead III (LIII) of the electrocardiogram, carotid pulse tracing (CT), echocardiogram and left ventricular pressure curves (LV PRESS.) in a 41-year-old patient with idiopathic hypertrophic subaortic stenosis. The first sinus beat is followed by a ventricular premature contraction (VPC). In the sinus beat the first and second heart sounds are normal and there is a low frequency, high amplitude systolic ejection murmur. Contour of the carotid pulse tracing in the sinus beats which precede and follow the premature contraction shows a small, late systolic bulge. Following the ventricular premature contraction there is a marked increase in amplitude of the systolic ejection murmur. The typical configuration of the carotid pulse tracing includes a rapid upstroke time followed by a mid-systolic retraction (SR) and a late systolic bulge. The echocardiogram shows increased thickness of the interventricular septum (IVS) to 2 cm and left ventricular posterior wall (LVPW) thickness measures 1 cm (asymmetrical septal hypertrophy). Following the ventricular premature contraction there is marked accentuation of the anterior systolic motion (SAM) of the mitral valve. The left ventricle (LV) measures 4.2 cm. AMV = anterior mitral valve, PMV = posterior mitral valve, RV = right ventricle.

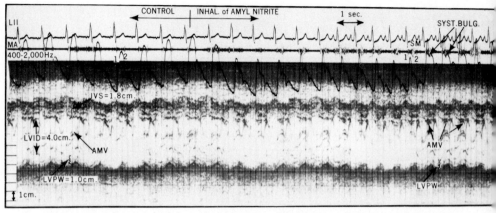

Fig. 5.48. Simultaneously recorded mitral area (MA) phonocardiogram, echocardiogram, carotid pulse tracing (CT) and lead II (LII) of the electrocardiogram before and during inhalation of amyl nitrite in a 52-year-old patient with idiopathic hypertrophic subaortic stenosis. The contour of the carotid pulse tracing is not compatible with the diagnosis of idiopathic hypertrophic subaortic stenosis in the control tracing. During inhalation of amyl nitrite the carotid pulse tracing shows the characteristic features of the disease as described in this chapter. Typical sinus tachycardia resulting from pharmacologic effects of the drug is seen. Note the increase in thickness of the interventricular septum (IVS) to 1.8 cm, and abnormal anterior mitral valve motion (AMV). LVID = left ventricular internal diameter, LVPW = left ventricular posterior wall, SM = systolic murmur.

contribute to the mid-cavity obstruction (figs. 5.45 and 5.47). In some patients, the degree of systolic anterior motion (SAM) of the anterior mitral valve may be so exaggerated that it will touch the interventricular septum (figs. 5.47 and 5.48). However, caution must be exercised in interpreting this finding. If the ultrasonic beam is pointed superiorly at the point where the mitral valve leaflet is seen, echoes from the mitral annulus are recorded and this structure may actually move anteriorly during ventricular contraction and false positive findings may be encountered in normal individuals. An index for degree of obstruction has been developed by several investigators and it takes into consideration the abnormal anterior mitral valve motion, separation of anterior mitral leaflet and the interventricular septum. It must be emphasized that the interventricular septum to posterior wall thickness ratio may be abnormal in children with congenital heart disease and associated right ventricular hypertrophy such as tetralogy of Fallot, transposition of the great vessels, ventricular septal defect, pulmonary stenosis and others. Abnormal motion of the aortic valve is seen in many patients with idiopathic hypertrophic subaortic stenosis, particularly those who have significant gradients at rest. In these patients, an early premature systolic closure of the aortic valve is seen and probably is due to the fact that most of the left ventricular stroke output is ejected into the aorta in the first third of the mechanical systole with the valve moving subsequently to a semiclosed position to reopen during late left ventricular systole.

Maneuvers and Pharmacologic Agents

Valsalva maneuver is important in the recognition of hypertrophic subaortic stenosis. This maneuver causes a decrease in left ventricular volume greatly increasing obstruction. Therefore, during the Valsalva maneuver, the systolic ejection murmur markedly increases in intensity as shown in figure 5.43.

The use of pharmacologic agents, such as inhalation of amyl nitrite, provokes an increase in the gradient across the outflow tract of the left ventricle and such agents are, therefore, useful in the diagnosis of this condition. As shown in figure 5.48, inhalation of amyl nitrite results in an exaggeration of the abnormalities in the echocardiogram as described above.

REFERENCES

1. Abelmann, W. H.: Aortic stenosis in older patients. N. Engl. J. Med., *281:* 1305, 1969.
2. Arani, D. T., and Carleton, R. A.: Assessment of aortic valvular stenosis from the aortic pressure pulse. Circulation, *36:* 30, 1967.
3. Bache, R. J., Wang, Y., and Greenfield, J. C. Jr.: Left ventricular ejection time in valvular aortic stenosis. Circulation, *47:* 527, 1973.
4. Benchimol, A., and Matsuo, S.: Ejection time before and after aortic valve replacement. Am. J. Cardiol., *27:* 244, 1971.
5. Bleich, A., Lewis, J., and Marcus, F. I.: Aortic regurgitation in the elderly. Am. Heart J., *71:* 627, 1966.
6. Bolteau, G. M., Libanoff, A. J., and Allenstein, B. J.: Upstroke time ratio in valvular aortic insufficiency. Am. J. Cardiol., *14:* 162, 1964.
7. Bonner, A. J. Jr., Sacks, H. N., and Tavel, M. E.: Assessing the severity of aortic stenosis by phonocardiography and external carotid pulse recordings. Circulation, *48:* 247, 1973.
8. Braunwald, E., Lambrew, C. T., Rockoff, S. D., Ross, J. Jr., and Morrow, A. G.: Idiopathic hypertrophic subaortic stenosis; I. A description of the disease based upon an analysis of 64 patients. Circulation, *30*(4): 3, 1964.
9. Caulfield, W. H., DeLeon, A. C. Jr., Perloff, J. K., and Steelman, R. B.: The clinical significance of the fourth heart sound in aortic stenosis. Am. J. Cardiol., *28:* 179, 1971.
10. Cohn, K. E., Flamm, M. D., and Hancock, E. W.: Amyl nitrite inhalation as a screening test for hypertrophic subaortic stenosis. Am. J. Cardiol., *21:* 681, 1968.
11. Cohn, K. E., Sandler, H., and Hancock, E. W.: Mechanisms of pulsus alternans. Circulation, *36:* 372, 1967.
12. Cohn, L. H. Mason, D. T., Ross, J. Jr., Morrow, A. G., and Braunwald, E.: Preoperative assessment of aortic regurgitation in patients with mitral valve disease. Am. J. Cardiol., *19:* 177, 1967.
13. Curtiss, E. I., Matthews, R. G., and Shaver, J. A.: Mechanism of normal splitting of the second heart sound. Circulation, *51:*(1): 157, 1975.
14. Danford, H. G., Danford, D. A., Mielke, J. E., and Peterson, L. F.: Echocardiographic evaluation of the hemodynamic effects of chronic aortic insufficiency with observations on left ventricular performance. Circulation, *48:* 253, 1973.
15. Dellocchio, T., Dolara, A., Salvatore, L., and Vergassola, R.: Left ventricular

hypertrophy with right ventricular outflow obstruction. Br. Heart J., *34:* 752, 1972.

16. Delman, A. J., Gordon, G. M., Eisenberg, R., Escher, D. J. W., and Rosenblum, R.: The direct brachial arterial pulse-pressure curve in the evalutation of patients with aortic valvular stenosis. Am. Heart J., *69:* 582, 1965.

17. Donnelly, G. L., and Vandenberg, E. A.: Early systolic sounds in aortic valve stenosis. Br. Heart J., *29:* 246, 1967.

18. Dressler, W., and Rubin, R.: Complex shape and variability of the diastolic murmur of aortic regurgitation. Am. J. Cardiol., *18:* 616, 1966.

19. Dressler, W., and Rubin, R.: Overlapping of ventricular filling and contraction. Am. Heart J., *69:* 599, 1965.

20. Eddleman, E. E. Jr., Bancroft, W. H. Jr., and Swatzell, R. H. Jr.: A contour study of the carotid pulse in normal subjects, aortic valvular disease, and hypertrophic subaortic stenosis. Comput. Biomed. Res., *3:* 274, 1970.

21. Eisenberg, R., Young, D., Jacobson, B., and Boito, A.: Familial supravalvular aortic stenosis. Am. J. Dis. Child., *108:* 341, 1964.

22. Epstein, E. J., Coulshed, N., Brown, A. K., and Doukas, N. G.: The 'A' wave of the apex cardiogram in aortic valve disease and cardiomyopathy. Br. Heart J., *30:* 591, 1968.

23. Fearon, R. E., Cohen, L. S., O'Hara, J. M., and Goodyer, A. V. N.: Diastolic murmurs due to two sequelae of atherosclerotic coronary artery disease; ventricular aneurysm and coronary artery stenosis. Am. Heart J., *76:* 252, 1968.

24. Feizi, O., Symons, C., and Yacoub, M.: Echocardiography of the aortic valve; I. Studies of normal aortic valve, aortic stenosis, aortic regurgitation, and mixed aortic valve disease. Br. Heart J., *36:* 341, 1974.

25. Feizi, O., Symons, C., and Yacoub, M.: Echocardiography of normal and diseased aortic valve. Br. Heart J., *35:* 560, 1973.

26. Finegan, R. E., Gianelly, R. E., and Harrison, D. C.: Aortic stenosis in the elderly; relevance of age to diagnosis and treatment. N. Engl. J. Med., *281:* 1261, 1969.

27. Fishleder, B. L.: *Exploracion Cardiovascular y Fonomecano-cardiografia Clinica.* La Prensa Medica Mexicana, Mexico, 1966.

28. Fischer, T., and Rona, G.: The clinical significance of presystolic gallop rhythm; preliminary communication. Cardiologia, *46:* 325, 1965.

29. Fleming, J. S.: The assessment of failure in aortic stenosis from the diastolic movements of the left ventricle. Am. Heart J., *76:* 235, 1968.

30. Fletcher, G. F., and Hurst, J. W.: An intermittent "cooing" diastolic murmur due to a torn aortic valve cusp. Am. Heart J., *75:* 537, 1968.

31. Folts, J. D., Young, W. P., and Rowe, G. G.: A study of Duroziez's murmur of aortic insufficiency in man utilizing an electromagnetic flowmeter. Circulation, *38:* 426, 1968.

32. Frank, S., and Braunwald, E.: Idiopathic hypertrophic subaortic stenosis; clinical analysis of 126 patients with emphasis on the natural history. Circulation, *37:* 759, 1968. 759, 1968.

33. Giles, T. D., Martinez, E. C., and Burch, G. E.: Gallavardin phenomenon in aortic stenosis; a possible mechanism. Arch. Intern. Med., *134:* 747, 1974.

34. Giulani, M. G., and Gould, L.: The pitfalls of the brachial arterial pressure curve in the evaluation of valvular aortic stenosis. Jap. Heart J., *10:* 467, 1969.

35. Gottlieb, S., Khuddus, S. A., Balook, H., Dominquez, A. E., and Myerburg, R. J.: Echocardiographic diagnosis of aortic valve vegetations in candida endocarditis. Circulation, *50:* 826, 1974.

36. Gould, L., and Lyon, A. F.: Postural changes in the brachial artery first derivative in the normal and pathologic state. Dis. Chest, *53:* 476, 1968.

37. Gramiak, R., Shah, P. M.: Echocardiography of the aortic root. Invest. Radiol., *3:* 356, 1968.

38. Gyulai, F., and Walsh, Z.: The Q-A2 interval during exercise in assessing severity of aortic stenosis. Acta Paediatr. Scand. Suppl., *177:* 34, 1967.

39. Halloran, K. H., Talner, N. S., and Browne, M. J.: A study of ventricular septal defect associated with aortic insufficiency. Am. Heart J., *69:* 320, 1965.

40. Hancock, E. W., and Eldridge, F.: Muscular subaortic stenosis; reversibility with varying cardiac cycle length. Am. J. Cardiol., *18:* 515, 1968.
41. Harris, A. M., Sleight, P., and Drew, C. E.: The diagnosis and treatment of aortic stenosis complicated by heart block. Br. Heart J., *27:* 560, 1965.
42. Henry, W. L., Clark, C. E., and Epstein, S. E.: Asymmetric septal hypertrophy; echocardiographic identification of the pathognomonic anatomic abnormality of IHSS. Circulation, *47:* 225, 1973.
43. Herbert, W. H.: Atrial transport and aortic insufficiency. Br. Heart J., *29:* 559, 1967.
44. Hernberg, J., Weiss, B., and Keegan, A.: The ultrasonic recording of aortic valve motion. Radiology, *94:* 361, 1970.
45. Hurwitz, L. E., and Roberts, W. C.: Quadricuspid semilunar valve. Am. J. Cardiol., *31:* 623, 1973.
46. Johnson, A. M.: Aortic stenosis, sudden death, and left ventricular baroceptors. Br. Heart J., *33:* 1, 1971.
47. Johnson, S. L., Baker, D. W., and Lute, R. A.: Transcutaneous Doppler echocardiographic measurements of proximal aortic blood velocity in man. Bibl. Cardiol., *34:* 12, 1974.
48. Jonsson, B., Szamosi, A., and Tornell, G.: Presystolic mitral regurgitation in severe aortic incompetence observed by cineangiography. Cardiology, *58*(6): 347, 1973.
49. Joyner, C. R., Harrison, F. S., and Gruber, J. W.: Diagnosis of hypertrophic subaortic stenosis with a Doppler velocity flow detector. Ann. Intern. Med., *74:* 692, 1971.
50. Judge, T. P., and Kennedy, J. W.: Estimation of aortic regurgitation by diastolic pulse wave analysis. Circulation, *41:* 659, 1970.
51. Lakier, J. B., Lewis, A. B., Heymann, M. A., Stanger, P., Hoffman, J. I. E., and Rudolph, A. M.: Isolated aortic stenosis in the neonate. Natural history and hemodynamic considerations. Circulation, *50:* 801, 1974.
52. Lewis, R. P., Bristow, J. D., Farrehi, C., Kloster, F. E., and Griswold, H. E.: Idiopathic left ventricular hypertrophy; a hemodynamic reappraisal. Am. J. Med., *38:* 842, 1965.
53. Lillehei, C. W., Bonnabeau, R. C. Jr., and Sellers, R. D.: Subaortic stenosis; diagnostic criteria, surgical approach, and late follow-up in 25 patients. J. Thorac. Cardiovasc. Surg., *55:* 94, 1968.
54. Linhart, J. W.: Aortic regurgitation; clinical, hemodynamic, surgical and angiographic correlations. Ann. Thorac. Surg., *11:* 27, 1971.
55. Lochaya, S., Igarashi, M., and Shaffer, A. B.: Late diastolic mitral regurgitation secondary to aortic regurgitation; its relationship to the Austin Flint murmur. Am. Heart J., *74:* 161, 1967.
56. Lyle, D. P., Bancroft, W. H. Jr., Tucker, M., and Eddleman, E. E. Jr.: Slopes of the carotid pulse wave in normal subjects, aortic valvular disease and hypertrophic subaortic stenosis. Circulation, *43:* 374, 1971.
57. Macieira-Coelho, E., Faleiro, L. L., and Santos, A. L.: Evaluation of aortic stenosis by noninvasive techniques. Acta Cardiol., *27:* 680, 1972.
58. Marcus, F. I., and Jones, R. C.: The use of the Valsalva maneuver to differentiate fixed-orifice aortic stenosis from muscular subaortic stenosis. Am. Heart J., *69:* 473, 1965.
59. Marcus, F. I., Perloff, J. K., and DeLeon, A. C.: The use of amyl nitrite in the hemodynamic assessment of aortic valvular and muscular subaortic stenosis. Am. Heart J., *68:* 468, 1964.
60. Mason, D. T., Braunwald, E., and Ross, J. Jr.: Effects of changes in body position on the severity of obstruction to left ventricular outflow in idiopathic hypertrophic subaortic stenosis. Circulation, *33:* 374, 1968.
61. Mason, D. T., Braunwald, E., Ross, J. Jr., and Morrow, A. G.: Diagnostic value of the first and second derivatives of the arterial pressure pulse in aortic valve disease and in hypertrophic subaortic stenosis. Circulation, *30:* 90, 1964.
62. Morrow, A. G., Fort, L. III, Roberts, W. C., and Braunwald, E.: Discrete subaortic stenosis complicated by aortic valvular regurgitation; clinical, hemodynamic, and pathologic studies and the results of operative treatment. Circulation, *31:* 163, 1971.

63. Moskowitz, R. L., and Wechsler, B. M.: Left ventricular ejection time in aortic and mitral valve disease. Am. J. Cardiol., *15:* 809, 1965.
64. Moyeryra, E., Klein, J. J., Shimada, H., and Segal, B. L.: Idiopathic hypertrophic stenosis diagnosed by reflected ultrasound. Am. J. Cardiol., *23:* 32, 1969.
65. Nanda, N. C., Gramiak, R., Manning, J., Mahoney, E. B., Lipchik, E. O., and DeWeese, J. A.: Echocardiographic recognition of the congenital bicuspid aortic valve. Circulation, *49:* 870, 1974.
66. Nanda, N. C., Gramiak, R., Shah, P. M., Stewart, S., and DeWeese, J. A.: Echocardiography in the diagnosis of idiopathic hypertrophic subaortic stenosis co-existing with aortic valve disease. Circulation, *50:* 752, 1974.
67. Nasser, W., Tavel, M. E., Feigenbaum, H., and Fisch, C.: Austin-Flint murmur versus the murmur of organic mitral stenosis. N. Engl. J. Med., *275:* 1007, 1966.
68. Oliver, G. C. Jr., Gazetopoulos, N., and Deuchar, D. C.: Reversed mitral diastolic gradient in aortic incompetence. Br. Heart J., *29:* 239, 1967.
69. Page, H. L., Vogel, J. H. K., Pryor, R., and Blount, S. G.: Supravalvular aortic stenosis; unusual observations in three patients. Am. J. Cardiol., *23:* 270, 1969.
70. Parisi, A. F., Salzman, S. H., and Schechter, E.: Systolic time intervals in severe aortic valve disease; changes with surgery and hemodynamic correlations. Circulation, *44:* 539, 1971.
71. Park, S. C., Steinfeld, L., and Dimich, I.: Systolic time intervals in infants with congestive heart failure. Circulation, *47:* 1281, 1973.
72. Parker, E., Craige, E., and Hood, W. P. Jr.: The Austin Flint murmur and the A wave of the apexcardiogram in aortic regurgitation. Circulation, *43:* 349, 1971.
73. Pasyk, S., and Dubiel, J.: The external carotid pulse wave in aortic stenosis. Cor Vasa, *9:* 48, 1967.
74. Paulus, H. E., Pearson, C. M., and Pitts, W. Jr.: Aortic insufficiency in five patients with Reiter's syndrome; a detailed clinical and pathologic study. Am. J. Med., *53:* 464, 1972.
75. Perloff, J. K.: Clinical recognition of aortic stenosis. The physical signs and differential diagnosis of the various forms of obstruction to left ventricular outflow. Prog. Cardiovasc. Dis., *10:* 323, 1968.
76. Popp, R. L., and Harrison, D. C.: Ultrasound in the diagnosis and evaluation of therapy of idiopathic hypertrophic subaortic stenosis. Circulation, *40:* 905, 1969.
77. Preston, T. A.: A simple clinical method of estimating arterial pulse rise time. Am. Heart J., *80:* 475, 1970.
78. Pridie, R. B. P.: Mitral valve in aortic regurgitation. Br. Heart J., *31:* 797, 1969.
79. Pridie, R. B. P., Benham, R., and Oakley, C. M.: Echocardiography of the mitral valve in aortic valve disease. Br. Heart J., *33:* 296, 1971.
80. Rich, L. L., and Tavel, M. E.: Arterial "triple hump" of idiopathic hypertrophic subaortic stenosis. Chest, *60:* 595, 1971.
81. Roberts, W. C., Perloff, J. K., and Costantino, T.: Severe valvular aortic stenosis in patients over 65 years of age; a clinicopathologic study. Am. J. Cardiol., *27:* 497, 1971.
82. Rogers, W. M., Harrison, J. S., and Blanchard, S.: Contour spectral phonocardiography in the assessment of aortic valve disease. Ann. N. Y. Acad. Sci., *147:* 690, 1969.
83. Rothbaum, D. A., DeJospeh, R. L., and Tavel, M.: Diastolic heart sound produced by mid-diastolic closure of the mitral valve. Am. J. Cardiol., *34:* 367, 1974.
84. Rowe, G. G., Afonso, S., Castillo, C. A., and McKenna, D. H.: The mechanism of the production of Duroziez's murmur. N. Engl. J. Med., *272:* 1207, 1965.
85. Sainani, G. S., Luisada, A. A., and Gupta, P.: Mapping of the precordium; II. Murmurs and abnormal sounds. Acta Cardiol., *23:* 152, 1968.
86. Sarewitz, A. B., and Muehsam, G. E.: Aortic insufficiency simulating combined aortic stenosis and insufficiency. Dis. Chest, *48:* 291, 1965.
87. Schlant, R. C.: Calcific aortic stenosis. Am. J. Cardiol., *27:* 581, 1971.
88. Schwab, R. H., and Killough, J. H.: The phonocardiographic differentiation of pulmonic and aortic insufficiency. Circulation, *32:* 352, 1965.
89. Segal, B. L., Likoff, W., and Kaspar, A. J.: "Silent" rheumatic aortic regurgitation. Am. J. Cardiol., *14:* 628, 1964.

90. Sell, S., and Scully, R. E.: Aging changes in the aortic and mitral valves. Histologic and histochemical studies, with observations on the pathogenesis of calcific aortic stenosis and calcification of the mitral annulus. Am. J. Pathol., *46:* 345, 1965.
91. Shah, P. M., Gramiak, R., Adelman, A. G., and Wigle, E. D.: Echocardiographic assessment of the effects of surgery and propranolol on the dynamics of outflow obstruction in hypertrophic subaortic stenosis. Circulation, *45:* 516, 1972.
92. Shah, P. M., Gramiak, R., Adelman, A. G., and Wigle, E. D.: Role of echocardiography in diagnostic and hemodynamic assessment of hypertrophic subaortic stenosis. Circulation, *44:* 891, 1971.
93. Shah, P. M., Gramiak, R., and Kramer, D. H.: Ultrasound localization of left ventricular outflow obstruction in hypertrophic obstructive cardiomyopathy. Circulation, *40:* 3, 1969.
94. Shibuya, M.: Ausculatory findings of heart sounds and murmurs in congenital heart anomalies and acquired valvular diseases; special reference to the determination of the severity of the condition on the basis of phonocardiography. Jap. J. Thorac. Surg., *18:* 1008, 1965.
95. Starr, I., Ambrosi, C., Manchester, J. H., and Shelburne, J. C.: Diagnosis of aortic stenosis from the carotid pulse and its derivative. Br. Heart J., *35:* 1062, 1973.
96. Stefadouros, M. A., and Witham, A. C.: Systolic time intervals by echocardiography. Circulation, *51*(1): 114, 1975.
97. Stein, P. D., and Munter, W. A.: New functional concept of valvular mechanics in normal and diseased aortic valves. Circulation, *44:* 101, 1971.
98. Stott, D. K., Marpole, D. G. F., Bristow, J. D., Kloster, F. E., and Griswold, H. E.: The role of left atrial transport in aortic and mitral stenosis. Circulation, *41:* 1031, 1970.
99. Surawicz, B., Mercer, C., Chlebus, H., Reeves, J. T., and Spencer, F. C.: Role of the phonocardiogram in evaluation of the severity of mitral stenosis and detection of associated valvular lesions. Circulation, *34:* 795, 1966.
100. Tafur, E., Cohen, L. S., and Levine, H. D.: The apex cardiogram in left ventricular outflow tract obstruction. Circulation, *30:* 392, 1964.
101. Tajik, A. J., Gau, G. T., and Schattenberg, T. T.: Echocardiographic "pseudo-IHSS" pattern in atrial septal defect. Chest, *62:* 324, 1972.
102. Tajik, A. J., Gau, G. T., Ritter, D. G., and Schattenberg, T. T.: Illustrative echocardiograms; mitral valve motion in severe aortic regurgitation. Chest, *63:* 271, 1973.
103. Talbot, S.: Clinical features and prognosis of dissecting aneurysms and ruptured saccular aneurysms. Chest, *66:* 252, 1974.
104. Tavel, M. E.: Clinical phonocardiography. Reversed (paradoxic) splitting of the second heart sound in aortic stenosis. Dis. Chest, *54:* 55, 1968.
105. Tavel, M. E., and Nasser, W. K.: Murmur alternans in aortic stenosis. Chest, *57:* 176, 1970.
106. Ueda, H., Sakamoto, T., and Kawai, N.: The Austin Flint murmur; phonocardiographic and patho-anatomical study. Jap. Heart J., *6:* 294, 1965.
107. Urschel, C. W., Covell, J. W., Sonnenblick, E. H., Ross, J. Jr., and Braunwald, E.: Myocardial mechanics in aortic and mitral valvular regurgitation; the concept of instantaneous impedance as a determinant of the performance of the intact heart. J. Clin. Invest., *47:* 867, 1968.
108. Usher, B. W., Goulden, D., and Murgo, J. P.: Echocardiographic detection of supravalvular aortic stenosis. Circulation, *49:* 1257, 1974.
109. Vogel, J. H. K., and Blount, S. G. Jr.: Clinical evaluation in localizing level of obstruction to outflow from left ventricle; importance of early systolic ejection click. Am. J. Cardiol., *15:* 782, 1965.
110. Vogelpole, L., Nellen, M., Beck, W., and Schrire, V.: The value of squatting in the diagnosis of mild aortic regurgitation. Am. Heart J., *77:* 709, 1969.
111. Whittaker, A. V., Shaver, J. A., Gray, S. III, and Leonard, J. J.: Sound-pressure correlates of the aortic ejection sound; an intracardiac sound study. Circulation, *39:* 475, 1969.

112. Wigle, E. D., Auger, P., and Marquis, Y.: Muscular subaortic stenosis; the direct relation between the intraventricular pressure difference and the left ventricular ejection time. Circulation, *36:* 36, 1967.
113. Winsberg, F., Gabor, G. E., Hernberg, J. G., and Weiss, B.: Fluttering of the mitral valve in aortic insufficiency. Circulation, *41:* 225, 1970.
114. Yeh, H. C., Winsberg, F., and Mercer, E. N.: Echographic aortic valve orifice dimension; its use in evaluating aortic stenosis and cardiac output. J. Clin. Ultrasound, *1:* 182, 1973.

chapter 6

Tricuspid Valvular Disease

Primary involvements of the tricuspid valve, either stenosis or insufficiency secondary to congenital or acquired heart diseases, are uncommon entities. Tricuspid insufficiency, however, may be present in the late stage of valvular lesions, myocardial disease, coronary artery disease or any other conditions associated with heart failure.

The auscultatory and phonocardiographic signs in patients with tricuspid stenosis or insufficiency grossly simulate the ones seen in patients with mitral valvular disease as described in Chapter 4.

TRICUSPID STENOSIS

Auscultation and Phonocardiography

Heart Sounds and Murmurs

The first heart sound may be accentuated and is best heard at the tricuspid area. With thickening or calcification of the tricuspid valve, the first heart sound progressively decreases in amplitude in proportion to the decrease in mobility of the valve (fig. 6.1). The second heart sound is usually normal. Right ventricular third or fourth heart sounds are not present unless there is associated tricuspid insufficiency. The tricuspid opening snap is heard in early diastole, 0.04–0.10 sec after the second heart sound and it corresponds to the time of tricuspid valve opening. If the second heart sound is split, the 2-OS interval should be measured from the pulmonary component of the second heart sound to the opening snap corresponding to the time of isovolumic relaxation of the right ventricle. If present, the diastolic murmur of tricuspid stenosis starts after right ventricular isovolumic relaxation and with the opening snap. This low frequency diastolic rumble (50–500 Hz) reaches maximal peak in mid-diastole, coinciding to the maximal velocity of flow across the stenotic tricuspid valve (fig. 6.1). Subsequently the murmur diminishes in amplitude, terminating prior to atrial contraction. With the onset of atrial contraction, a second diastolic murmur is heard if the patient is in

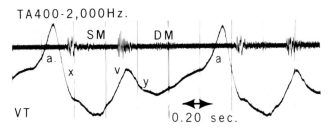

Fig. 6.1. Simultaneously recorded tricuspid area phonocardiogram (TA) and jugular venous tracing (VT) in a patient with tricuspid stenosis. A prominent A wave precedes the first heart sound by 0.12 sec. The X descent is normal on the jugular venous tracing. The peak of the V wave shortly after the second heart sound is followed by a slow X descent and a continuous slow rise prior to the fall of the atrial wave. The phonocardiogram shows a diminished first heart sound. A high frequency, low amplitude systolic regurgitant murmur (SM) begins with the first heart sound and terminates before the second heart sound. Note the presence of a medium frequency, medium amplitude, mid-diastolic murmur (DM) which terminates prior to atrial contraction. The atrial systolic murmur in this patient with sinus rhythm is not well recorded.

sinus rhythm. This atrial systolic murmur (pre-systolic accentuation of the diastolic murmur) has the same characteristics as described for the murmur of mitral stenosis, with the maximal peak at the time of inscription of the P wave of the electrocardiogram. It terminates with the first heart sound. The atrioventricular diastolic and atrial systolic m urmurs both increase during inspiration (Carvallo's sign) corresponding to augmented venous return and increased flow across the stenotic tricuspid valve during that phase of the respiratory cycle.

Carotid Pulse Tracing

The carotid pulse tracing in tricuspid stenosis is normal unless the patient is in congestive heart failure.

Jugular Venous Pulse Tracing

The jugular venous pulse tracing is quite helpful in the diagnosis of tricuspid stenosis, particularly if the patient is in sinus rhythm. The tracing shows a large A wave representing forceful right atrial contraction against the stenotic tricuspid valve (fig. 6.1). The A wave to V wave ratio may be as high as 5:1. Following the A wave the X descent is recorded during systole and has normal characteristics. This is followed by the V wave which has a normal configuration and amplitude. The peak of the V wave usually corresponds to the opening snap of the tricuspid valve. After the V wave the Y descent is inscribed. It is characteristically slow due to the decreased rate of emptying of the right atrium into the right ventricle (fig. 6.1).

Apexcardiogram

The apexcardiogram of the left ventricle is normal. However, in some patients with tricuspid stenosis, a right ventricular apexcardiogram may be recorded. A technically satisfactory tracing will show a small A wave, sharp E point and rapid systolic retraction. The O point may coincide with the opening snap of the tricuspid valve. It is followed by a shallow or absent rapid filling wave and terminates with a slow filling wave.

Systolic Time Intervals

Measurement of these intervals does not contribute significantly to the diagnosis of this condition.

Echocardiogram

Good echocardiographic recordings of the tricuspid valve in normal subjects or in patients with tricuspid valvular disease are not easy to record as compared with mitral valve echocardiograms. The normal pattern of tricuspid valve motion is seen in figure 6.2. The waveform configuration is very similar to the echocardiogram of normal mitral valve motion (see Chapter 4). Abnormalities of tricuspid valve motion in tricuspid stenosis are similar to those described for mitral stenosis (see Chapter 4), i.e. decrease in E-F slope of the anterior leaflet and paradoxical motion of the posterior leaflet. Multiple and disorganized echoes derived from this structure indicate calcification or thickening of the tricuspid valve. In addition, there is abnormal closure of the valve if right ventricular hypertrophy is present. Elevation of right ventricular end-diastolic pressure, which is indicative of poor late right ventricular end-diastolic compliance, results in prolongation of the A-C interval. As seen in patients with mitral stenosis, measurements of the PR interval of the electrocardiogram minus the A-C interval of the echocardiogram shorten considerably.

TRICUSPID INSUFFICIENCY

Organic tricuspid insufficiency secondary to rheumatic fever is rare. However, tricuspid insufficiency is not uncommon in patients with long standing rheumatic heart disease involving the mitral or aortic valves, coronary artery disease, primary myocardial disease or cor pulmonale. In these patients, long standing pulmonary hypertension results in dilatation of the right ventricule and tricuspid annulus causing separation of the tricuspid leaflets and tricuspid insufficiency.

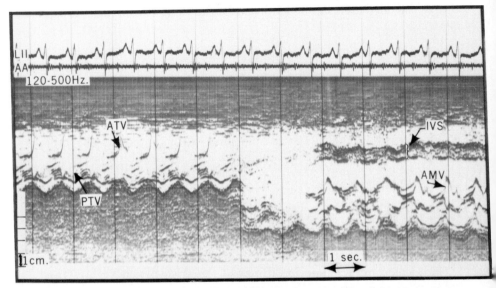

Fig. 6.2. Simultaneously recorded echocardiogram, lead II (LII) of the electrocardiogram and aortic area (AA) phonocardiogram in a 48-year-old patient demonstrating
a normal tricuspid valve. The anterior (ATV) and posterior tricuspid valve (PTV) is
well demonstrated. Note the normal diastolic descent shown by a normal E-F slope,
in this patient with sinus rhythm. The right side of this tracing is the scan toward the
mitral valve showing the interventricular septum (IVS) motion and the normal
anterior mitral valve (AMV). Note the similar motion of the mitral and tricuspid
valves.

Heart Sounds and Murmurs

The first heart sound is diminished due to decreased excursion of the
tricuspid leaflets. The second heart sound is normal or diminished. If the
second heart sound is split and both aortic and pulmonary valve
components are clearly identified, the pulmonary valve closure sound
may be accentuated, reflecting the presence of pulmonary hypertension.
The pulmonary valve closure sound may be well transmitted to the
mitral and aortic areas. Paradoxical splitting of the second heart sound
due to an early closure of the pulmonic valve has been described, but is
very rare. Systolic ejection clicks, recorded in approximately 20% of
patients with tricuspid insufficiency, are seen in patients with marked
dilatation of the pulmonary arteries. The third heart sound is part of the
auscultatory and phonocardiographic findings in tricuspid insufficiency.
It reflects augmented right ventricular filling due to a large volume of
blood crossing the insufficient tricuspid valve in early diastole. A fourth
heart sound may also be recorded if the patient is in sinus rhythm.

The systolic murmur of tricuspid insufficiency starts during the period of isovolumic contraction, i.e., with the first heart sound. It is a high frequency regurgitant murmur with the maximum peak in early systole. It then reaches a plateau throughout mid-systole and terminates prior to or with the second heart sound (figs. 6.3 and 6.4). This high frequency murmur, best recorded at the tricuspid area, transmits well to the right side of the precordium and spine. In patients with severe tricuspid insufficiency, a low frequency, short, mid-diastolic, rumbling murmur is present representing diastolic augmentation of flow across the tricuspid valve. Patients with atrial septal defect and large left-to-right shunts usually have this type of murmur which is called relative tricuspid

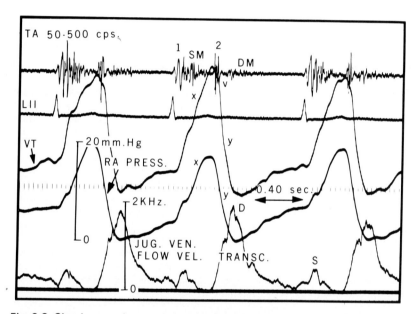

Fig. 6.3. Simultaneously recorded tricuspid area phonocardiogram (TA) lead II (LII) of the electrocardiogram, jugular venous tracing (VT), right atrial pressure (RA PRESS.) and transcutaneous jugular venous flow velocity (VT) in a 63-year-old patient with mitral stenosis and mitral and tricuspid insufficiencies. The rhythm is atrial fibrillation. There is a high frequency, low amplitude systolic regurgitant murmur (SM) on the phonocardiogram. The first and second heart sound are normal. There is a short, atrioventricular diastolic murmur (DM) which follows the peak of the V wave on the jugular venous tracing. The short, high frequency vibration on this tracing probably represents an opening snap of the tricuspid valve. A sustained systolic wave, followed by a rapid Y descent is seen on the transcutaneous jugular venous tracing and simultaneous recording of the right atrial pressure curve. Both tracings show a prominent V wave, sustained systolic (S) wave, and rapid Y descent. The transcutaneous jugular venous flow tracing shows a prominent diastolic (D) wave indicative of diastolic augmentation of flow velocity during diastole.

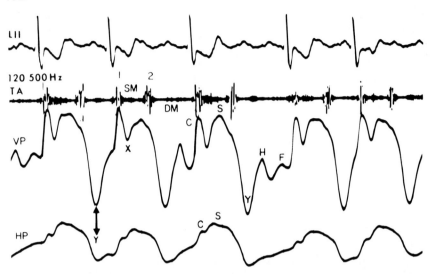

Fig. 6.4. Simultaneously recorded lead II of the electrocardiogram (LII), tricuspid area phonocardiogram (TA) jugular venous (VP) and hepatic pulse tracing (HP) in a patient with severe tricuspid insufficiency. The rhythm is atrial fibrillation with a varying ventricular response. The phonocardiogram shows a high frequency, medium amplitude systolic regurgitant murmur (SM) which starts with the first heart sound and terminates prior to the second heart sound. There is also a low frequency, atrioventricular diastolic murmur (DM). Its maximal intensity precedes the peak of the H wave on the jugular venous tracing (VP). The jugular venous tracing shows a sharp C point followed by a small X descent and a sustained systolic wave (S). This is followed by a rapid diastolic Y descent. A prominent H wave follows the Y decent. A secondary wave (F) may be seen in patients with atrial fibrillation. The etiology of this wave is unknown. The hepatic pulse tracing (HP) shows a sustained systolic wave followed by a prominent Y descent. The configuration of this tracing is similar to the transcutaneous jugular venous pulse. The varying configuration of the jugular venous and hepatic pulse is due to atrial fibrillation with variable cycle length.

stenosis. The murmur of tricuspid insufficiency characteristically increases in the early phase of inspiration. Arterial diastolic murmurs sometimes heard in patients with tricuspid insufficiency represent either aortic or pulmonic insufficiencies and the differentiation between the two is difficult to make during auscultation or phonocardiography.

Carotid Pulse Tracing

The carotid pulse tracing has a normal configuration in tricuspid insufficiency.

Jugular Venous and Hepatic Pulse Tracings

Recording the jugular venous pulse tracing and pulsation over the liver area is quite helpful in recognizing tricuspid insufficiency. If the patient is in sinus rhythm, the A wave has increased amplitude but not to the degree seen in tricuspid stenosis. The X descent is obliterated by a sustained systolic plateau representing marked increase in the right atrial pressure during right ventricular systole (figs. 6.3 and 6.4). This systolic plateau terminates at the time of the second heart sound, followed by the peak of a prominent V wave which, in many situations, is not clearly identified (fig. 6.4). As soon as the tricuspid valve opens near the peak of the V wave, the Y descent begins. The Y descent is characteristically very rapid and terminates 0.08–0.16 sec after the peak of the V wave (figs. 6.3 and 6.4). Following the Y descent, the tracing continues to rise, reaching a plateau during mid-diastole and terminating with a sharp H wave (fig. 6.4) or with the A wave of the diastolic cycle. On the jugular venous and hepatic pulse tracings these findings reflect the changes in pressure and flow in the right atrium, superior vena cava and jugular vein (fig. 6.3). In patients with tricuspid insufficiency the right ventricle ejects blood into both the pulmonary artery and right atrium. As a result, there is "ventricularization" of right atrial pressure during systole. As the tricuspid valve opens, this large volume of blood is ejected from the right atrium into the right ventricle causing a rapid Y

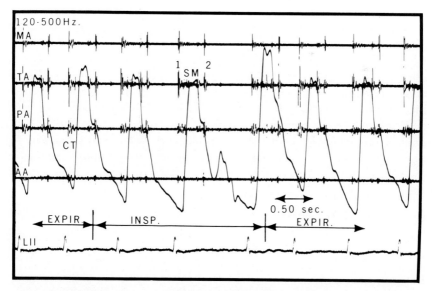

Fig. 6.5. Simultaneously recorded phonocardiogram at the mitral (MA), tricuspid (TA) pulmonic (PA) and aortic (AA) areas, carotid pulse tracing (CT) and lead II (LII) of the electrocardiogram in a 45-year-old patient with mitral stenosis, tricuspid insufficiency and atrial fibrillation. Note the increase in amplitude of the high frequency, systolic regurgitant murmur during inspiration (INSP.).

descent. The abnormalities described for the jugular venous pulse and hepatic pulse tracings are exaggerated during inspiration because of increased augmentation of the regurgitant fraction across the insufficient tricuspid valve (fig. 6.5).

The configuration of the jugular venous pulse tracing in patients with isolated atrial fibrillation, without tricuspid insufficiency, is nearly identical to tracings of patients with tricuspid insufficiency and atrial fibrillation. This is due to the lack of a period of atrial relaxation in patients with this type of cardiac arrhythmia. Isolated atrial fibrillation without associated tricuspid insufficiency may cause a diminution of the X descent and a slight increase in the Y descent. Therefore, caution must be exercised in interpreting jugular venous pulse tracing abnormalities in patients with atrial fibrillation. In this instance recording of transcutaneous jugular vein velocity, using the Doppler flowmeter technique, is useful to differentiate between the two conditions (fig. 6.3) because it records only the velocity of blood crossing the transducer. The lack of the period of isovolumic relaxation of the atria is unimportant. Caution should be exercised in interpreting abnormalities of the jugular venous pulse tracing in patients with other types of cardiac arrhythmias. Recordings of several cardiac cycles must be obtained in order to properly interpret the abnormalities displayed as shown in figure 6.6.

Apexcardiogram

The apexcardiogram of the left ventricle in patients with tricuspid insufficiency is normal. At times, it is possible to record a right ventricular apexcardiogram. If a technically satisfactory tracing is obtained, the abnormalities noted are: (1) the A wave will be slightly accentuated, if the patient is in sinus rhythm; (2) the E point is not well recognized since it usually merges with a sustained, round systolic wave representing right ventricular hypertrophy or overloading; (3) the O point usually coincides with the opening snap of the tricuspid valve; (4) the rapid filing wave is quite accentuated and its peak corresponds to the time of inscription of the right ventricular third heart sound; and (5) the slow filling wave is normal.

Systolic Time Intervals

The systolic time intervals are not altered significantly in patients with tricuspid insufficiency.

Echocardiography

In tricuspid insufficiency, echocardiography is useful for measurement of diameter of the right ventricle, which is quite frequently increased above the normal upper limit of 2.6 cm (fig. 6.7). In addition, this tech-

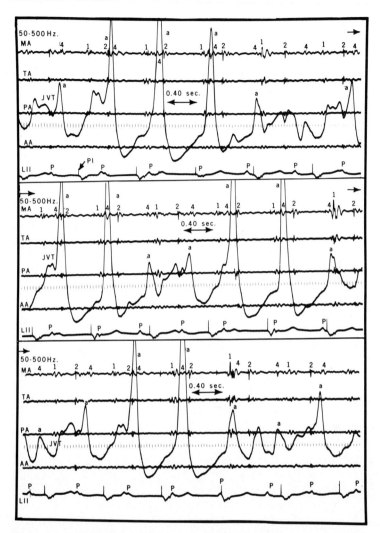

Fig. 6.6. Simultaneously recorded phonocardiogram at the mitral (MA), tricuspid (TA), pulmonic (PA), and aortic areas (AA), jugular venous tracing (VT) and lead II (LII) of the electrocardiogram in a 68-year-old patient with complete heart block and a permanent pacemaker (PI = pacemaker impulse). When the P wave (P) is inscribed during systole, a "cannon" wave is recorded on the jugular venous tracing, representing summation of the A and C waves (atrial contraction against a closed tricuspid valve). However, when the P wave is inscribed during diastole and near the QRS complex, the jugular venous tracing has a normal configuration (see text).

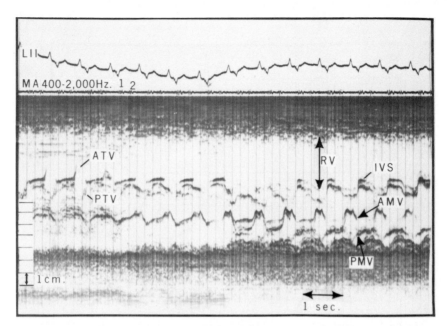

Fig. 6.7. Simultaneously recorded echocardiogram, lead II (LII) of the electrocardiogram and phonocardiogram at the mitral area (MA) in a 59-year-old man with tricuspid insufficiency. Anterior tricuspid (ATV) and posterior tricuspid valve (PTV) motions are well shown. The interventricular septum (IVS) is shown in the scan from the tricuspid valve to the mitral valve area. Note increase in size of the right ventricular diameter to 3.5 cm. RV = right ventricle, PMV = posterior mitral valve.

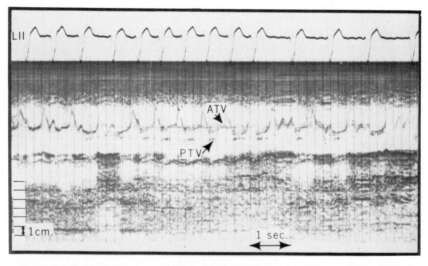

Fig. 6.8. Simultaneously recorded echocardiogram of the tricuspid valve in a 73-year-old man with tricuspid insufficiency and atrial fibrillation of varying cycle length. Note the fine fibrillatory waves seen in the motions of the anterior (ATV) and posterior tricuspid valve (PTV).

nique is useful to detect the presence of pulmonary hypertension frequently seen in patients with tricuspid insufficiency. If right ventricular end-diastolic pressure is elevated, abnormalities of tricuspid valve motion are essentially the same as described earlier in this chapter (see "Tricuspid Stenosis"). Recording of pulmonic valve motion using echocardiography shows a diminished or absent A wave.

Abnormalities of tricuspid valve motion are frequently noted with various cardiac arrhythmias such as coarse fibrillation waves seen in patients with atrial fibrillation (fig. 6.8). Fine fibrillatory movements of the tricuspid valve in patients with pulmonic insufficiency are the same as those described for abnormalities of the mitral valve motion in patients with aortic insufficiency.

REFERENCES

1. Abinader, E. G.: Systolic venous reflux sounds. Am. Heart J., 85: 452, 1973.
2. Ainsworth, R. P., Hartman, A. F., Jr., Aker, U., and Schad, N.: Tricuspid valve prolapse with late systolic tricuspid insufficiency. Radiology, 107: 309, 1973.
3. Ali, N.: Pulsations of arm veins in the absence of tricuspid insufficiency. Chest, 63: 41, 1973.
4. Aravanis, C.: Clinical phonocardiography. Confusion with murmurs of tricuspid insufficiency with mitral insufficiency in the presence of tight mitral stenosis. Dis. Chest, 55: 426, 1969.
5. Aravanis, C., and Michaelides, G.: Tricuspid insufficiency masquerading as mitral insufficiency in patients with severe mitral stenosis. Am. J. Cardiol., 20: 417, 1967.
6. Benchimol, A., Barreto, E. C., and Tio, S.: Phasic right atrium and superior vena cava flow velocity in patients with tricuspid insufficiency. Am. Heart J., 79: 603, 1970.
7. Boicourt, O. W., Nagle, R. E., and Mounsey, J. P.: The clinical significance of systolic retraction of the apical impulse. Br. Heart J., 27: 379, 1965.
8. Brito, A. H. de, Sekeff, J. A., Toledo, A. N., Zaniola, W., Sniteowsky, R., DeLucena Costa, C. A., and Decarvalho Azeuedo, A.: Early stage of t ˈuspid stenosis. Am. J. Cardiol., 18: 57, 1966.
9. Cairns, K. B., Kloster, F. E., Bristlow, J. D., Lees, M. H., and Griswold, H. E.: Problems in the hemodynamic diagnosis of tricuspid insufficiency. Am. Heart J., 75: 173, 1968.
10. Eisenberg, S., and Suyemoto, J.: Rupture of a papillary muscle of the tricuspid valve following acute myocardial infarction; report of a case. Circulation, 30: 588, 1964.
11. Facci, M., Lipparini, R., and Puvianai, G.: Extrensic tricuspid stenosis due to chronic calcified pericarditis; clinical case. Minerva Cardioangiol., 13: 299, 1965.
12. Fiege, J. G., Jr., Vlad, P., and Ehrenhaft, J. L.: Aneurysm of the tricuspid valve causing infundibular obstruction. Ann. Thorac. Surg., 3: 446, 1967.
13. Galvis, E. L., and Bouchard, F.: Tricuspid insufficiency and congenital cardiopathies. Arch. Mal. Couer, 58: 100, 1965.
14. Gooch, A. S., Maranhao, V., Scampardonis, G., Cha, S. D., and Yang, S. S.: Prolapse of both mitral and tricuspid leaflets in systolic murmur-click syndrome. N. Engl. J. Med., 287: 1218, 1972.
15. Gorinina, N. K., and Shcherba, S. G.: Phonocardiography in the diagnosis of tricuspid stenosis. Kardiologia, 4: 25, 1964.
16. Joyner, C. R., Jr., Hey, E. B., Jr., Johnson, J., and Reid, J. M.: Reflected ultrasound in the diagnosis of tricuspid stenosis. Am. J. Cardiol., 19: 66, 1967.
17. Kavanagh-Gray, D., and Gerien, A.: The preoperative assessment of multiple valve disease. Can. Med. Assoc. J., 91: 887, 1964.
18. Kawashima, U., Nakano, S., and Manabe, H.: Tricuspid insufficiency; a study of hemodynamics. Am. J. Physiol., 74: 853, 1974.

19. Keefe, J. F., Wolk, M. J., and Levine, H. J.: Isolated tricuspid valvular stenosis. Am. J. Cardiol., *25:* 252, 1970.
20. Leon, D. F., Leonard, J. J., Lancaster, J. F., Kroetz, F. W., and Shaver, J. A.: Effect of respiration on pansystolic regurgitant murmurs as studied by biatrial intracardiac phonocardiography. Am. J. Med., *39:* 429, 1965.
21. Lisa, C. P., and Tavel, M. E.: Tricuspid stenosis; graphic features which help in its diagnosis. Chest, *61:* 291, 1972.
22. Luisada, A. A.: Internal and external phonocardiography; mitral stenosis, pulmonary hypertension, pulmonary and tricuspid insufficiency. Dis. Chest, *54:* 461, 1968.
23. Luisada, A. A.: Phonocardiography and venous tracings; pulmonary heart disease and tricuspid insufficiency in a drug addict. Dis. Chest, *54:* 140, 1968.
24. Mahaim, C., and Mahaim, I.: Gallops, "snaps" and the apex cardiogram. Cardiologia (Basel), *48:* 169, 1966.
25. Morgan, J. R., and Forker, A. D.: Isolated tricuspid insufficiency. Circulation, *43:* 559, 1971.
26. Pieroni, D. R., Homcy, E., and Freedom, R. M.: Echocardiography in atrioventricular canal defect; a clinical spectrum. Am. J. Cardiol., *35:* 54, 1975.
27. Rios, J. C., Massumi, R. A., Breesmen, W. T., and Sarin, R. K.: Auscultatory features of acute tricuspid regurgitation. Am. J. Cardiol., *23:* 4, 1969.
28. Rubeiz, G. A., Nassar, M. E., and Dagher, I.K.: Study of the right atrial pressure pulse in functional triscupid regurgitation and normal sinus rhythm. Circulation, *30:* 190, 1964.
29. Sanders, C. A., Harthorne, J. W., DeSanctis, R. W., and Austen, W. G.: Tricuspid stenosis, a difficult diagnosis in the presence of atrial fibrillation. Circulation, *33:* 26, 1966.
30. Sinclair-Smith, B. C., Bloomfield, D. A., and Newman, E. V.: Venous hypertension, tricuspid valve function and congestive cardiac failure. Trans. Assoc. Am. Physicians, *78:* 292, 1965.
31. Takabatake, Y., and Iizuka, M.: Pathophysiology of tricuspid insufficiency—clinical and experimental study. Am. J. Physiol., *74:* 843, 1974.
32. Toso, M., and Innocien, P.: The Rivero-Carvallo maneuver in the diagnosis of tricuspid insufficiency; conventional and intracavitary phonocardiographic study. Cuore Circ., *50:* 94, 1966.
33. Upshaw, C. B., Jr.: Precordial honk due to tricuspid regurgitation. Am. J. Cardiol., *35:* 85, 1975.
34. Wada, O.: Detection of the tricuspid lesion by the ultrasound cardiogram (abstract). Jap. Circ. J., *36:* 1277, 1972.

chapter 7

Prosthetic Cardiac Valves

Three basic types of prosthesis can be used to replace diseased cardiac valves: (1) caged ball, (2) caged disc, and (3) hetero- and homograft. Each of these implanted valves present a variety of auscultatory, phonocardiographic, pulse wave, and echocardiographic findings. Only the most commonly used valves will be described in this chapter. At the end of this chapter several types of prostheses in use throughout the country are illustrated (see Figs. 7.50 and 7.51).

The earliest models of caged, ball type prostheses, used in patients with severe aortic insufficiency were the Hufnagel, placed in the descending aorta, and the Harken, implanted in the subcoronary position. More recent types include the Starr-Edwards, and Cutter-Smeloff which has a ball made of silicone placed in a double open cage structure; the Braunwald-Cutter, which has a silastic ball with an open cage; the DeBakey, a sutureless valve; and the Cooley-Liotta-Cromie, a titanium valve.

The most commonly used caged disc prostheses are the Kay-Shiley, a silastic caged disc protected with muscle guard; the Kay-Suzuki, a Teflon discoid valve with four small protrusions within the orifice; the Cross-Jones caged lens which has a titanium frame, a silicone lens-shaped disc, and a woven Teflon fixation ring; the Wada-Cutter, which has a tilting disc and a titanium ring; the Beall disc valve; and the Björk-Shiley and Lillehei-Kaster valves with tilting discs.

Homografts, implanted in the mitral, tricuspid, or aortic position, are valves preserved from human cadavers. Other types of homografts are made from stented fascia lata, pericardium, or human dura mater. The most common type of heterograft is the stented Hancock-Porcine valve which can be implanted in the mitral, triscuspid, aortic, and pulmonary positions. Hancock-Porcine conduits are used in the Rastelli and Fontan procedures for correction of pulmonary and tricuspid atresia.

MITRAL VALVE PROSTHESES

Most of our experience has been in patients with a Starr-Edwards ball valve, Beall disc valve and, more recently, the Björk-Shiley tilting disc and Hancock-Porcine valves.

Ball Valves
Clicks and Murmurs

Normally functioning ball valve prostheses usually produce high frequency opening and closing clicks (fig. 7.1) which are the result of sudden impact of the ball against the cage. The amplitude of these vibrations is approximately the same, however, the opening click may be higher than the closing click in some patients. The opening click of the prosthetic ball occurs at the time the mitral valve normally opens. After the closing click, ventricular systole, as recorded on the phonocardiogram, should be free of any clicks since the ball should remain in a closed position against the cage. The time interval from onset of the Q wave of the electrocardiogram to the onset of valve closure is 40 msec or less in patients with sinus rhythm, 54 msec if the rhythm is atrial fibrillation, and to the final closure, 80–90 msec. The interval from the aortic valve

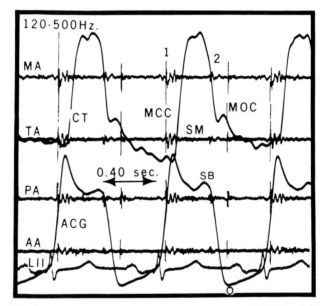

Fig. 7.1. Simultaneously recorded phonocardiogram at the mitral (MA) tricuspid (TA), pulmonic (PA) and aortic areas (AA), carotid pulse tracing (CT), apexcardiogram (ACG), and lead II (LII) of the electrocardiogram in a 38-year-old patient with a Starr-Edwards mitral ball valve prosthesis. High frequency, high amplitude mitral opening (MOC) and closing clicks (MCC) of the prosthetic valve are recorded in all precordial areas. The second sound-opening click interval is approximately 0.13 sec. The high frequency, low amplitude systolic regurgitant murmur (SM), best recorded at the tricuspid area, is due to a mild degree of tricuspid insufficiency. The carotid pulse tracing is normal. The apexcardiogram shows a small, late systolic bulge (SB) and an inconspicuous rapid filling wave. Note that the mitral opening click coincides with the O point of the apexcardiogram.

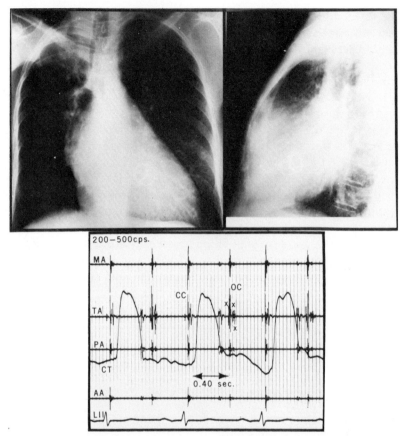

Fig. 7.2. (Top panel) Chest X-ray in the anteroposterior and lateral positions in a 44-year-old patient with a No. 2 Starr-Edwards mitral ball valve prosthesis. The chest X-ray reveals the position of the prosthesis and a moderate degree of cardiomegaly. (Bottom panel) Simultaneously recorded phonocardiogram at the mitral (MA), tricuspid (TA), pulmonic (PA) and aortic areas (AA), carotid pulse tracing (CT), and lead II (LII) of the electrocardiogram showing several diastolic opening clicks (OC). This is a frequent finding in patients with mitral ball valve prostheses and is due to motion of the ball against the cage during left ventricular filling. Amplitude of the closing (CC) and opening clicks is identical. The carotid pulse tracing is normal.

closure sound to the opening click ranges from 80 to 160 msec with a mean of 110 msec. In most patients this interval is fairly constant and quite independent of variation in cycle length, as seen in patients with atrial fibrillation. Amplitude of the closing click should be identical in several consecutive beats providing the patient is in sinus rhythm and has consistently regular RR intervals. Minor variations in amplitude of the closing click may be seen in patients with a varying RR interval such as in atrial fibrillation, atrial tachycardia with varying degree of AV block, etc., but this is not an indication of valve malfunction.

A prosthetic third heart sound can be heard in approximately 60% of patients. Multiple diastolic clicks are common and they are a normal feature in patients with this type of prosthesis as shown in figure 7.2.

A prosthetic fourth heart sound (fig. 7.3) seen in 30–40% of patients in sinus rhythm, may have two components. The first component will have low amplitude, occurring 0.06–0.11 sec after the P wave of the electrocardiogram. The second and most prominent component occurs 0.12–0.18 sec after the onset of the P wave on the electrocardiogram.

All prosthetic valve sounds, which may be heard over the entire precordium, are most prominent at the mitral area and are well transmitted to the spine. They have a click-like characteristic and short duration.

Patients with normally functioning prosthetic mitral valves should not present with systolic regurgitant murmurs. However, many patients with mitral valve disease who have been subjected to mitral valve replacement may have tricuspid insufficiency. In this setting, a high frequency,

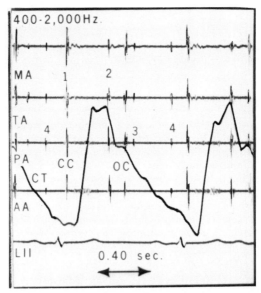

Fig. 7.3. Simultaneously recorded phonocardiogram at the mitral (MA), tricuspid (TA), pulmonic (PA) and aortic areas (AA), lead II (LII) of the electrocardiogram and a carotid pulse tracing (CT) in a 39-year-old patient with a normally functioning Starr-Edwards ball valve prosthesis. Note the opening (OC) and closing clicks (CC) of the prosthetic valve. There is an early diastolic prosthetic valve sound and a prosthetic fourth heart sound which occurs shortly after inscription of the P wave of the electrocardiogram. The carotid pulse tracing is normal.

high amplitude systolic regurgitant murmur may be heard or recorded at the mitral and/or tricuspid areas. If tricuspid insufficiency is excluded by other diagnostic techniques (see Chapter 6, "Tricuspid Valve Disease"), the systolic murmur has important clinical implications since it is usually due to prosthetic valve malfunction.

Disc Valves
Clicks and Murmurs

Disc valves, with the exception of the Björk-Shiley and Lillehei-Kaster, always present with the same auscultatory and phonocardiographic findings. The closing click is well recorded in most precordial areas. The time interval from the aortic valve closure sound to the opening click is shown in figure 7.4. Both of these intervals are fairly constant and do not change significantly with variations in cycle length. The opening and

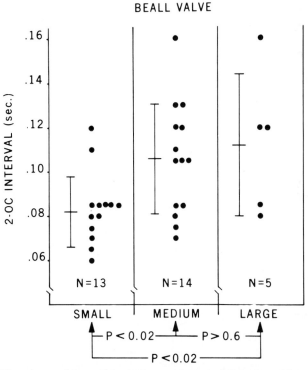

Fig. 7.4. Time interval from the aortic component of the second heart sound to the opening click (OC) interval measured on the phonocardiogram at the tricuspid area in a group of patients with normally functioning Beall mitral prostheses of small, medium, and large valve sizes. The range and mean values for this interval are indicated. In patients with the small valve prostheses, the 2-OC interval averages 0.83 sec, for the medium size, 0.11 sec and for the large prostheses, the 2-OC interval averages 0.11 sec. N = number of patients.

closing click amplitude should be essentially identical. Amplitude of the closing click is inversely proportional to the preceding cycle length, i.e., the longer the preceding diastolic cycle, the smaller the amplitude of the opening click and vice versa (figure 7.5). This is a normal feature of most prosthetic disc valves in the mitral position; however, the opening click remains fairly constant in a wide range of cycle lengths in patients with Beall valve prostheses. Multiple clicks, during mid-diastole or atrial contraction, in patients with sinus rhythm are not part of the normal auscultatory and phonocardiographic findings in patients with prosthetic disc valves. The auscultatory and phonocardiographic features of the Björk-Shiley prosthesis in the mitral position are illustrated in figure 7.6.

Carotid Pulse Tracing
Ball and Disc Prostheses

The carotid pulse tracing should have a normal contour and ejection time should be normal providing that the patient is not in heart failure (figs. 7.1–7.3).

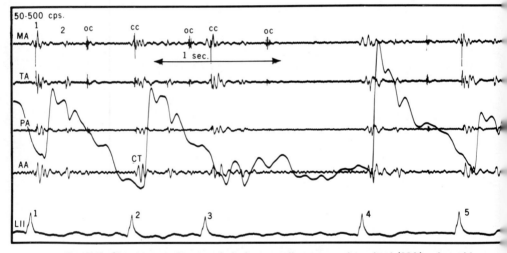

Fig. 7.5. Simultaneously recorded phonocardiogram at the mitral (MA), tricuspid (TA), pulmonic (PA) and aortic areas (AA), carotid pulse tracing (CT), and lead II (LII) of the electrocardiogram in a 52-year-old patient with a Beall mitral valve prosthesis. The opening (OC) and closing clicks (CC) of the prosthesis are well recorded at the mitral area. There are no murmurs. In patients with this type of prosthesis, variations in amplitude of the closing click are related to the preceding cycle length. In beat 4, which is preceded by a long diastolic cycle length, amplitude of the prosthetic closing click, well seen at the mitral area, is less as compared with beats 1, 2, and 3. This is not a sign of disc valve malfunction. The carotid pulse tracing is normal.

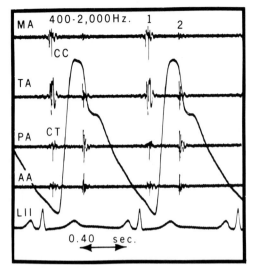

Fig. 7.6. Simultaneously recorded phonocardiogram at the mitral (MA), tricuspid (TA), pulmonic (PA), and aortic areas (AA), carotid pulse tracing (CT), and lead II (LII) of the electrocardiogram in a 49-year-old patient with a No. 29 Björk-Shiley prosthesis implanted in the mitral position. The closing click (CC) of the prosthesis is well recorded, particularly at the mitral area and there is no opening click. The second heart sound is normal. There are no systolic or diastolic murmurs. The carotid pulse tracing is normal.

Jugular Venous Pulse Tracing
Ball and Disc Prostheses

The jugular venous pulse tracing cannot be utilized to determine normal or abnormal prosthetic valve function. It does help, at times, to determine the presence of tricuspid insufficiency in patients who present with systolic murmurs at the mitral and/or tricuspid areas. It is particularly valuable in patients with sinus rhythm, but is not a reliable indicator in patients with atrial fibrillation (see Chapter 6, "Tricuspid Valve Disease").

Apexcardiogram

The apexcardiogram usually exhibits a small rapid filling wave of short duration, or this wave may not be present (fig. 7.1). The systolic wave is normal providing the patient does not have left ventricular dyskinesis. The apexcardiogram is valuable in determining the time of inscription of the first opening click in patients with prosthetic ball valves. The opening click should coincide with or occur shortly before the O point of the apexcardiogram.

Homograft and Heterograft Valves
Mitral Position

The auscultatory and phonocardiographic features of these valves include the presence of two components of the first heart sound. The first component occurs approximately 30–40 msec after the Q wave of the electrocardiogram and is probably due to systolic ballooning of the valve when it comes to a sudden stop. The second component occurs a few msec later and may be the result of a sudden backward movement of the leaflets to the base of the heart at the onset of ventricular ejection (fig. 7.7). The second component may be obscured in patients with mitral insufficiency.

Third heart sounds which may be present in these patients are not an indicator of heart failure. The interval from the aortic component of the second sound to the third heart sound is in the range of 0.12–0.18 sec.

Carotid and jugular venous pulse tracings, apexcardiogram, and systolic time intervals have not proven to be valuable in the early recognition of normal or abnormal function of homografts or heterografts.

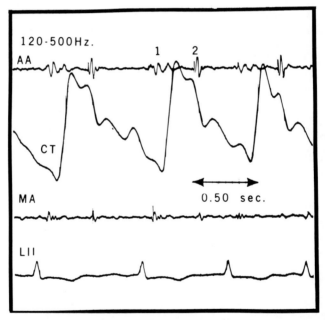

Fig. 7.7. Simultaneously recorded phonocardiogram at the aortic (AA) and mitral areas (MA), carotid pulse tracing (CT), and lead II (LII) of the electrocardiogram in a 50-year-old patient with a Hancock-Porcine prosthetic mitral valve. Note the low frequency transients recorded at the time of inscription of the first heart sound. A definite opening click of the prosthetic valve or a murmur were not recorded. The carotid pulse tracing is normal.

AORTIC VALVE PROSTHESES

Ball and Disc—Clicks and Murmurs

Normally functioning aortic ball valve prostheses such as the Starr-Edwards result in high frequency, high amplitude opening and closing clicks which are transmitted to multiple precordial areas including the suprasternal notch area (fig. 7.8). The opening click has higher amplitude than the closing click and the normal aortic opening-aortic closing click ranges from 0.5–1.2 sec (fig. 7.9) as recorded at the tricuspid area. This ratio is independent of variations in cycle length. It is not uncommon to observe multiple systolic clicks (fig. 7.10), particularly in early systole. They are probably the result of turbulent motion of the ball within the cage.

High frequency systolic ejection murmurs are uniformly present in patients with prosthetic aortic ball valves (figs. 7.8–7.10). The character-

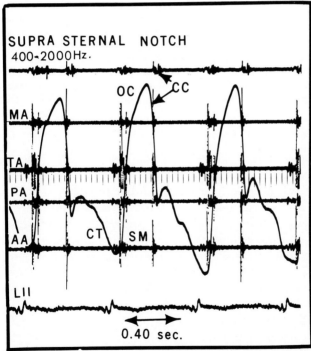

Fig. 7.8. Simultaneously recorded phonocardiogram at the mitral (MA), tricuspid (TA), pulmonic (PA), aortic (AA) and suprasternal notch areas, carotid pulse tracing (CT), and lead II (LII) of the electrocardiogram in a 46-year-old patient with a prosthetic Starr-Edwards aortic valve. The opening (OC) and closing clicks (CC) of the prosthetic valve have normal amplitude and are transmitted to the suprasternal area. There is a high frequency, low amplitude systolic murmur (SM) best recorded at the aortic area. The carotid pulse tracing is normal.

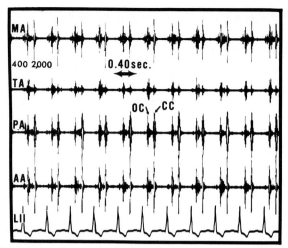

Fig. 7.9. Simultaneously recorded phonocardiogram at the mitral (MA), tricuspid (TA), pulmonic (PA) and aortic areas (AA), and lead II (LII) of the electrocardiogram in a 47-year-old patient with a Starr-Edwards aortic valve prosthesis. Note the consistent ratio of the opening (OC) to closing clicks (CC) of the prosthetic valve during several cardiac cycles. Phonocardiograms in patients with prosthetic valves should be recorded at a fast paper speed such as 150–200 mm/sec as well as a slow paper speed of 25 mm/sec. On the slow speed recording, one can appreciate the reproducibility of this ratio. The normal opening to closing click ratio measured at the tricuspid area should be greater than 0.5. In this patient, the ratio is approximately 2:1.

istics of the systolic ejection murmurs vary with the size of the prosthesis. Small ball valves usually produce a prominent systolic ejection murmur, Grade II–IV/VI, heard over most precordial areas but very prominent at the mitral and aortic areas. This murmur is well transmitted to both carotid arteries and to the spine. The smaller the valve, the higher the amplitude of the systolic ejection murmur. The larger the ball, the smaller the amplitude of the murmur. This is because patients with small aortic ball valves have higher pressure gradients between the left ventricle and aorta as opposed to smaller gradients in patients with large ball valves.

Arterial diastolic murmurs resulting from prosthetic valve insufficiency are not uncommon in patients with a normally functioning Cutter-Smeloff ball valve prosthesis but are rare in patients with a Starr-Edwards valve.

The disc valves most commonly used are the Björk-Shiley and Lillehei-Kaster prostheses. They usually produce very soft opening and closing sounds similar to the characteristics of normal heart sounds (fig. 7.11). Systolic ejection clicks are rare (fig. 7.12). Systolic ejection

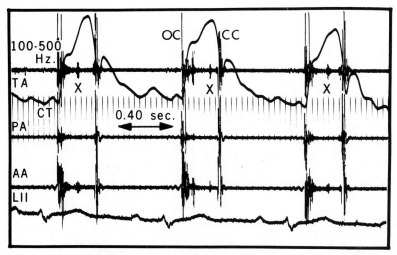

Fig. 7.10. Simultaneously recorded phonocardiogram at the tricuspid (TA), pulmonic (PA) and aortic areas (AA), carotid pulse tracing (CT), and lead II (LII) of the electrocardiogram in a 54-year-old patient with a Starr-Edwards aortic ball valve prosthesis. Note the high amplitude opening (OC) and closing clicks (CC) of the prosthetic aortic valve. Multiple systolic clicks occurring in early, mid and late systole are particularly well recorded at the tricuspid area. Multiple clicks are not uncommon in patients with any type of ball valve prosthesis and they do not represent valve malfunction. The amplitude ratio of the opening click to the closing click of approximately 1:1 measured at the tricuspid area, is in the normal range. The carotid pulse tracing is normal.

murmurs usually have low amplitude (Grade I-II/VI) and high frequency characteristics (figs 7.11 and 7.12) similar to those seen in patients with a mild degree of aortic valvular stenosis. These murmurs are heard best at the aortic and mitral areas. Arterial diastolic murmurs are rare in patients with aortic disc prostheses and when present suggest the possibility of prosthetic valve malfunction.

Carotid Pulse Tracing
Aortic Ball Valve Prosthesis

The carotid pulse tracing usually shows normal upstroke time and a quite prominent dicrotic notch.

Jugular Venous Pulse Tracing

The jugular venous pulse tracing is useful only when the patient develops valve malfunction, congestive heart failure or pulmonary hypertension in which case it will show the characteristic findings seen in patients with pulmonary hypertension (see Chapter 9, "Congenital Heart Disease").

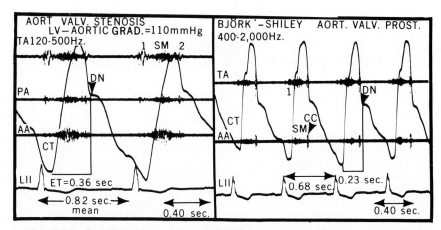

Fig. 7.11. Simultaneously recorded phonocardiogram at the tricuspid (TA), pulmonic (PA) and aortic areas (AA), carotid pulse tracing (CT), and lead II (LII) of the electrocardiogram in a 65-year-old patient with severe aortic valvular stenosis and a left ventricular aortic pressure gradient of 110 mm Hg (left panel). The first heart sound is normal. The second heart sound is single and markedly diminished. A high frequency, high amplitude systolic ejection murmur (SM) is best recorded at the aortic area. The carotid pulse tracing shows a slow upstroke time, inconspicuous dicrotic notch (DN) and prolonged ejection time to 0.36 sec. (Right panel) Simultaneously recorded phonocardiogram at the tricuspid and aortic areas, carotid pulse tracing and lead II of the electrocardiogram following aortic valve replacement with a Björk-Shiley prosthesis. There is no opening click, which is not uncommon in patients with this type of prosthesis. The closing click (CC) is well recorded and coincides with the dicrotic notch of the carotid pulse tracing. There are marked alterations in the configuration of the carotid pulse tracing. It shows a rapid upstroke time, sharp dicrotic notch, and decreased ejection time to 0.23 sec.

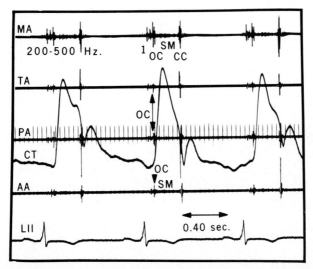

Fig. 7.12. Simultaneously recorded phonocardiogram at the mitral (MA), tricuspid (TA), pulmonic (PA) and aortic areas (AA), carotid pulse tracing (CT), and lead II (LII) of the electrocardiogram in a 60-year-old patient with a Björk-Shiley aortic valve prosthesis showing opening (OC) and closing clicks (CC). Patients with Björk-Shiley prostheses may or may not present with an opening click. In this case, the opening click has essentially the same amplitude as the closing click as recorded at the mitral area. There is a short, high frequency, low amplitude systolic ejection murmur (SM) representing turbulent flow across the prosthesis. This murmur terminates prior to the second heart sound. The carotid pulse tracing is normal.

Apexcardiogram

The apexcardiogram is of some value in evaluating patients with prosthetic aortic ball valves. Abnormalities usually present are of the type seen in patients with left ventricular hypertrophy, including a prominent A wave, inconspicuous E point, round and sustained systolic wave and a small rapid filling wave (fig. 7.13).

Systolic Time Intervals

Patients with aortic valvular disease have increased ejection time. Following aortic valve replacement systolic ejection time decreases considerably. The pre-ejection period and left ventricular ejection time ratio tends to normalize following valve replacement.

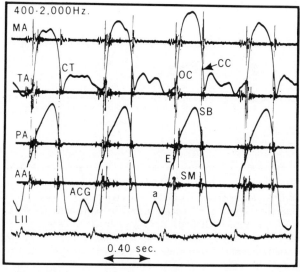

Fig. 7.13. Simultaneously recorded phonocardiogram at the mitral (MA), tricuspid (TA), pulmonic (PA) and aortic areas (AA), carotid pulse tracing (CT), apexcardiogram (ACG), and lead II (LII) of the electrocardiogram in a 46-year-old patient with a prosthetic Starr-Edwards aortic ball valve. The opening (OC) and closing clicks (CC) of the prosthetic valve are well recorded. There is a short, high frequency, low amplitude systolic ejection murmur (SM) representing turbulent flow across the prosthetic aortic valve. The carotid pulse tracing is normal. The apexcardiogram is abnormal showing marked accentuation of the late systolic bulge (SB) with its peak near the aortic closing click. This is usually seen in patients with left ventricular hypertrophy or left ventricular dyskinesis.

HOMOGRAFT AND HETEROGRAFT VALVES

Aortic Position

Homograft valves usually do not exhibit opening or closing clicks. However, low amplitude, high frequency systolic ejection murmurs are frequently noted due to turbulent flow across the prosthesis, or calcification of the valve as shown in figure 7.14. An ejection sound is usually present. The time interval from the Q or R wave of the electrocardiogram to the ejection sound with a range of 0.12–0.17 sec is probably due to motion of the valve and/or ring.

Arterial diastolic murmurs may be heard at varying times following valve replacement and are due to a mild degree of aortic valve insufficiency.

The auscultatory and phonocardiographic findings in patients with heterograft valves such as the Hancock-Porcine have not been definitely established. In our experience with 15 cases we find that the majority of patients do not have any significant arterial diastolic murmurs but systolic ejection murmurs are observed frequently (figs. 7.15 and 7.16).

The carotid and jugular venous pulse tracings, apexcardiogram and systolic time intervals have not proven to be of diagnostic value in determining valve malfunction.

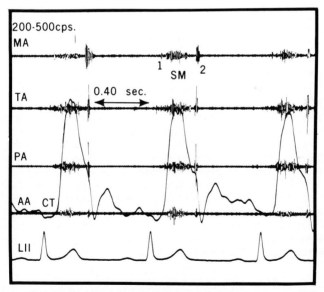

Fig. 7.14. Simultaneously recorded phonocardiogram at the mitral (MA), tricuspid (TA), pulmonic (PA) and aortic areas (AA), carotid pulse tracing (CT), and lead II (LII) of the electrocardiogram in a 13-year-old patient with a homograft aortic valve. There was mild calcification of the valve at the time of this recording, approximately 2 years after aortic valve replacement for aortic valvular stenosis. The first heart sound is normal. The second heart sound is single, with normal amplitude. There is a high frequency, high amplitude systolic ejection murmur (SM) recorded in all precordial areas. The carotid pulse tracing is normal.

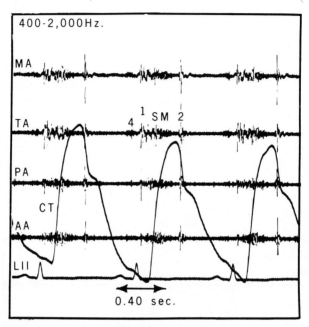

Fig. 7.15. Simultaneously recorded phonocardiogram at the mitral (MA), tricuspid (TA), pulmonic (PA) and aortic areas (AA), carotid pulse tracing (CT), and lead II (LII) of the electrocardiogram in a 61-year-old patient with a No. 23 Hancock-Porcine aortic valve prosthesis. The first heart sound is normal. No definite opening clicks are recorded. The second heart sound is single and probably due to the prosthetic aortic valve closure sound which precedes the dicrotic notch in the carotid pulse tracing. There is a high frequency, high amplitude, "noisy" systolic ejection murmur (SM) which has maximal amplitude in mid-systole and terminates prior to the aortic closure sound. The series of vibrations which correspond with the time of inscription of the fourth heart sound probably represent a prosthetic valve fourth heart sound. No diastolic murmurs are recorded. The carotid pulse tracing has an inconspicuous dicrotic notch and is otherwise within normal limits.

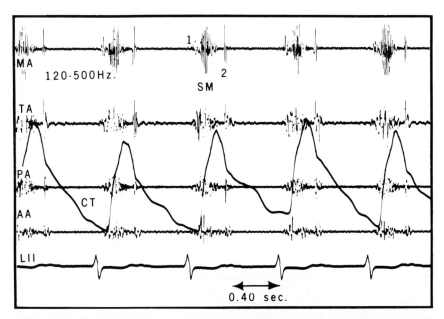

Fig. 7.16. Simultaneously recorded phonocardiogram at the mitral (MA), tricuspid (TA), pulmonic (PA) and aortic areas (AA), carotid pulse tracing (CT), and lead II (LII) of the electrocardiogram in a 63-year-old patient with a No. 19 Hancock-Porcine aortic valve prosthesis. The recording at the mitral area shows normal first and second heart sounds. There is a high frequency, high amplitude, muscial systolic murmur (SM) best recorded at the mitral area. The carotid pulse tracing shows an inconspicuous dicrotic notch and the upstroke time is normal. Most patients with prosthetic Hancock-Porcine valves do not present with a systolic murmur but its presence does not necessarily indicate prosthetic valve malfunction.

TRICUSPID VALVE

Tricuspid valve replacement is uncommon, therefore, the auscultatory and phonocardiographic findings are not well known. However, opening and closing clicks of the prosthetic ball or disc are usually similar to the ones seen when prostheses are implanted in the mitral position. An example of our findings in a patient with a Beall prosthesis in the tricuspid position is shown in figure 7.17.

Our limited experience with the Hancock-Porcine valve prosthesis in the tricuspid position indicates that the opening and closing clicks are not clearly identifiable.

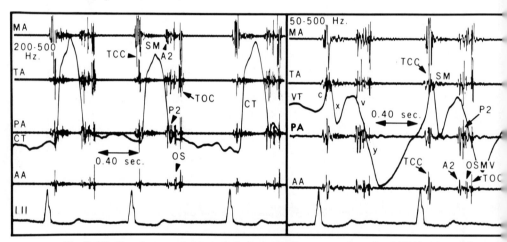

Fig. 7.17. Simultaneously recorded phonocardiogram at the mitral (MA), tricuspid (TA), pulmonic (PA) and aortic areas (AA), carotid pulse tracing (CT), and lead II (LII) of the electrocardiogram in a 53-year-old patient with a Beall prosthetic tricuspid valve. (Left panel) The opening (TOC) and closing clicks (TCC) of the tricuspid prosthetic valve have essentially the same amplitude at the mitral and tricuspid areas. An opening snap (OS) is recorded in all precordial areas. The second heart sound is split by 0.04 sec and the pulmonic component is slightly accentuated. A short, high frequency, low amplitude systolic regurgitant murmur (SM) is best recorded at the mitral area. (Right panel) Simultaneously recorded phonocardiogram at the mitral, tricuspid, pulmonic and aortic areas and jugular venous tracing (VT) on the same patient. The jugular venous tracing shows a normal X descent with the V wave peaking at the level of the second heart sound. The Y descent is normal. The patient's rhythm is atrial fibrillation in both recordings. MV = mitral valve.

MULTIPLE VALVE REPLACEMENT

Patients subjected to multiple valve replacement will exhibit the findings outlined for the types of prostheses implanted (fig. 7.18).

PROSTHETIC MITRAL VALVE MALFUNCTION

Valve variance is defined as valvular dysfunction secondary to physical and chemical alterations in the silastic disc or ball of the

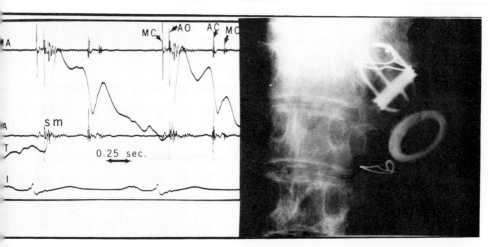

Fig. 7.18. Simultaneously recorded phonocardiogram at the mitral (MA) and tricuspid areas (TA), carotid pulse tracing (CT), and lead II (LII) of the electrocardiogram in a 44-year-old patient with a Cutter prosthetic aortic valve and a Beall mitral valve prosthesis. (Left panel) The mitral closing click (MC) has a higher amplitude than the mitral opening click (MO), well seen at the mitral area. This is followed by an aortic opening click (AO) and a high frequency, low amplitude systolic ejection murmur (SM) which terminates in mid-systole. This murmur represents turbulent flow across the prosthetic aortic valve. The aortic closing click (AC), well recorded at the mitral area, has about half the amplitude of the opening click. The carotid pulse tracing is normal. (Right panel) Chest x-ray demonstrating normal position of the prosthetic valves.

prosthesis. It results in increased or decreased diameter of the ball or disc and changes of the poppet core, causing either peri- or intravalvular insufficiency. Other causes of malfunction include fragmentation of the ball, thrombus formation around the cage or disc, and lipid infiltration which leads to increased hydrostatic pressure. We have also observed that, even when the prosthesis appears to be functioning well, the disproportionate increase in left atrial internal dimension as related to left ventricular diameter may create an increase in the pressure gradient between the two chambers which could be responsible for significant impairment of left ventricular filling and, therefore, may result in the development of heart failure.

Delayed, short, erratic, and absent opening clicks (figs. 7.19–7.23) are the phonocardiographic criteria for mitral ball or disc variance. The relative amplitude of the opening and closing clicks is not always helpful.

Peri- and Intravalvular Insufficiency

A reduced A2-OC interval, diminished intensity of the opening click OC/CC <0.35, a pansystolic murmur at the mitral area (fig. 7.24) and

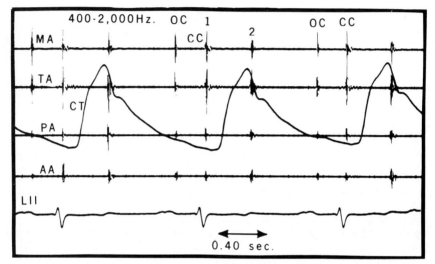

Fig. 7.19. Simultaneously recorded phonocardiogram at the mitral (MA), tricuspid (TA), pulmonic (PA) and aortic areas (AA), carotid pulse tracing (CT), and lead II (LII) of the electrocardiogram in a 70-year-old patient with a prosthetic mitral Beall valve. The second heart sound is normal. The closing click (CC) has normal characteristics. The opening click (OC) of the mitral valve prosthesis occurs late in diastole after inscription of the P wave on the electrocardiogram. The long second sound-aortic click interval is usually indicative of prosthetic valve malfunction. Heart murmurs were not recorded during systole or diastole. The contour of the carotid pulse tracing is normal.

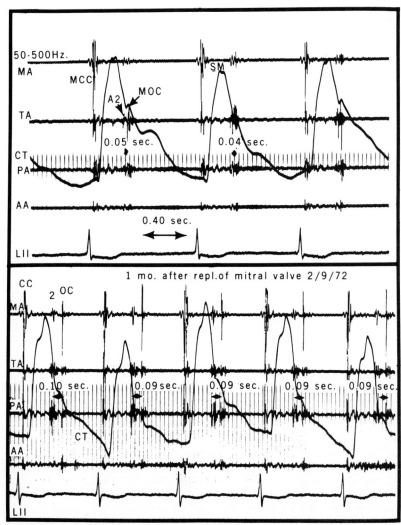

Fig. 7.20. Simultaneously recorded phonocardiogram at the mitral (MA), tricuspid (TA), pulmonic (PA), and aortic areas (AA), carotid pulse tracing (CT), and lead II (LII) of the electrocardiogram in a 42 year old patient with a medium size Beall mitral valve prosthesis showing malfunction (upper panel). Note the marked shortening of the second sound-opening click interval to 0.04–0.05 sec. (Bottom panel) Simultaneously recorded phonocardiogram at the mitral, tricuspid, pulmonic and aortic areas, carotid pulse tracing, and lead II of the electrocardiogram one month after replacement of the mitral valve prosthesis. Note a normal closing click (CC) in this recording. The second sound-opening click (OC) interval, within the normal range for this type of prosthesis, averages 0.09 sec. The patient's rhythm is atrial fibrillation. The carotid pulse tracing is normal. M = mitral.

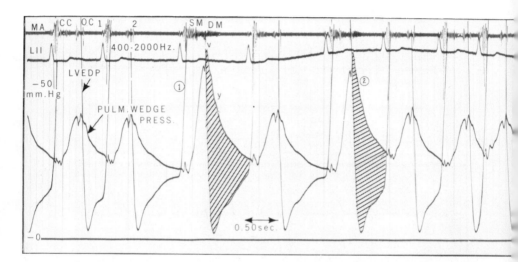

Fig. 7.21. Simultaneously recorded mitral area (MA) phonocardiogram, lead II (LII) of the electrocardiogram, pulmonary "wedge" pressure curve and magnified left ventircular pressure curve in a 53-year-old patient with a large malfunctioning Beall mitral valve prosthesis. In the phonocardiogram, beats with a short cycle length show normal amplitude of the opening (OC) and closing clicks (CC) of the prosthetic valve. Beats preceded by a long cycle length (1 and 2), show a high frequency, high amplitude systolic regurgitant murmur (SM) as well as a diastolic murmur (DM) which follows the second heart sound, and absence of the opening click. In these beats, note the very prominent V wave in the pulmonary "wedge" pressure curve followed by a slow Y descent. The diastolic gradient between the pulmonary "wedge" and the left ventricle is a result of the obstructive lesion caused by deformity of the disc. The gradient is high in beats 1 and 2 which are preceded by a long diastolic cycle length. LVDP = left ventricular end-diastolic pressure.

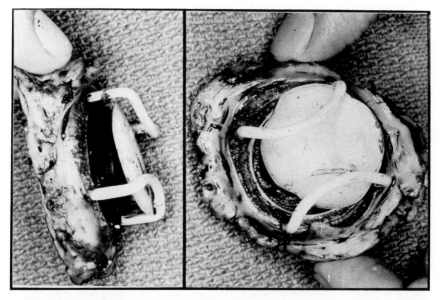

Fig. 7.22. Prosthetic Beall valve which was removed at time of surgery showing marked deformity of the disc structure which caused significant obstruction of flow from the left atrium to the left ventricle. The abnormal configuration of the valve allowed the disc to remain in a semi-closed position during ventricular systole and diastole causing mitral insufficiency as well as obstruction during ventricular diastole as shown in the phonocardiogram in figure 7.21.

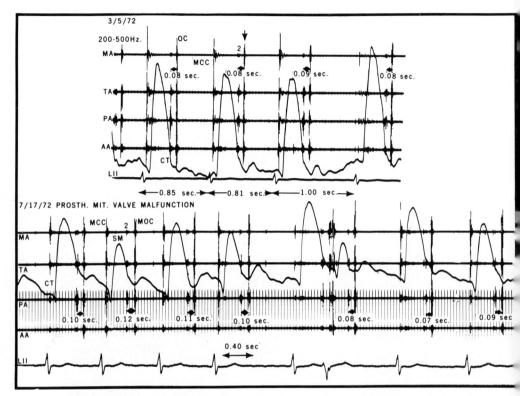

Fig. 7.23. Simultaneously recorded phonocardiogram at the mitral (MA), tricuspid (TA), pulmonic (PA), and aortic areas (AA), carotid pulse tracing (CT) and lead II (LII) of the electrocardiogram in a 54-year-old patient with a medium size Beall valve prosthesis in the mitral position. (Top panel) The patient's rhythm is atrial fibrillation with a slight variation in cycle length. Despite the variation, the time interval from the aortic component of the second heart sound to the opening click (OC) is essentially the same. However, amplitude of the closing click in this patient, as well as in most patients with disc valve prostheses is dependent on the preceding cycle length. In the last beat, which has a preceding cycle length of 1 sec, the closing click is practically absent. This can be seen at the tricuspid area. It is not an indication of valve malfunction, but the explanation for this finding is not known. It seems that disc prostheses, due to their hemodynamic profile, will float slowly during a long diastolic pause. When the valve is in a completely closed position it just barely touches the ring causing a low amplitude vibration which at times may be inaudible. The bottom tracing was recorded 4 months post-operatively when the patient developed prosthetic valve malfunction. The tracing shows marked variations in the second sound-opening click interval ranging from 0.07 to 0.12 sec. which is suggestive of prosthetic valve malfunction. The carotid pulse tracing is normal. M = mitral.

reduced left ventricular ejection time are all indicative of perivalvular insufficiency. The systolic murmur is usually soft and of short duration in patients with a mild degree of insufficiency and holosystolic in moderate to severe mitral insufficiency. A mid-diastolic murmur may infrequently be present (fig. 7.24). A third heart sound is usually associated with severe perivalvular leak. Dehiscence of mitral valve prostheses usually results in absence of the opening click and a very prominent systolic regurgitant murmur.

Mechanical obstruction may be due to thrombus formation or tissue ingrowth. Absence of the opening click, prolongation of the A2-OC interval (0.16–0.22 sec with a mean of 0.20), and less frequently, shortening of the A2-OC interval and a mid-diastolic murmur are indicative of mechanical obstruction.

Cocking of the disc may be defined as tilting of the disc in a fixed position (figs. 7.21 and 7.22) and usually occurs in the presence of severe aortic insufficiency. It results in absence of the opening and closing clicks and a loud systolic regurgitant murmur at the mitral area.

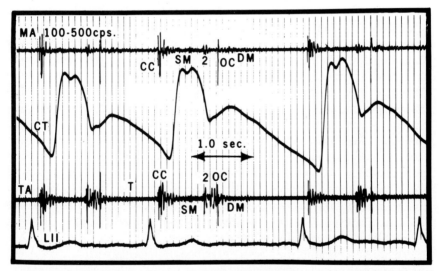

Fig. 7.24. Simultaneously recorded phonocardiogram at the mitral (MA) and tricuspid areas (TA), carotid pulse tracing (CT) and lead II (LII) of the electrocardiogram in a 47-year-old patient with prosthetic mitral Beall valve malfunction. Amplitude of the closing (CC) and opening clicks (OC) is within normal range. Note the presence of a high frequency, low amplitude systolic regurgitant murmur (SM) representing peri-prosthetic mitral insufficiency. Following the opening click there is a low frequency, medium amplitude atrioventricular diastolic murmur (DM) usually seen in patients with prosthetic valve malfunction. This is usually indicative of a significant gradient between the left atrium and left ventricle secondary to thrombus formation around the disc resulting in obstruction of flow across the valve. The contour of the carotid pulse tracing is normal.

HOMOGRAFT AND HETEROGRAFT
MALFUNCTION—MITRAL POSITION

Reported findings on the use of non-invasive techniques in patients with these prostheses are scarce. Investigators have found that these patients do not have opening clicks. The presence of prominent mitral systolic regurgitant or diastolic murmurs should be taken as possible evidence of mitral valve malfunction. However, this has not been proven.

A third heart sound is sometimes present and the time interval from aortic valve closure to the third heart sound (A2-S3) is 0.10–0.12 sec.

There have not been any reports on the value of carotid or jugular venous pulse tracings, the apexcardiogram or systolic time intervals to determine normal or abnormal function of these prostheses.

AORTIC VALVE MALFUNCTION

When malfunction is caused by lipid infiltration, cracking of the valve, ingrowth tissue formation, thrombus formation, or partial detachment of the valve, several findings can be detected by auscultation or phonocardiography. There is a progressive diminution in amplitude of the opening click (figs. 7.25 and 7.26) up to the point where the click is intermittently or completely absent. The opening to closing click ratio decreases to less than 0.5 on a high frequency (250–500 Hz) phonocardiogram recorded at the tricuspid area. In addition, there is prolongation of the time interval from the first, high frequency component of the first heart sound to the aortic opening click above 0.08 sec. The quality of the opening click changes significantly. It sounds like a thud rather than a click and, therefore, becomes a low frequency transient. The systolic ejection murmur may increase or decrease in amplitude and may vary from beat to beat. High frequency, high amplitude arterial diastolic murmurs of aortic insufficiency suggest aortic valve malfunction due to periprosthetic insufficiency, particularly when they are associated with the above findings. Figure 7.27 shows the prosthetic ball removed from the patient whose phonocardiogram was shown in figure 7.26.

Pseudo ball variance has been described in patients with left ventricular dyskinesis associated with low cardiac output, elevated left ventricular end-diastolic pressure and poor left ventricular performance.

Carotid Pulse Tracing

The carotid pulse tracing is useful only in the presence of thrombus formation around the cage. A significant left ventricular-aortic pressure gradient accompanies thrombus formation, causing an increase in ejection and upstroke times and an inconspicuous dicrotic notch. These findings are similar to what is seen in patients with aortic valvular stenosis. In patients with periprosthetic insufficiency, however, the

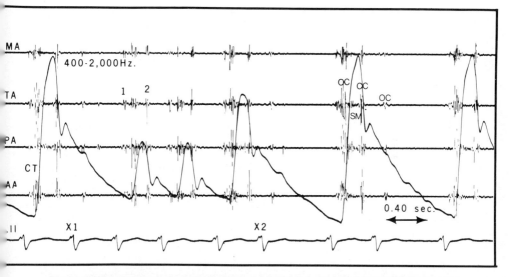

Fig. 7.25. Simultaneously recorded phonocardiogram at the mitral (MA), tricuspid (TA), pulmonic (PA) and aortic areas (AA), carotid pulse tracing (CT) and lead II (LII) of the electrocardiogram in a 60-year-old patient with a Cutter-Smeloff aortic ball valve prosthesis. The patient was found to have prosthetic valve malfunction at cardiac catheterization. The rhythm is atrial fibrillation with a variable ventricular rate. The opening (OC) and closing clicks (CC) of the aortic valve prosthesis are well appreciated in the first, third, fourth, and fifth beats. Beat X1 shows a small opening click and a very small, low amplitude sound at the end of systole. Beat X2 shows a small opening click and a very small closing click. After beat X2 the opening and closing clicks are quite apparent, and in the following beat the opening click is present but the closing click is absent. There is a high frequency, low amplitude systolic ejection murmur recorded best at the tricuspid area. The carotid pulse tracing has a normal contour and a short ejection time.

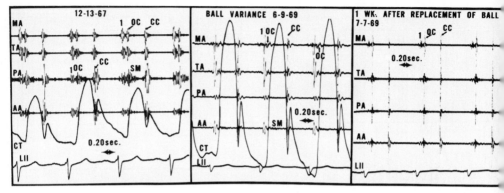

Fig. 7.26. Simultaneously recorded phonocardiogram at the mitral (MA), tricuspid (TA), pulmonic (PA) and aortic areas (AA), carotid pulse tracing (CT), and lead II (LII) of the electrocardiogram in a 52-year-old patient with a Magovern aortic ball valve prosthesis. Left panel: Amplitude of the opening (OC) and closing click (CC) ratio is approximately 0.07 sec, measured at the tricuspid area. A high frequency, low amplitude systolic ejection murmur (SM) is best recorded at the pulmonic area. The carotid pulse tracing is normal. Approximately 2 years later, the patient developed prosthetic valve malfunction (middle panel) and the phonocardiogram demonstrates marked diminution of the opening click in relation to the closing click. The valve was replaced and the recording in the right panel demonstrates a normal opening click ratio. The valve which was removed at the time of surgery is shown in figure 7.27.

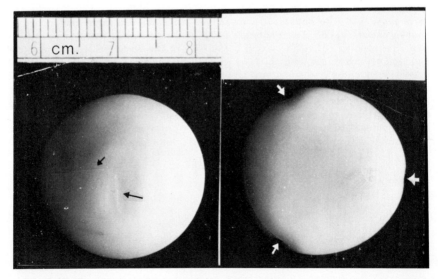

Fig. 7.27. Prosthetic ball removed from the patient whose phonocardiogram is shown in figure 7.26. Cracking of the ball in three areas is indicated by arrows.

carotid pulse tracing assumes the characteristics described for patients with aortic insufficiency such as rapid upstroke time, pulse bisferiens and a low placed and conspicuous dicrotic notch.

Jugular Venous Pulse Tracing

The jugular venous pulse tracing is useful to determine the presence of right heart failure and pulmonary hypertension. It will exhibit a quite prominent A wave and other abnormalities if the patient develops tricuspid insufficiency.

HOMOGRAFT AND HETEROGRAFT MALFUNCTION—AORTIC POSITION

Very little has been described regarding the use of non-invasive techniques in detecting malfunction of these prostheses. On the phonocardiogram, patients with homografts (preserved cadaver valves) and heterografts (Hancock-Porcine valves) present with high frequency, musical systolic murmurs with varying amplitude from beat to beat, unrelated to the preceding cycle length. This is due to the fact that these valves have a tendency to become calcified, therefore, the murmur will be similar to the one described for patients with calcific aortic valvular stenosis (see Chapter 5, "Aortic Valvular Disease"). However, the presence of musical systolic murmurs is not always a definite indicator of valve malfunction since they may also be recorded in patients with normally functioning homograft or heterograft valves.

High frequency, high amplitude (Grade III–IV/VI) arterial diastolic murmurs are usually significant and should make the examiner suspect the presence of prosthetic valve insufficiency. Murmurs similar to the Austin Flint murmur have been described in these patients and probably represent a regurgitant jet of insufficiency against the mitral valve. Prominent third and fourth heart sounds are frequently noted.

Carotid Pulse Tracing

The carotid pulse tracing shows the abnormalities seen in patients with aortic insufficiency or aortic stenosis.

Jugular Venous Pulse Tracing

The jugular venous pulse tracing is useful in the diagnosis of homograft valve malfunction only when the patient presents with the clinical picture of right ventricular failure.

Apexcardiogram

The apexcardiogram usually exhibits a prominent A wave and a prominent rapid filling wave which coincides with the prominent third heart sound.

Systolic Time Intervals

The systolic time intervals are essentially identical to the ones described for patients with aortic valvular disease and patients with heart failure.

PROSTHETIC TRICUSPID VALVE MALFUNCTION

Replacement of the tricuspid valve is uncommon and there are only a few reports of the normal and abnormal characteristics of tricuspid valve prostheses. These reports indicate that malfunction due to thrombus formation around the prosthesis results in findings similar to the ones seen in patients with tricuspid stenosis or insufficiency. On the phono-cardiogram, these patients show a decrease in amplitude and wandering of the tricuspid opening click, and a low frequency, high amplitude atrioventricular diastolic murmur similar to what is seen in patients with tricuspid stenosis. When the valve does not close properly, the typical phonocardiographic features of tricuspid insufficiency are seen, such as a high frequency, high amplitude systolic regurgitant murmur, decrease in amplitude of the first heart sound, and a prominent third heart sound. Although the basic mechanism for this type of dysfunction has not been established, it has been suggested that it is the result of impingement of the valve cage or disc against the right ventricular myocardium or interventricular septum. In addition, there may be laceration of the myocardium or bacterial and fungal endocarditis. This is particularly common in patients with a prosthetic Cutter-Smeloff valve.

Carotid Pulse Tracing

The carotid pulse tracing shows decreased ejection time, probably secondary to a decrease in left ventricular stroke volume.

Jugular Venous Pulse Tracing

The jugular venous pulse tracing is valuable in determining the presence of tricuspid valve prosthesis malfunction. If the malfunction is primarily stenosis, it shows the typical features of tricuspid stenosis such as a very prominent A wave and a normal X descent followed by a V wave with a very slow Y descent. If the malfunction results in insufficiency, the findings for tricuspid insufficiency will be evident (see Chapter 6, "Tricuspid Valvular Disease").

Systolic Time Intervals

In patients with tricuspid valve prostheses the systolic time intervals are non-specific and are only indicative of right and left ventricular failure.

ECHOCARDIOGRAPHY IN NORMAL AND ABNORMAL PROSTHETIC VALVE FUNCTION

It is important to obtain a baseline echocardiogram for each patient subjected to valve replacement prior to discharge from the hospital in order to determine normal values and the characteristics of the prosthesis implanted. This is very valuable because disc or ball excursions, diameters, and opening and closing velocities vary according to individual valve design and size. A technically satisfactory echocardiogram in the immediate post-operative period serves as each patient's control and any subsequent changes in the above parameters may be helpful in identifying valve malfunction. Transducer angulation and position for the baseline recording should be recorded and subsequent tracings be obtained utilizing the same technique.

Ball Valve Prosthesis
Mitral Position

Normal echocardiographic features of a Starr-Edwards mitral ball valve are shown in figures 7.28 and 7.29. The findings usually include (1) opening and closing of the valves are related to approximate crossover pressure changes of the left atrium and left ventricle and (2) the ball moves to the open position (D-E slope) and to the closed position (B-C slope). The remainder of the echocardiographic recording is due to move-

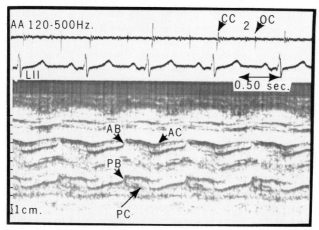

Fig. 7.28. Simultaneously recorded aortic area (AA) phonocardiogram, lead II of the electrocardiogram and echocardiogram in a 38-year-old patient with a normally functioning Starr-Edwards mitral ball valve prosthesis. The anterior ball (AB), anterior cage (AC), posterior ball (PB), and posterior cage (PC) echoes are well seen. The ball moves to a closed position starting with the closing click (CC) period and opens to full excursion at the time of the opening click (OC) of the phonocardiogram.

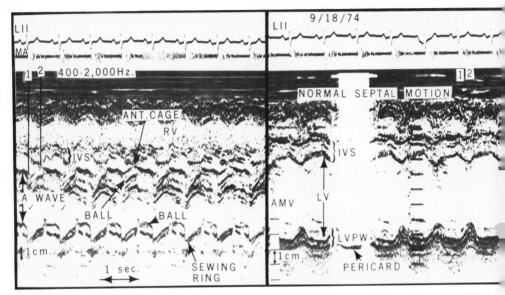

Fig. 7.29. Simultaneously recorded mitral (MA) area phonocardiogram, lead II (LII) of the electrocardiogram and echocardiogram in a 39-year-old patient with a prosthetic Starr-Edwards mitral ball valve. (Left panel) Echocardiogram showing the anterior cage. The ball moves to a closed position and nearly reaches the anterior cage during ventricular systole and remains in a wide open position during ventricular diastole. Strong echoes are recorded from the sewing ring. Right panel: Recording of the interventricular septum (IVS) demonstrating normal motion. Normal septal motion can be seen in patients with normally functioning prosthetic mitral valves and does not necessarily indicate prosthetic valve malfunction. The left ventricular (LV) internal diameter measures 5.5 cm which is within the normal limits. The tracing was recorded at damping settings. AMV = anterior mitral valve. LVPW = left ventricular posterior wall, and RV = right ventricle.

ment of the cage while the ball remains against the apex or the valve ring. The rest of the movement, apart from the B-C and D-E slopes is due to the cage, since the ball moves with the cage. The stenotic E-F slope of the prosthetic mitral ball valve resembles the E-F slope seen in patients with mitral stenosis; i.e., there is no significant rapid movement toward the right during ventricular filling. The exact mechanism for this finding is not known. It has been postulated that it may be due to the absence of movement of the prosthetic ball, independent of the cage, during that phase of the cardiac cycle, somewhat similar to the findings in mitral stenosis where there is absence of the "vortex" mechanism (a whirlpool behind the cusps and left ventricle).

In vitro physiological methods have been described to measure the diameter of the opening and closing velocities and excursion of the ball valve during ventricular systole. For the various Starr-Edwards models the figures are: diameter—dimension of the valve is multipled by a correction factor of 0.64. For Model 2M, the diameter averages 2.05 cm with a range of 2–2.1 cm. Excursion of the valve during systole averages 0.83 cm with a range of 0.8–0.90 cm. For Model 3M, diameter averages 2.21 cm (range 2.2–2.30 cm) and the excursion, 0.86 cm (range 0.8–0.9 cm). The Model 4M diameter averages 2.44 cm (range 2.4–2.5 cm) and the excursion averages 0.94 cm.

Silastic and metallic balls have specific gravity slightly greater than the blood. Hence, gravity affects the opening speed of the prosthetic valve and the closing is greater than the opening velocity. Opening velocity has been reported to be approximately 26 cm/sec and the closing velocity, 46 cm/sec. There have not been any reports of significant differences in the average values for patients in sinus rhythm or atrial fibrillation.

Echocardiography has not been established as a tool in the definite diagnosis of prosthetic valve malfunction. However, a few reports have indicated that it is valuable in patients with normally functioning prosthetic mitral ball valves where the interventricular septum usually moves paradoxically. This finding can also be seen in patients with mild-to-moderate periprosthetic insufficiency. In patients with severe periprosthetic insufficiency, the interventricular septum will show normal anterior motion. The mechanism of paradoxical septal motion in patients with normally functioning prostheses is not well known. Possible mechanisms for this phenomenon include: (1) abnormal diastolic filling of the left ventricle as the normally functioning prosthetic valve is obstructive in early diastole, and filling of the right ventricle is more rapid as compared to the left ventricle, resulting in posterior movement of the septum, (2) a relative volume overload of the right ventricle, and (3) anatomical proximity of the prosthetic valve close to the interventricular septum. Caution should be exercised in interpreting this finding since many patients with normal functioning valves may have normal septal motion (fig. 7.29). The usual echocardiographic features of patients with prosthetic valve malfunction include multiple echoes derived from within the prosthesis, indicating the presence of thrombus formation. This causes obstruction of flow from the left atrium to left ventricle resulting in an increase in left atrial pressure and an increase in left atrial internal diameter.

In the Cutter-Smeloff mitral ball prosthesis, delayed opening of the ball as well as delayed cage motion have been described in patients with valve malfunction. At operation, ingrowth of fibroid tissue or clot

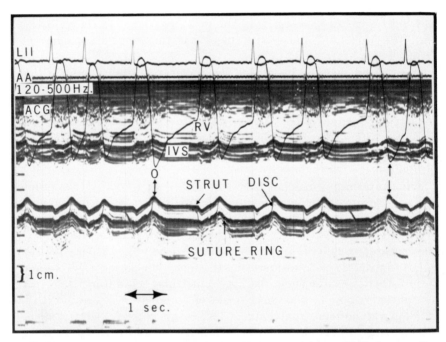

Fig. 7.30. Simultaneously recorded echocardiogram, aortic area (AA) phonocardiogram, apexcardiogram (ACG), and lead II (LII) of the electrocardiogram in a
44-year-old patient with a Beall mitral valve prosthesis. The rhytym is atrial
fibrillation. The disc moves to an open position at the end of isovolumic relaxation,
which coincides with the O point of the apexcardiogram. The valve remains fully open
during ventricular diastole and closes during ventricular systole, shortly after the
onset of the QRS complex of the electrocardiogram. The echocardiographic recording
of the strut and suture ring is shown. This patient has a normal functioning valve.
Recording of the interventricular septum (IVS) is shown but left ventricular posterior
wall motion is not recorded because of the necessity for increased damping to obtain
good echocardiographic recordings in patients with this type of prosthesis. RV =
right ventricle.

formation has been identified and this is most likely the mechanism which prevents proper ball excursion.

Ball Valve Prosthesis
Aortic Position

The following features have been described for normally functioning Starr-Edwards prostheses in the aortic position: (1) motion of opening and closing of the ball valve and cage appear to be related to the appropriate crossover pressure changes between the aorta and left ventricle, (2) movement of the cage is much less evident in the aortic position as compared with the mitral position. Rocking movement of the cage during diastole has been observed in patients with partial valve detachment, and (3) the normal average opening velocity of the valve is 40 cm/sec and closing velocity is 43 cm/sec.

Beall Disc Valves—Mitral Position

Most disc valve prostheses present with nearly identical echocardiographic patterns. Our experience has been primarily in patients with a Beall prosthesis. The normal echocardiographic pattern of the Beall prosthesis in the mitral position is shown in figure 7.30. The first echo arises from the anterior surface of one of the struts; the second echo from the anterior disc, which moves rapidly away from the anterior strut to the closed position. The third echo represents the suture ring. Another faint echo can be seen during systole and is located behind the anterior strut. During systole, all three echoes move synchronously and this represents movement of the mitral annulus.

Disc excursion and opening and closing velocities vary according to model and size (Table 7.1). Normal opening velocity ranges from 210–590 mm/sec and closing velocity from 250–750 mm/sec. In patients with prosthetic disc malfunction these figures are reduced. The decrease in disc excursion is due to incomplete valve closure.

Failure of the anterior echo of the disc to merge with the strut echo is usually indicative of incomplete disc opening and a 1-mm decrease in

Table 7.1. Disc Excursions in Centimeters of Beall Valves as Measured by Echocardiography

Beall Valve	Model No. 103	Model No. 104
Small	0.56 ± 0.02*	0.65 ± 0.02
Medium	0.67 ± 0.03	0.73 ± 0.02
Large	0.79 ± 0.01	

* Number to the right of the ± sign represents 1 standard deviation of mean.

disc excursion is almost always an indicator of malfunction due to thrombus formation. An example of a malfunctioning mitral Beall valve prosthesis is shown in figure 7.31.

Dehiscence of the suture ring can be detected through echocardiography if the valve cage changes its motion pattern as compared with a previous echocardiogram, but disc motion may show a normal pattern in perivalvular insufficiency (fig. 7.32). A few reports have also indicated that significant perivalvular insufficiency may be recognized by a sudden or progressive increase in left atrial and left ventricular internal diameters. Figure 7.33 illustrates markedly increased left atrial internal diameter due to malfunction of a Starr-Edwards valve in the mitral position.

Björk-Shiley Tilting Disc Valve
Mitral and Aortic Positions

The Björk-Shiley prosthetic disc valve can be implanted in the mitral (figs. 7.34–7.36) or aortic (fig. 7.37) position. The valve is asymmetrical along the X (right-left), Y (superior-inferior) and Z axis (anterior-posterior) and the disc pivots about 60 degrees during ventricular ejection.

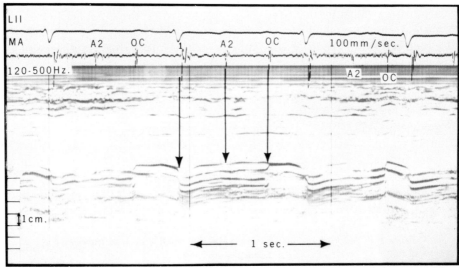

Fig. 7.31. Simultaneously recorded mitral area (MA) phonocardiogram, lead II (LII) of the electrocardiogram, and echocardiogram in a 70-year-old patient with a Beall mitral valve prosthesis, which was malfunctioning. The tracing was taken at a paper speed of 100 mm/sec. The rhythm is sinus with first degree atrioventricular block. Note marked prolongation of the second sound-opening click (OC) interval. The echocardiogram shows the stenotic slope of the valve. Timing of the opening click of the prosthetic mitral valve coincides with the opening click of the phonocardiogram and occurs late in diastole at the time of inscription of the P wave of the electrocardiogram.

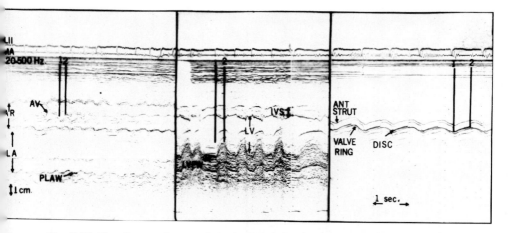

Fig. 7.32. Simultaneously recorded mitral area (MA) phonocardiogram, lead II (LII) of the electrocardiogram, and echocardiogram of a 55-year-old patient with a prosthetic mitral Beall valve. This patient had periprosthetic insufficiency. (Left panel) Echocardiographic recording of the left atrium (LA) and aortic root (AR) showing marked enlargement of the left atrium as compared with the aortic root. (Middle panel) Recording of the interventricular septum (IVS) and left ventricle (LV) showing slight exaggeration of left ventricular posterior wall (LVPW) motion. (Right panel) Recording of the anterior and posterior structures of the prosthetic valve are well seen. The transducer was placed at the apex to record the prosthetic mitral valve echoes with maximal damping to obtain a better recording of the valve structures.

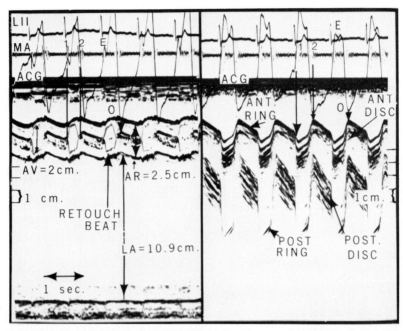

Fig. 7.33. Simultaneously recorded echocardiogram, apexcardiogram (ACG), mitral area (MA) phonocardiogram, and lead II (LII) of the electrocardiogram in a 57-year-old patient with a Starr-Edwards mitral valve prosthesis. (Left panel) Echocardiogram of the aortic valve showing normal configuration of the valve structure. Observe the markedly increased left atrial (LA) internal diameter of 10.9 cm as compared with the aortic root (AR) of 2.5 cm. The aortic valve (Av) opening is within the normal range at 2 cm. In patients with aortic valve prostheses, marked increase in left atrial size is a suggestive indirect sign of prosthetic valve malfunction. (Right panel) Recording of the prosthetic valve showing normal motion of the anterior and posterior ring and disc. Other structures are not seen because of the necessity to increase damping to record prosthetic valve structures. On the phonocardiogram, the opening click coincides with opening of the prosthetic valve as the disc moves anteriorly toward the anterior ring. The disc remains fully open during ventricular diastole. The typical stenotic diastolic slope of the valve is seen, but this is not always an indication of valve malfunction.

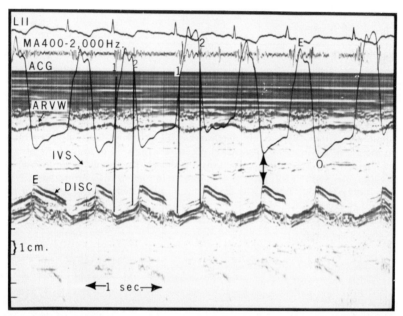

Fig. 7.34. Simultaneously recorded echocardiogram, mitral area (MA) phono-cardiogram, apexcardiogram (ACG), and lead II (LII) of the electrocardiogram in a 63-year-old patient with a No. 25 Björk-Shiley mitral valve prosthesis. The rhythm is atrial fibrillation. Time of inscription of the opening and closing of the prosthetic valve is indicated. The disc moves to an anterior position with a wide open excursion during diastole and to a closed position during systole. The O point of the apexcardiogram follows the second heart sound and coincides with the E point of the echocardiogram. Echoes from the interventricular septum (IVS) are shown as well as the anterior right ventricular wall motion (ARVW).

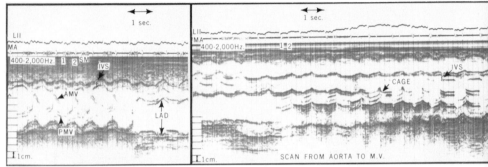

Fig. 7.35. Simultaneously recorded mitral area (MA) phonocardiogram, lead II (LII) of the electrocardiogram and echocardiographic recording prior to (left panel), and following mitral valve replacement (right panel) with a Björk-Shiley prosthesis in a 53-year-old patient with mitral insufficiency. (Left panel) Echocardiographic scan from the mitral valve to the aorta. Note an increase in left atrial internal diameter (LAD) to 5 cm. The phonocardiogram shows a high amplitude, high frequency systolic regurgitant murmur (SM) at the mitral area. (Right panel) Echocardiographic scan from the aorta to the mitral valve (MV) prosthesis showing echoes of the prosthetic Björk-Shiley valve. The poppet structures are shown. Compare the flat motion of the interventricular septum (IVS) in the post-operative tracing with normal motion in the pre-operative tracing. AMV = anterior mitral valve and PMV = posterior mitral valve.

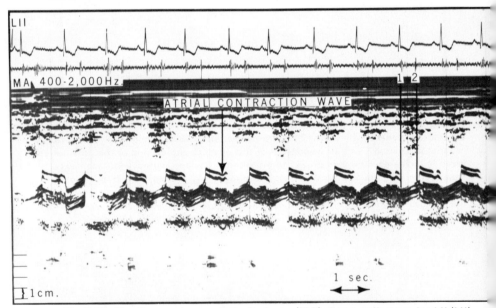

Fig. 7.36. Simultaneously recorded mitral area (MA) phonocardiogram, lead II (LII) of the electrocardiogram, and echocardiogram in a 57-year-old patient with a Björk-Shiley mitral valve prosthesis. Note a stenotic, diastolic E-F slope. Following inscription of the P wave of the electrocardiogram with subsequent atrial contraction, there is anterior motion of the valve.

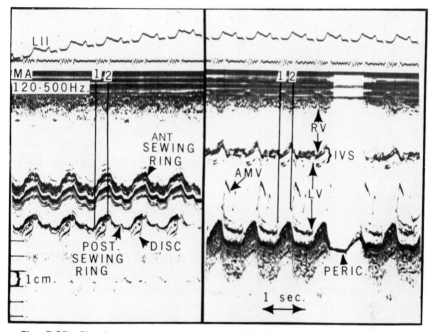

Fig. 7.37. Simultaneously recorded echocardiogram, phonocardiogram at the mitral area (MA) and lead II (LII) of the electrocardiogram in a 47-year-old patient with a Björk-Shiley aortic valve prosthesis. (Left panel) Echocardiogram of the Björk-Shiley valve showing the anterior and posterior rings, and the disc which is appreciated in the posterior aspect of the sewing ring. (Right panel) Echocardiogram of the mitral valve and interventricular septum (IVS). Note normal mitral valve motion. The pericardium and interventricular septum are well seen and there is abnormal interventricular septal motion. This tracing was taken at various degrees of damping. RV = right ventricle, LV = left ventricle, and AMV = anterior mitral valve.

The values for maximum disc excursion for the greater curvature of various size valves are shown in Table 7.2. During ventricular ejection the larger segment of the disc exhibits greater excursion as compared with the lesser segment.

Table 7.2. Dimensions and Maximal Disc Excursion of Björk-Shiley Prosthetic Valves

Tissue Annulus Size (mm)	17	19	21	23	25	27	29	31
Orifice Diameter (mm)	12	14	16	18	20	22	24	24
Excursion (mm)	9	10	11	13	14	16	17	17

Optimal alignment of the transducer in relation to the valve for detecting maximal disc excursion, which occurs when the ultrasonic beam is perpendicular to the maximally opened disc, varies from patient to patient, e.g., 2 to 8 o'clock position in X-Z planes. It is usually possible to obtain satisfactory excursion of the lesser and greater curvatures of the disc with the transducer placed at the second or third intercostal space at the left sternal border and directed medially and inferiorly. However, many other transducer positions and angulations have been described.

Definite criteria for detection of Björk-Shiley valve malfunction have not been established. However, the presence of strong and disorganized echoes within the valve structure may suggest clot formation. This is illustrated in a prosthesis implanted in the mitral position in figure 7.38 and the valve removed from this patient showing large clots around the disc is shown in figure 7.39. Figure 7.40 shows a Björk-Shiley prosthesis in the aortic position which is malfunctioning and figure 7.41 is the valve removed from this patient illustrating multiple clots.

In a few reported cases of aortic valve malfunction diagnosed pre-operatively by echocardiography, the records revealed absence of disc motion and the aortic root was filled with dense and disorganized echoes. After surgical removal of clots, a post-operative echocardiogram will show the findings usually seen in patients with normally functioning prostheses.

Lillehei-Kaster Tilting Disc Valve
Mitral and Aortic Positions

Echocardiographic features of the Lillehei-Kaster valve have been described in a series of patients with normally functioning prostheses (fig. 7.42). The opening velocity ranges from 28 to 59 cm/sec with a mean of 37.7 cm/sec. Closing velocity ranges from 39 to 99 cm/sec with a mean of 59.8 cm/sec. Amplitude of valve movement varies from 7 to 12 mm. Valve excursion, opening, and closing velocities decrease with aging, and the valve velocity is not uniform. Considerable variation has been noted in patients who have apparently normal functioning prostheses. The average opening and closing velocities of Lillehei-Kaster valves exceed those of the Starr-Edwards and Beall valves.

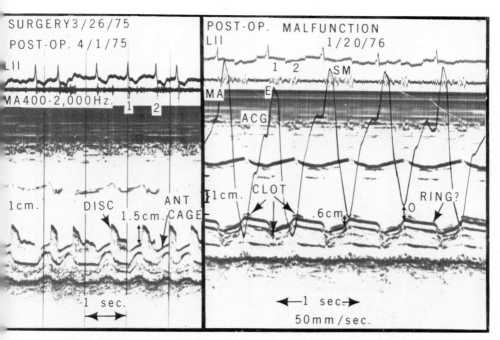

Fig. 7.38. Echocardiogram in a 53-year-old patient who had a No. 29 Björk-Shiley prosthesis implanted in the mitral position and developed prosthetic valve malfunction. (Left panel) Simultaneously recorded echocardiogram, mitral area (MA) phonocardiogram, and lead II (LII) of the electrocardiogram obtained approximately 10 days following mitral valve replacement. Note the motion of the disc excursion (DISC) which is 1.5 cm. The patient subsequently developed congestive heart failure and prosthetic valve malfunction was suspected prior to surgery. (Right panel) Simultaneously recorded echocardiogram, mitral area phonocardiogram, apexcardiogram (ACG), and lead II of the electrocardiogram on the same patient. Note the presence of heavy and disorganized echoes which seems to indicate the presence of clot formation (CLOT). At time of surgery, the valve was found to have multiple clots around the disc. This valve which was removed at time of surgery is shown in figure 7.39. ANT CAGE = anterior cage and SM = systolic murmur.

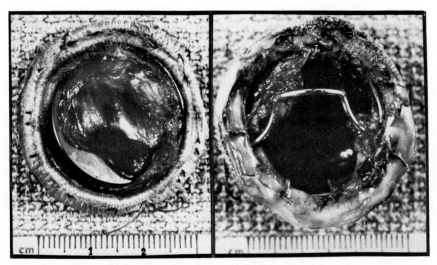

Fig. 7.39. Björk-Shiley prosthesis removed from the patient shown in figure 7.38 showing the presence of large clots around the disc which prevented a normal, full excursion of the valve during ventricular systole and diastole.

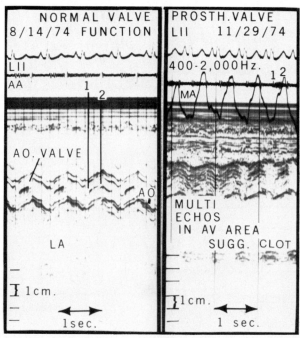

Fig. 7.40. (Left panel) Simultaneously recorded aortic area (AA) phonocardio-gram, lead II (LII) of the electrocardiogram and echocardiogram of a 54-year-old patient with a normally functioning Björk-Shiley prosthetic aortic valve implanted on 8/14/74. Note the box-like structure of the valve. (Right panel) Simultaneously recorded mitral area (MA) phonocardiogram, lead II of the electrocardiogram, echocardiogram, and carotid pulse tracing of the same patient recorded on 11/29/74. At the time of this recording, the patient was in congestive heart failure. The echocardiogram demonstrates multiple echoes originating from the aortic (AO) valve area suggestive of clot formation. The patient was re-operated and the valve was replaced with another Björk-Shiley valve. The operative findings revealed multiple clots around the disc. A picture of the valve which was removed is shown in figure 7.41. LA = left atrium.

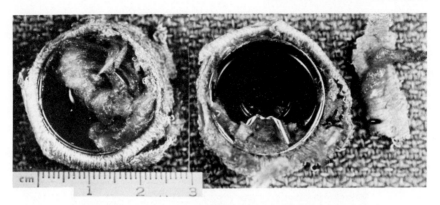

Fig. 7.41. Prosthetic valve removed from the patient described in figure 7.40 showing the presence of multiple clots around the disc and at the base of the valve.

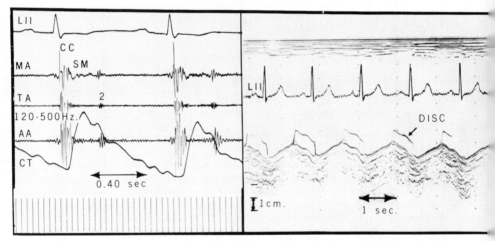

Fig. 7.42. (Left panel) Simultaneously recorded phonocardiogram at the mitral (MA), tricuspid (TA), and aortic areas (AA), carotid pulse tracing (CT), and lead II (LII) of the electrocardiogram in a patient with a Lillehei-Kaster mitral valve prosthesis. The high frequency vibration following the QRS complex of the electrocardiogram probably represents the closing click (CC) of the prosthesis. This is followed by a high frequency, low amplitude, short decrescendo systolic murmur (SM) which terminates in mid-systole. The second heart sound is single and normal. There are no opening clicks in diastole. The carotid pulse tracing is normal. (Right panel) Simultaneously recorded lead II of the electrocardiogram and echocardiogram on the same patient showing the disc (DISC) motion. The disc has a decreased E-F slope. The echocardiographic features for this type of valve are quite similar to the ones described in patients with Björk-Shiley prostheses. (Courtesy of Anis L. Obeid, M.D., State University Hospital of Upstate Medical Center, Syracuse, N. Y.)

Heterograft Valves

The most commonly used heterograft is the stented Hancock-Porcine, a chemically preserved aortic valve of a pig, which can be implanted in the mitral (figs. 7.43 and 7.44), tricuspid (fig. 7.45), or aortic positions (figs. 7.46–7.48). There has not been a large series of reported echocardiographic findings for this prosthesis. In our experience, the valve exhibits the features seen in normally functioning human valves in the mitral, tricuspid, or aortic positions. Definite patterns for recognition of malfunction have not been established. The Hancock-Porcine valve is also used for the Rastelli (fig. 7.49) and Fontan procedures for surgical correction of pulmonary and tricuspid atresia.

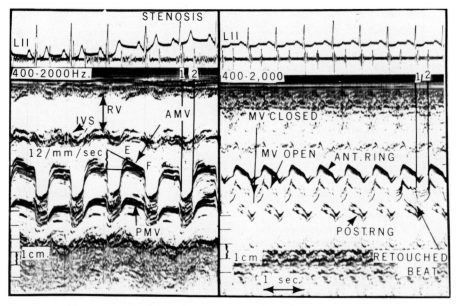

Fig. 7.43. Simultaneously recorded phonocardiogram, lead II (LII) of the electrocardiogram and echocardiogram in a 35-year-old patient with severe mitral stenosis. (Left panel) Echocardiogram of the mitral valve showing the typical features seen in patients with mitral stenosis; namely decrease in E-F slope to 12 mm/sec, anterior motion of the posterior mitral valve (PMV) and multiple echoes from the mitral valve indicating the presence of fibrosis or calcification of the valve. (Right panel) The patient was operated and the mitral valve was replaced with a Hancock-Porcine valve. Observe the motion of the mitral valve which moves to a fully open (MV OPEN) position during diastole. The recording of the anterior ring (ANT RING) and the posterior ring (POST RING) is indicated. A retouched beat is seen at the last beat of this recording. IVS = interventricular septum, AMV = anterior mitral valve, and RV = right ventricle.

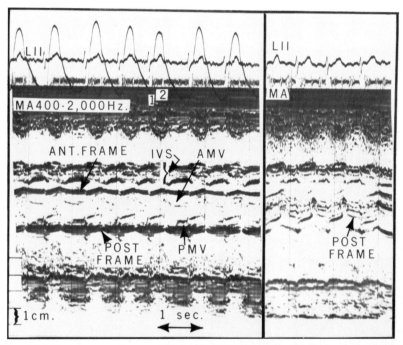

Fig. 7.44. Simultaneously recorded mitral area (MA) phonocardiogram, lead II (LII) of the electrocardiogram and echocardiogram in a 68-year-old patient with a Hancock-Porcine valve implanted in the mitral position. (Left panel) Echocardiographic recording of the anterior and posterior frames of the valve is best appreciated at the level of the mid-left ventricular cavity. This prosthetic valve has a motion similar to a normally functioning mitral valve with the exception of the E-F slope which is decreased. The interventricular septum (IVS) has a flat motion. (Right panel) Echocardiogram demonstrating a better recording of the posterior frame of the valve. The transducer was angulated from the apex to the base of the heart. AMV = anterior mitral valve and PMV = posterior mitral valve.

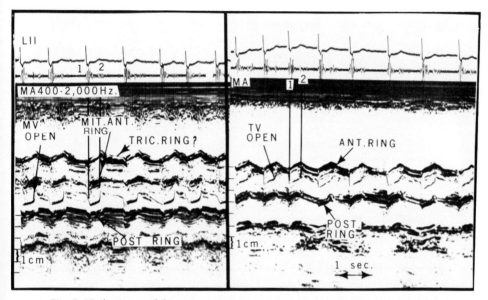

Fig. 7.45. (Left panel) Simultaneously recorded mitral area (MA) phonocardiogram lead II (LII) of the electrocardiogram and echocardiogram in a 58-year-old patient with a No. 31 Hancock-Porcine valve implanted in the mitral position. Time of inscription of the opening and closing of the prosthetic valve is indicated. Note a decrease in the E-F slope of the anterior valve structures. Recordings of the mitral anterior ring (MIT ANT RING) and posterior ring (POST RING) are shown. The other echoes recorded may be tricuspid (TRIC) ring echoes. (Right panel) Echocardiogram of the same patient who had a No. 33 Hancock-Porcine valve implanted in the tricuspid position for correction of severe tricuspid insufficiency. Recordings of the anterior (ANT RING) and posterior ring (POST RING) of the valve are well seen. Time of inscription of the first and second heart sounds is indicated. Note that the echocardiographic features of the mitral and tricuspid prosthetic valves are essentially identical.

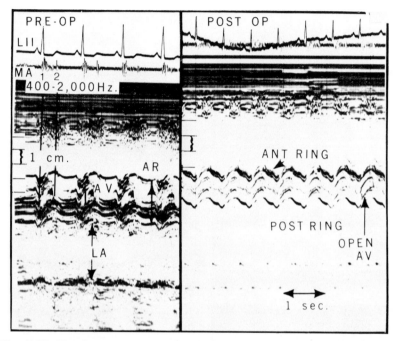

Fig. 7.46. Simultaneously recorded echocardiogram, mitrol area (MA) phonocardiogram and lead II (LII) of the electrocardiogram in a 61-year-old patient who
had severe aortic stenosis and aortic insufficiency. The electrocardiogram shows
sinus rhythm. (Left panel) The pre-operative tracing shows multiple and disorganized
echoes derived from the aortic valve (AV) with a small aortic valve opening indicating
a calcified valve. This was confirmed at the time of cardiac catheterization and
surgery. The left atrial (LA) internal diameter is 4 cm which is within normal limits. At
cardiac catheterization, the patient had a 55-mm gradient across the heavily calcified
aortic valve. (Right panel) Echocardiogram of the same patient after aortic valve
replacement with a No. 23 Hancock-Porcine prosthetic aortic valve. The valve has a
wide open excursion during ventricular systole and echoes are also recorded during
diastole simulating a normally functioning aortic valve. For recording an aortic valve
prosthesis of this type, the echocardiographic transducer is usually placed at the apex
of the heart and increased damping is necessary to eliminate certain structures.
Therefore, recording of the interventricular septum and posterior wall of the left
ventricle are not possible to obtain from that position and intracardiac internal
diameter measurements cannot be made from those recordings. This valve has a
box-like structure similar to what one sees in a patient with a normally functioning
aortic valve. The anterior and posterior ring recordings are indicated. AR = aortic
root.

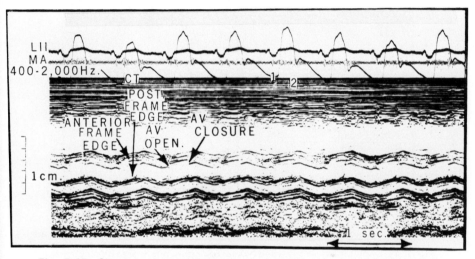

Fig. 7.47. Simultaneously recorded echocardiogram, phonocardiogram at the mitral area (MA), carotid pulse tracing (CT) and lead II (LII) of the electrocardiogram in a 39-year-old patient with a Hancock-Porcine aortic valve prosthesis. In this tracing, one can appreciate the echoes derived from the anterior and posterior frames of the prosthesis as well as timing of the opening and closing of the prosthetic valve. The box-like structure of the valve is similar to what is seen in patients with normally functioning aortic valves. It is wide open during systole, with a single diastolic echo during diastole beginning at the time of aortic valve closure.

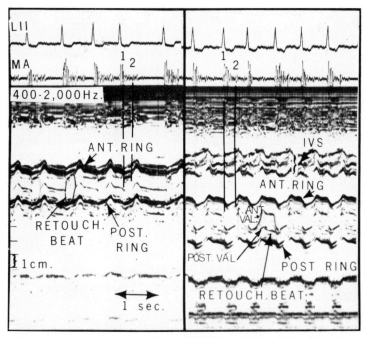

Fig. 7.48. Simultaneously recorded echocardiogram, mitral area (MA) phonocardiogram and lead II (LII) of the electrocardiogram in a 53-year-old patient with aortic and mitral valve prostheses. (Left panel) The aortic valve was replaced with a No. 25 Hancock-Porcine valve. The typical box-like structure of this valve is similar to what is seen in patients with normally functioning aortic valves. The valve moves to a wide open excursion in early systole and remains open and in close contact with the anterior and posterior wall of the aorta during systole. It comes to a closed position at the time of the second heart sound. There is a single diastolic echo as is seen in a normally functioning aortic valve. The anterior and posterior rings are indicated. The phonocardiogram shows a systolic ejection murmur (SM) and normal first and second heart sounds at the mitral area. The rhythm is atrial fibrillation. (Right panel) The mitral valve was replaced with a No. 32 Hancock-Porcine prosthesis. Time of inscription of the first and second heart sounds is indicated. In the mitral position, the prosthesis will have a motion similar to a normally functioning mitral valve except that the diastolic E-F slope is decreased similar to what is seen in patients with a mild degree of mitral stenosis. IVS = interventricular septum.

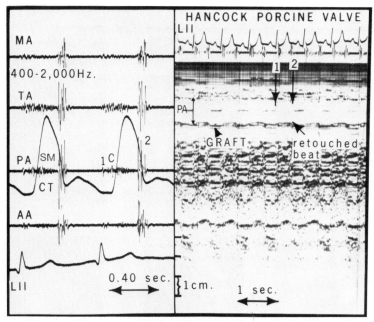

Fig. 7.49. (Left panel) Phonocardiogram at the mitral (MA), tricuspid (TA), pulmonic (PA) and aortic areas (AA), carotid pulse tracing (CT), and lead II (LII) of the electrocardiogram in a 8-year-old patient who had a Rastelli procedure for palliative correction of pulmonary atresia by implanting a right ventricle to pulmonary artery graft with a Hancock-Porcine prosthetic valve inserted in the graft near the right ventricle. The phonocardiogram shows a normal first heart sound followed by a systolic ejection click (C) and a systolic ejection murmur (SM) best recorded at the pulmonic area. The second heart sound is slightly accentuated. This murmur probably represents turbulent flow across the right ventricular-pulmonary artery graft. (Right panel) Echocardiogram showing a recording of the pulmonary artery (PA) and graft.

Homograft Valves

Echocardiograms of patients with stented fascia lata grafts in the mitral position have been reported. The diastolic closure rate (E-F slope) of the cusps revealed significant correlation with the effective valve area as calculated by standard formulas for valve area measurements using invasive techniques.

Autograft valves, made of human dura mater, have been used for mitral, aortic, and tricuspid valve replacement. The echocardiographic features are not well known, but the findings seem to be similar to the ones described for the heterograft Hancock-Porcine valve.

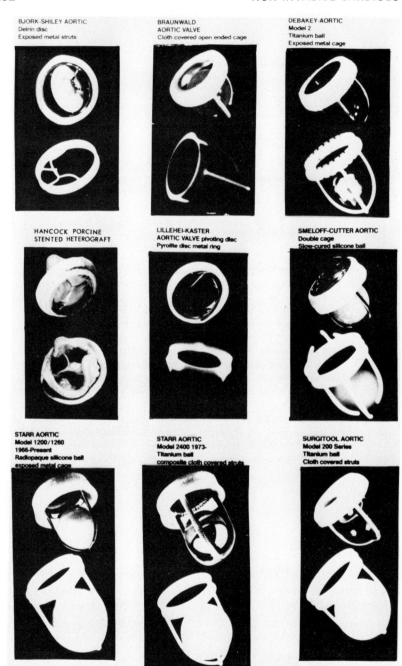

Fig. 7.50. Prosthetic mitral valves. (Reproduced, Courtesy of Dryden Morse, M.D., Deborah Heart and Lung Center, Browns Mills, New Jersey.)

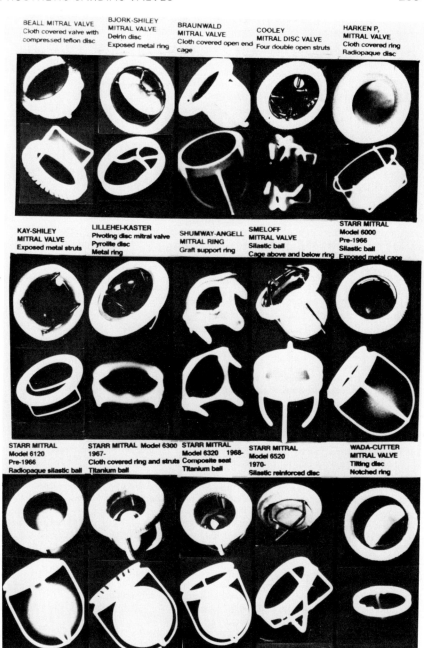

Fig. 7.51. Prosthetic aortic valves. (Reproduced, Courtesy of Dryden Morse, M.D., Heart and Lung Center, Browns Mills, New Jersey.)

REFERENCES

1. Angell, W. W., deLanerolle, P., and Shumway, N. E.: Valve replacement; present status of homograft valves. Prog. Cardiovasc. Dis., *15:* 589, 1973.
2. Aravanis, C., Toutouzas, P., and Stavrou, S.: Disappearance of opening sound of Starr-Edwards mitral valve due to valvular detachment. Br. Heart J., *34:* 1314, 1972.
3. Assad-Morell, J. L., Tajik, A. J., Anderson, M. W., Tancredi, R. G., Wallace, R. B., and Giuliani, E. R.: Malfunctioning tricuspid valve prosthesis; clinical, phonocardiographic, echocardiographic, and surgical findings. Mayo Clin. Proc., *49:* 443, 1974.
4. Aston, S. J., and Mulder, D. G.: Cardiac valve replacement; a seven-year follow up. J. Thorac. Cardiovasc. Surg., *61:* 547, 1971.
5. Bain, W. H., Turner, M. A., and Thomson, R. M.: Early experience with Björk-Shiley tilting disc prosthesis. Br. Heart J., *35:* 556, 1973.
6. Balkoura-Christopoulos, M. H., Resnekov, L., and Kittle, C. F.: Malfunction of a disc mitral valve prosthesis; detection by phonocardiography. Chest, *63:* 624, 1973.
7. Barratt-Boyes, B. G.: Long-term follow-up of aortic valvular grafts. Br. Heart J., *33* (Suppl.): 60, 1971.
8. Beall, A. C. Jr., and Sheely, C. H., II: Current status of prosthetic valve replacement. Cardiovasc. Clin. 5(2): 319, 1973.
9. Behrendt, D. M., and Austen, W. G.: Current status of prosthetics for heart valve replacement. Prog. Cardiovasc. Dis., *15:* 369, 1973.
10. Belenkie, I.L., Carr, M., Schlant, R. C., Nutter, D. O., and Symbas, P. N.: Malfunction of a Cutter-Smeloff mitral ball valve prosthesis; diagnosis by phonocardiography and echocardiography. Am. Heart J., *86:* 399, 1973.
11. Bellhouse, B. J.: Fluid mechanics of model aortic and mitral valves. Proc. R. Soc. Med., *63:* 996, 1970.
12. Bellhouse, B. J., Bellhouse, F. H., and Gunning, A. J.: Studies of a model mitral valve with three cusps. Br. Heart J., *35:* 1075, 1973.
13. Ben-Zvi, J., Hildner, F. J., Chandraratna, P. A., and Samet, P.: Thrombosis on Björk-Shiley aortic valve prosthesis; clinical, arteriographic, echocardiographic, and therapeutic observations in seven cases. Am. J. Cardiol., *34:* 538, 1974.
14. Björk, V. O.: Aortic valve replacement with Björk-Shiley tilting disc valve prosthesis. Br. Heart J., *33* (Suppl.): 42, 1971.
15. Björk, V. O., and Henze, A.: Encapsulation of the Björk-Shiley aortic disc valve prosthesis caused by the lack of anticoagulant treatment. Scand. J. Thorac. Cardiovasc. Surg. *7:* 17, 1973.
16. Boicourt, O. W., Bristow, J. D., Starr, A., and Griswold, H. E.: A phonocardiographic study of patients with multiple Starr-Edwards prosthetic valves Br. Heart J., *28:* 531, 1966.
17. Brown, D. F.: Decreased intensity of closure sound in a normally functioning Starr-Edwards mitral valve prosthesis; observations on presystolic mitral valve closure. Am. J. Cardiol., *31:* 93, 1973.
18. Clark, R. E., and Surtera, S. P.: Methods of design of leaflet valvular prosthesis; stresses in mitral valve leaflets in health and disease. J. Thorac. Cardiovasc. Surg., *65:* 890, 1973.
19. Cleland, J., and Molloy, P. J.: Thrombo-embolic complications of the cloth-covered Starr-Edwards prostheses no. 2300 and no. 6300 mitral. Thorax, *28:* 41, 1973.
20. Cohen, A. I., Benchimol, A., and Brown, L. B.: Clinical and phonocardiographic recognition of prosthetic aortic valve ball variance. Ariz. Med., *27:* 90, 1970.
21. Connolly, D. C., Harrison, C. E., and Ellis, F. H. Jr.: Ball variance in a Starr-Edwards prosthetic mitral valve causing acute pulmonary edema (diagnosis by auscultation before onset of symptoms). Mayo Clin. Proc., *45:* 20, 1970.
22. Dayem, M. K., and Raftery, E. B.: Mechanisms of production of heart sounds: based on records of sounds after valve replacement. Am. J. Cardiol., *18:* 837, 1966.
23. Dayem, M. K., and Raftery, E. B.: Phonocardiogram of the ball and cage aortic valve prosthesis. Br. Heart J., *29:* 446, 1967.
24. Delman, A. J.: Aortic ball variance. Am. Heart J., *83:* 291, 1972.
25. Delman, A. J., Attai, L. A., Naidu, S., and Robinson, G.: Limitations of phonocardio-

graphic assessment of ball variance. Ann. Thorac. Surg., *10:* 278, 1970.

26. Douglas, J. E., and Williams, G. D.: Echocardiographic evaluation of the Björk-Shiley prosthetic valve. Circulation, *50:* 52, 1974.

27. Fernandez, J., Morse, D., Maranhao, V., and Gooch, A. S.: Results of use of the pyrolytic carbon tilting disc Björk-Shiley aortic prosthesis. Chest, *65:* 640, 1974.

28. Fishman, N. H., Hutchinson, J. C., Massengale, M. M., and Roe, B. B.: Follow-up evaluation of 100 consecutive mitral prosthesis implants. Arch. Surg., *97:* 691, 1968.

29. Fleming, J., Hamer, J., Hayward, G., Hill, I., and Tubbs, O. S.: Long-term results of aortic valve replacement. Br. Heart J., *31:* 388, 1969.

30. Folts, J. D., Young, W. P., and Rowe, G. G.: Phasic flow through normal and prosthetic mitral valves in unanesthetized dogs. J. Thorac. Cardiovasc. Surg., *61:* 235, 1971.

31. Gibson, D. G., Broder, G., and Sowton, E.: Assessment of left ventricular function in patients with aortic Starr-Edwards prostheses. Br. Heart J., *31:* 388, 1969.

32. Gibson, D. G., Broder, G., and Sowton, E.: Phonocardiographic method of assessing changes in left ventricular function after Starr-Edwards replacement of aortic valve. Br. Heart J., *32:* 142, 1970.

33. Hamby, R. I., Aintablian, A., and Wisoff, B. G.: Mechanics of closure of the mitral prosthetic valve and the role of atrial systole; phonocardiographic and cinefluorographic study. Am. J. Cardiol., *31:* 616, 1973.

34. Hildner, F. J.: Detection of prosthetic valve dysfunction by bedside and laboratory evaluation. Cardiovasc. Clin., *5:* 289, 1973.

35. Hylen, J. C., Kloster, F. E., Herr, R. H., Starr, A., and Griswold, H. E.: Sound spectrographic diagnosis of aortic ball variance. Circulation, *39:* 849, 1969.

36. Hylen, J. C., Kloster, F. E., Starr, A., and Griswold, H. E.: Aortic ball variance; diagnosis and treatment. Ann. Intern. Med., *72:* 1, 1970.

37. Ionescu, M. I.: Mitral valvular grafts. Br. Heart J., *33* (Suppl.): 56, 1971.

38. Isom, O. W., Williams, C. D., Falk, E. A., Glassman, E., and Spencer, F. C.: Long-term evaluation of cloth-covered metalic ball prostheses. J. Thorac. Cardiovasc. Surg., *64:* 354, 1972.

39. Jarcho, S.: Experiments on the mitral valve (Stricker, 1883). Am. J. Cardiol., *33:* 550, 1974.

40. Johnson, M. L., Holmes, J. H., and Paton, B. C.: Echocardiographic determination of mitral disc valve excursion. Circulation, *47:* 1274, 1973.

41. Johnson, M. L., Paton, B. C., and Holmes, J. H.: Ultrasonic evaluation of prosthetic valve motion. Circulation, *41* (Suppl. II): 3, 1970.

42. Kawai, N., Segal, B. L., and Linhart, J. W.: Delayed opening of Beall mitral valve prosthetic valve detected by echocardiography. Chest, *67:* 239, 1975.

43. Kellebrew, E., and Cohn, K.: Observations on murmurs originating from incompetent heterograft mitral valves. Am. Heart J., *81:* 490, 1971.

44. Laniado, S., Yellin, E., Kolter, M., Levy, L., Stadler, J., and Terdiman, R.: A study of the dynamic relations between the mitral valve echogram and phasic mitral flow. Circulation, *51:* 104, 1975.

45. Leachman, R. D., and Cokkinos, D. V. P: Absence of opening click in dehiscence of mitral valve prosthesis. N. Eng. J. Med., *281:* 461, 1969.

46. Levy, M. J., Vidne, B., Salomon, J., and Eshkol, D.: Long-term follow-up (one to four years) of heart valve prostheses (102 consecutive patients). Dis. Chest, *56:* 440, 1969.

47. Martinez-Lopez, J. I.: Heart sounds following prosthetic valve replacement. J. La. State Med. Soc., *121:* 133, 1969.

48. Mary, D. A. S., Pakrashi, B. C., Catchpole, R. W., and Ionescu, M. I.: Echocardiographic studies of stented fascia lata grafts in the mitral position. Circulation, *49:* 237, 1974.

49. Miller, H. C., Stephens, J., and Gibson, D.: Echocardiographic features of mitral Starr-Edwards paraprosthetic regurgitation. Br. Heart J., *35:* 560, 1973.

50. Morrow, A. G.: Prosthetic replacement of the mitral valve: an assessment of the clinical and hemodynamic results of operation. Calif. Med., *111:* 498, 1969.

51. Najmi, M., and Segal, B. L.: Auscultatory and phonocardiographic findings in patients with prosthetic ball-valves. Am. J. Cardiol., *16:* 794, 1965.

52. Parisi, A. F., and Milton, B. G.: Relation of mitral valve closure to the first heart sound in man; echocardiographic and phonocardiographic assessment. Am. J. Cardiol., *32:* 779, 1973.

53. Pileggi, F., Sosa, E. A., Bellotti, G., DelNero, E. Jr., Verginelli, G., Tranchesi, J., Puig, L. B. and Decourt, L. V.: O fonomecanocardiograma da valva de dura-mater em posicao mitral. Arq. Bras. Cardiol., *28*(3): 267, 1975.

54. Pohost, G. M., Dinsmore, R. E., Rubenstein, J. J., O'Keefe, D. D., Grantham, R. N., Scully, H. E., Beierholm, E. A., Frederiksen, J. W., Weisfeldt, M. L., and Daggett, W. M.: The echocardiogram of the anterior leaflet of the mitral valve; correlation with hemodynamic and cineroentgenographic studies in dogs. Circulation, *51:* 88, 1975.

55. Raftery, E. B.: Origin of the third heart sound. Br. Med. J., *3:* 598, 1969.

56. Roberts, W. C., Bulkley, B. H., and Morrow, A. G.: Pathologic anatomy of cardiac valve replacement: a study of 224 necropsy patients. Prog. Cardiovasc. Dis., *15:* 539, 1973.

57. Ross, D. N.: Aortic valve replacements. Br. Heart J., *33* (Suppl.): 39, 1971.

58. Ross, D. N., Yates, A. K., and Wright, J. E. C.: Replacement of aortic valve with unsupported fascia lata: report on technique and results in 43 cases. Br. Heart J., *33:* 611, 1971.

59. Rubenstein, J. J., Pohost, G. M., Dinsmore, R. E., and Harthorne, J. W.: The echocardiographic determination of mitral valve opening and closure; correlation with hemodynamic studies in man. Circulation, *51:* 98, 1975.

60. Schelbert, H. R., and Muller, O. F.: Detection of fungal vegetations involving a Starr-Edwards mitral prosthesis by means of ultrasound. Vasc. Surg., *6:* 20, 1972.

61. Shaw, T. R. D., Gunstensen, J., and Turner, R. W. D.: Sudden mechanical malfunction of Hammersmith mitral valve prostheses due to wear of polypropylene. J. Thorac. Cardiovasc. Surg., *67:* 579, 1974.

62. Smith, G. H., and Chandra, K.: Massive aortic incompetence associated with the Bjork-Shiley prosthesis. Thorax, *28:* 627, 1973.

63. Starr, A.: Mitral valve replacement with ball-valve prostheses. Br. Heart J., *33* (Suppl.): 47, 1971.

64. Stein, P. D., and Munter, W. A.: New functional concept of valvular mechanics in normal and diseased aortic valves. Circulation, *44:* 101, 1971.

65. Stimmel, B., Stein, E., Katz, A. M., Litwak, R. S., and Donoso, E.: Phonocardiographic manifestations of heterograft valve dysfunction in mitral area. Br. Heart J., *34:* 936, 1972.

66. Stross, J. K., Willis, P. W., and Kahn, D. R.: Diagnostic features of malfunction of disc mitral valve prostheses. J.A.M.A., *217:* 305, 1971.

67. Swanson, W. M., and Clark, R. E.: Aortic valve leaflet motion during systole; numerical-graphical determination. Circ. Res., *32:* 42, 1973.

68. Thomas, T. V.: Diagnosis of disrupted prosthetic valves. J. Thorac. Cardiovasc. Surg., *62:* 27, 1971.

69. VonBernuth, G., Tsakiris, A. G., and Wood, E. H.: Effects of variations in the strength of the left ventricular contraction on aortic valve closure in the dog. Circ. Res., *28:* 705, 1971.

chapter 8

Coronary Artery Disease

Selective coronary arteriography, biplane left ventricular angiography, right and left heart catheterization, exercise stress testing, vectorcardiography and other techniques used for evaluation of patients with coronary artery disease have resulted in significant improvements in our diagnostic skills. The definition of abnormal ventricular function in this condition, documented by invasive techniques, has made possible a much better understanding of the abnormal findings seen in noninvasive, graphic techniques.

HEART SOUNDS AND MURMURS

The first heart sound is normal (fig. 8.1). The second heart sound is normal or may show a fixed or paradoxical (reverse) splitting, particularly during episodes of angina pectoris. These findings are most consistently present when patients have right (fixed splitting) (fig. 8.2), or left bundle branch block (paradoxical splitting) (fig. 8.3). The pulmonary component of the second heart sound may be abnormally accentuated if the patient is in congestive heart failure and has pulmonary hypertension. Systolic ejection clicks, present in a small percentage of patients with coronary artery disease, are probably due to dilatation of the ascending aorta (fig. 8.3). The presence of a fourth heart sound in patients with coronary artery disease has been related to abnormalities of left ventricular function at the time of atrial contraction (figs. 8.1–8.3). During the past few years, however, several investigators have raised questions concerning the clinical importance of the fourth heart sound as an indicator of chronic coronary artery disease, or during episodes of angina pectoris (see Chapter 3). This is because a large number of normal subjects past age 40 have a fourth heart sound which is audible with a stethoscope and recorded on the phonocardiogram at the mitral or aortic areas. We have found it useful to record an apexcardiogram simultaneously with the phonocardiogram. If the A wave of the apexcardiogram exceeds the upper normal value of 15% of total amplitude of the apexcardiogram (distance from the E to the O point), the fourth heart sound may be of pathologic significance. The presence of a third heart

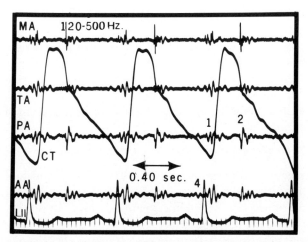

Fig. 8.1. Simultaneously recorded phonocardiogram at the mitral (MA), tricuspid (TA), pulmonic (PA) and aortic (AA) areas, carotid pulse tracing (CT), and lead II (LII) of the electrocardiogram in a 56-year-old patient with coronary artery disease. The first (1) and second (2) heart sounds are normal. There is a faint fourth (4) heart sound recorded in all precordial areas, including the aortic area. There are no murmurs. The configuration of the carotid pulse is normal.

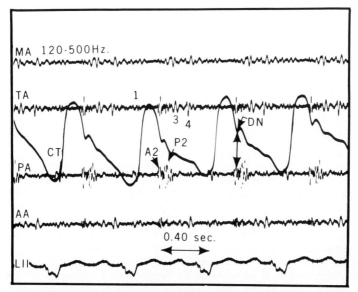

Fig. 8.2. Simultaneously recorded phonocardiogram at the mitral (MA), tricuspid (TA), pulmonic (PA) and aortic (AA) areas, carotid pulse tracing (CT), and lead II (LII) of the electrocardiogram in a 57-year-old patient with severe triple vessel coronary artery disease, dyskinesis of the anterior wall of the left ventricle, and complete right bundle branch block. The first (1) and second (2) heart sounds are diminished. The second heart sound is wide and has fixed splitting. There are prominent third (3) and fourth (4) heart sounds. The carotid pulse tracing shows a diminished ejection time. The presence of a third heart sound in patients with coronary artery disease is usually indicative of a moderate-to-marked degree of left ventricular dyskinesis and associated, elevated left ventricular end-diastolic pressure. DN = dicrotic notch.

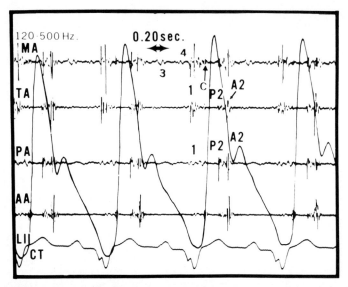

Fig. 8.3. Simultaneously recorded phonocardiogram at the mitral (MA), tricuspid (TA), pulmonic (PA) and aortic (AA) areas, carotid pulse tracing (CT), and lead II (LII) of the electrocardogram in a 53-year-old patient with triple vessel coronary artery disease, a marked degree of left ventricular dyskinesis, and complete left bundle branch block. The first heart sound is normal. The second heart sound is paradoxically split and both components precede the dicrotic notch on the carotid pulse tracing. The aortic component of the second heart sound has twice the amplitude of the pulmonic component and is well transmitted to all precordial areas. The pulmonic component of the second heart sound is well recorded in the mitral area. This is usually indicative of elevated pulmonary artery pressure secondary to left ventricular failure and dilatation of the right ventricle. There is a systolic ejection click (C) which is occasionally seen in patients with coronary artery disease. The carotid pulse tracing shows a diminished ejection time which is usually associated with diminished stroke volume.

sound is an abnormal finding in patients with coronary artery disease and usually indicates the presence of left ventricular dyskinesis and/or ventricular aneurysm with elevated left ventricular end-diastolic pressure, decreased cardiac output, stroke volume and ejection fraction.

Characteristic murmurs have not been described in patients with chronic coronary artery disease without papillary muscle dysfunction syndrome. It has been suggested, however, that some patients with obstructive disease of the left anterior descending artery may present with a continuous murmur along the left sternal border. This murmur has been attributed to a continuous flow through the stenotic lesion in the left anterior descending artery, best heard at the tricuspid area. This seems to be a rare occurrence and in our experience it has not proven to be of clinical importance.

High frequency, low amplitude systolic ejection murmurs frequently present in patients with coronary artery disease are usually of no clinical significance. The systolic ejection murmur which at times can be of high amplitude (Grade II–III/VI) and transmitted well to all precordial areas (fig. 8.4), is probably due to turbulent flow across a slightly sclerotic, thickened or calcified aortic valve. At cardiac catheterization, most patients do not have a significant gradient across the aortic valve.

Mitral insufficiency murmurs have also been described in this condition due to anterior and/or posterior papillary muscle dysfunction. The murmur of papillary muscle dysfunction usually starts shortly after the first heart sound, reaching a peak in mid- or late systole and terminating at the time of aortic valve closure (fig. 8.5). This murmur may

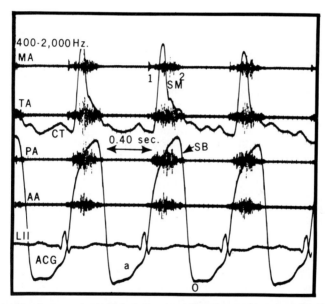

Fig. 8.4. Simultaneously recorded phonocardiogram at the mitral (MA), tricuspid (TA), pulmonic (PA) and aortic (AA) areas, carotid pulse tracing (CT), and lead II (LII) of the electrocardiogram and apexcardiogram (ACG). The patient was a 65-year-old woman who had mitral insufficiency secondary to papillary muscle dysfunction, a mild degree of aortic sclerosis, and a mild degree of calcification of the aortic valve without a significant systolic gradient between the left ventricle and aorta at left heart catheterization. The first (1) heart sound is normal. The second (2) heart sound is diminished. The phonocardiogram shows a high frequency, high amplitude, systolic murmur (SM) which has the characteristics of both an ejection and regurgitant murmur. The carotid pulse tracing shows a rapid ascending limb with a rapid systolic retraction. Ejection time is normal. The apexcardiogram shows a conspicuous A wave and a sustained systolic wave. The E point is not well recognized. This is the type of apexcardiogram that one sees in patients with coronary artery disease and associated left ventricular hypertrophy. SB = systolic bulge.

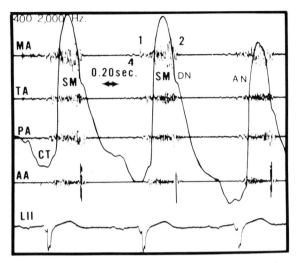

Figure 8.5. Simultaneously recorded phonocardiogram at the mitral (MA), tricuspid (TA), pulmonic (PA) and aortic (AA) areas, carotid pulse tracing (CT), and lead II (LII) of the electrocardiogram in a 68-year-old patient with coronary artery disease, and mitral insufficiency secondary to papillary muscle dysfunction. The characteristic murmur of papillary muscle dysfunction starts shortly after the first (1) heart sound and has maximal intensity at time of the second (2) heart sound. This murmur is best recorded at the mitral area but is transmitted to the tricuspid, pulmonic, and aortic areas. The carotid pulse tracing shows a high anacrotic notch (AN) and an inconspicuous dicrotic notch (DN). The ejection time is diminished in the carotid pulse tracing. SM = systolic murmur.

be preceded by an early systolic click in approximately 5% of cases. The systolic murmur of anterior papillary muscle dysfunction tends to radiate posteriorly and to the left of the axillary line, as opposed to the murmur of posterior papillary muscle dysfunction which radiates anteriorly and to the right sternal border. It is a high frequency murmur, usually Grade II–III/VI, heard best when the patient is placed in a left lateral decubitus position. The explanation for late systolic accentuation of this murmur is that the ischemic papillary muscle does not provide sufficient strength to pull the chordae tendineae together during late systole, thus allowing regurgitation to occur during that phase of the cardiac cycle. In most cases this murmur of mitral insufficiency does not have major hemodynamic significance and the regurgitant fraction seen during left ventricular angiography is small. In a small group of patients, however, mitral regurgitation is of such a degree that congestive heart failure occurs and mitral valve replacement may be required. In this situation the murmur is usually pansystolic and accompanied by prominent third and fourth heart sounds, with or without a soft, low frequency mid-diastolic rumble. At times, the murmur of papillary muscle dysfunction and the third heart sound may be heard only during acute episodes of coronary insufficiency.

Murmurs of a ruptured papillary muscle or chordae tendineae, seen during acute myocardial infarction, may resemble murmurs of mitral insufficiency due to rheumatic heart disease (see Chapter 4). The murmur is usually musical, of high amplitude and radiates to all precordial areas. It may be preceded by an ejection or mid-systolic click (fig. 8.6). Ruptured chordae tendineae is usually a catastrophic event during acute myocardial infarction and should be recognized immediately through auscultation or other non-invasive techniques. It requires aggressive medical or surgical therapy, since the mortality rate is very high. If rupture of the interventricular septum occurs, a prominent pansystolic murmur will be present. This murmur is the result of

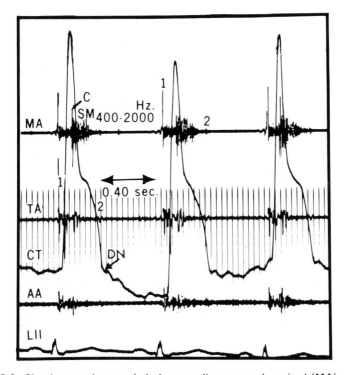

Fig. 8.6. Simultaneously recorded phonocardiogram at the mitral (MA), tricuspid (TA), pulmonic (PA) and aortic (AA) areas, carotid pulse tracing (CT), and lead II (LII) of the electrocardiogram in a 74-year-old patient with coronary artery disease and rupture of the chordae tendineae. A normal first (1) heart sound is followed by a systolic click (C): Following the systolic click in the early part of systole, there is a decrescendo systolic murmur (SM) which terminates at the second (2) heart sound. The carotid pulse tracing shows a rapid rise, rapid descending limb and a low placed dicrotic notch (DN).

turbulent flow across the acquired "ventricular septal defect" due to a left-to-right ventricular shunt and is identical to the murmur seen in patients with congenital ventricular septal defects. If the magnitude of the left-to-right shunt is large, pulmonary to systemic flow ratio exceeds 2:1, and third and fourth heart sounds and a low frequency mid-diastolic rumble are heard. These findings are due to increased rate of flow across a normal mitral valve (see Chapter 4).

CAROTID PULSE TRACING

The carotid pulse tracing is usually of normal contour (figs. 8.1 and 8.2) in patients with uncomplicated coronary artery disease. However, it may show slow upstroke time, a high anacrotic notch and an inconspicuous dicrotic notch which are probably related to decreased distensibility of the carotid artery with or without associated aortic sclerosis (fig. 8.7). Ejection time may be decreased (figs. 8.1–8.3) during periods of angina pectoris.

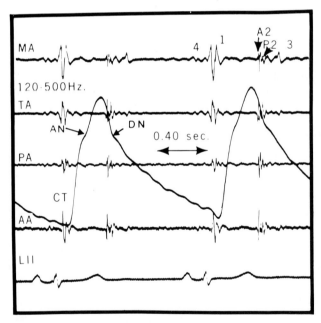

Fig. 8.7. Simultaneously recorded phonocardiogram at the mitral (MA), tricuspid (TA), pulmonic (PA) and aortic (AA) areas, carotid pulse tracing (CT), and lead II (LII) of the electrocardiogram in a 38-year-old patient with coronary artery disease. The first (1) and second (2) heart sounds are normal. Prominent third (3) and fourth (4) heart sounds are recorded in all precordial areas. The carotid pulse tracing shows a prominent anacrotic notch (AN) and an inconspicuous dicrotic notch (DN). The ejection time is normal.

JUGULAR VENOUS PULSE TRACING

The jugular venous pulse tracing is normal unless the patient develops congestive heart failure, pulmonary hypertension or tricuspid insufficiency. In those settings the tracing will exhibit the typical features seen in these conditions (see Chapter 6) (fig. 8.8).

APEXCARDIOGRAM

In 1969 we observed that a large A wave was recorded during spontaneous episodes of angina pectoris (fig. 8.9). As angina pectoris subsided, there was a progressive diminution in size of the A wave to the pre-angina level. Amplitude of the A wave at rest should not exceed 15% of total amplitude of the apexcardiogram, measured from the E to the O point (fig. 8.10). Since then, abnormalities of the A wave in the apexcardiogram have become a useful tool for diagnosis of coronary artery disease. This abnormality in the apexcardiogram was found not to

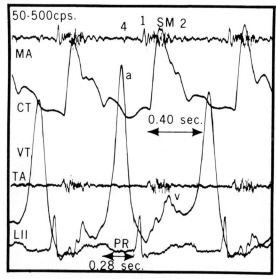

Fig. 8.8. Simultaneously recorded phonocardiogram at the mitral (MA) and tricuspid (TA) areas, carotid pulse tracing (CT), jugular venous tracing (VT), and lead II (LII) of the electrocardiogram in a 53-year-old patient with coronary artery disease, and first degree atrioventricular block in the electrocardiogram. The first (1) and second (2) heart sounds are normal. There is a high frequency, low amplitude, systolic ejection murmur (SM) best recorded at the mitral area, probably due to aortic sclerosis. The patient had no gradient across the aortic valve during cardiac catheterization. Note marked increase in amplitude of the A wave in the jugular venous tracing suggestive of elevated right atrial and right ventricular pressures. At catheterization, the patient had a moderate degree of pulmonary hypertension secondary to left ventricular failure.

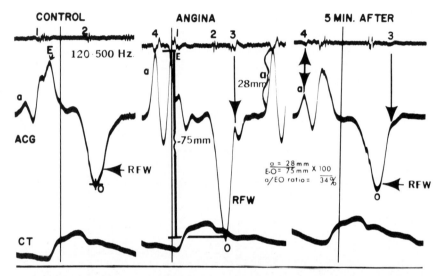

Fig. 8.9. Simultaneously recorded phonocardiogram, apexcardiogram (ACG), and carotid pulse tracing (CT) before, during and 5 minutes after a spontaneous episode of angina pectoris. Note the appearance of prominent third (3) and fourth (4) heart sounds which coincide with large A and rapid filling waves (RFW) on the apexcardiogram. Five minutes after the disappearance of angina pectoris there is diminution of the third and fourth heart sounds and the A and rapid filling waves have decreased markedly.

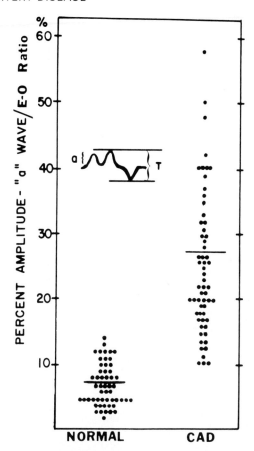

Fig. 8.10. Percent amplitude of the A wave to E-O ratio in normal subjects and in patients with coronary artery disease (CAD). The top diagram demonstrates how the ratio is measured. Note a significant difference in the percent of amplitude in normal subjects and patients with coronary artery disease.

be a reflection of aging, since amplitude of the A wave did not increase in various age groups at rest or after exercise, as shown in figures 8.11 and 8.12. A large A wave on the apexcardiogram was found to be a reflection of abnormal left ventricular function or compliance in patients with coronary artery disease and elevated left ventricular end-diastolic pressure (figs. 8.13 and 8.14). It must be emphasized that an increase in the amplitude of the A wave is not a specific finding in coronary artery disease since it may also be found in conditions associated with left ventricular hypertrophy, elevated left ventricular end-diastolic pressure, such as idiopathic hypertrophic subaortic stenosis, aortic stenosis, hypertension, congestive heart failure and others (see Chapter 5).

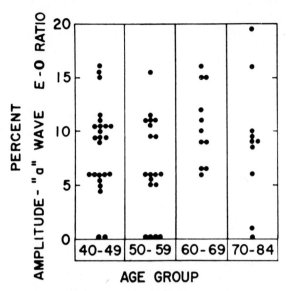

Fig. 8.11. Frequency distribution of A wave ratio of the apexcardiogram, at rest, in 64 normal subjects from different age groups. Note that the A wave ratio was below 20% in this particular population without significant increase in the older decades.

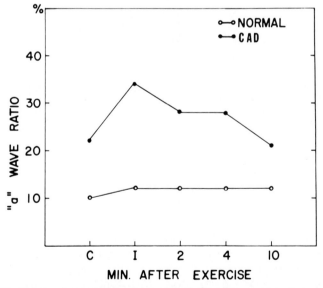

Fig. 8.12. Average A wave ratio on the apexcardiogram measured at rest and after double Masters two-step exercise test in various decades in 64 normal subjects. Note the absence of any major changes in the older decades. CAD = coronary artery disease.

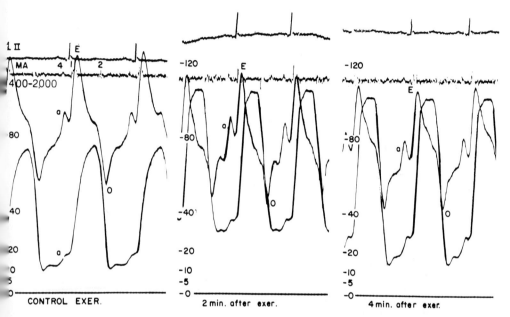

Fig. 8.13. Simultaneously recorded mitral (MA) area phonocardiogram, lead II (LII) of the electrocardiogram, apexcardiogram and left ventricular pressure at control, 2 and 4 minutes after bicycle exercise. The first (1) and second (2) heart sounds are normal. There is a fourth (4) heart sound which coincides with a slightly prominent A wave on the apexcardiogram. The left ventricular end-diastolic pressure is elevated at rest to 18 mm Hg. Two minutes after exercise, there is a marked increase in amplitude of the A wave on the apexcardiogram as well as on the left ventricular pressure curve. Left ventricular end-diastolic pressure is elevated to 38 mm Hg. Four minutes after exercise there is a decrease in amplitude of the A wave in both the apexcardiogram and the left ventricular pressure curve. Left ventricular end-diastolic pressure 4 minutes after exercise was 30 mm Hg.

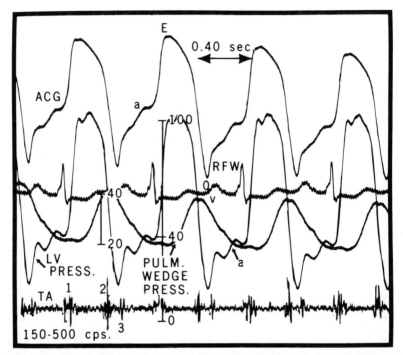

Fig. 8.14. Simultaneously recorded apexcardiogram (ACG), lead II (LII) of the electrocardiogram, left ventricular and pulmonary "wedge" pressure curves, and tricuspid (TA) area phonocardiogram in a 30-year-old patient with severe triple vessel coronary artery disease. The A wave in both the apexcardiogram and left ventricular pressure curve has increased amplitude. Note the marked elevation of the left ventricular end-diastolic pressure to 40 mm Hg. There is a prominent third (3) heart sound on the phonocardiogram. The patient had a marked degree of akinesis of the anterior wall of the left ventricle and total obstruction of the proximal left anterior descending coronary artery.

Further studies have shown that in addition to abnormalities of the A wave, the systolic component and rapid filling wave of the apexcardiogram are important in this disease state, as shown in figures 8.4, 8.9, 8.14–8.17, and Table 8.1. In patients with coronary artery disease and associated left ventricular hypertrophy, the E point on the apexcardiogram may be obscured and fused with the round, sustained systolic wave (figs. 8.14 and 8.15). The A wave may have normal amplitude. In patients with localized anterior left ventricular hypokinesis or akinesis, the E point is followed by a prominent systolic retraction and a late systolic bulge (figs. 8.18–8.21). In patients with a true ventricular aneurysm proven by left ventricular biplane angiography, the left ventricular akinetic segment moves paradoxically during left ventricular systole. This is reflected on the apexcardiogram by a late systolic wave which reaches its peak at the time of the second heart sound. The peak of the late systolic wave may exceed the E point. Various combinations of A, systolic and rapid filling wave abnormalities are shown in figure 8.21.

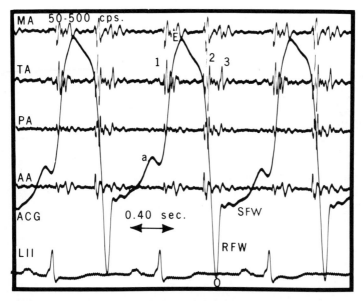

Fig. 8.15. Simultaneously recorded phonocardiogram at the mitral (MA), tricuspid (TA), pulmonic (PA) and aortic (AA) areas, apexcardiogram (ACG), and lead II (LII) of the electrocardiogram in a 33-year-old patient with severe triple vessel coronary artery disease. The first (1) and second (2) heart sounds are normal. Note the prominent third (3) heart sound recorded in all precordial areas. The apexcardiogram shows prominent A and rapid filling waves (RFW).

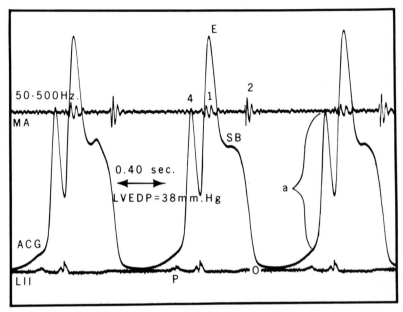

Fig. 8.16. Simultaneously recorded phonocardiogram at the mitral (MA) area, apexcardiogram (ACG), and lead II (LII) of the electrocardiogram in a 68-year-old patient with coronary artery disease and left ventricular dyskinesis. There is a fourth (4) heart sound on the phonocardiogram and normal first (1) and second (2) heart sounds. The apexcardiogram shows a marked increase in amplitude of the A wave. Left ventricular end-diastolic pressure (LVEDP) in this patient was 38 mm Hg. There is a small systolic bulge (SB) following the E point of the apexcardiogram. The rapid filling wave is inconspicuous.

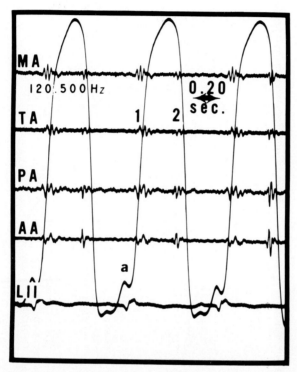

Fig. 8.17. Simultaneously recorded phonocardiogram at the mitral (MA), tricuspid (TA), pulmonic (PA) and aortic (AA) areas, and lead II (LII) of the electrocardiogram in a 64-year-old patient with coronary artery disease and left ventricular aneurysm. The precordial pulsations taken over the left ventricular aneurysm show a small A wave, inconspicuous E point, and a sustained systolic wave. This patient had a large aneurysm of the anterior wall of the left ventricle on the left ventricular angiogram.

Table 8.1. Apexcardiogram in Normal Subjects and in Patients with Coronary Artery Disease*

Subjects	Time†	"a" Ratio		"a" Duration		a-E Interval		RFW Ratio	
		Range	Average‡	Range	Average	Range	Average	Range	Average
		%	%	sec	sec	sec	sec	%	%
Normal patients (64)	C	2–19	10 ± 3.6	0.03–0.13	0.06	0.03–0.28	0.10	30–84	57
	1	2–33	12	0.03–0.12	0.06	0.03–0.13	0.09	35–85	59
	2	2–23	12	0.03–0.13	0.06	0.03–0.18	0.10	20–100	63
	4	2–40	12	0.02–0.14	0.06	0.04–0.16	0.10	40–89	62
	10	2–24	12	0.03–0.13	0.06	0.03–0.17	0.09	39–92	59
Patients with coronary artery disease (45)	C	8–48	22 ± 8.1	0.04–0.26	0.09	0.04–0.27	0.13	32–86	57
	1	8–146	34	0.04–0.24	0.09	0.04–0.24	0.14	19–121	69
	2	8–77	29	0.04–0.24	0.09	0.04–0.26	0.14	28–97	61
	4	9–77	29	0.04–0.24	0.09	0.05–0.26	0.14	35–88	59
	10	6–46	21	0.04–0.16	0.08	0.04–0.32	0.13	29–76	54

* Range and averages of the "a" wave ratio, its duration, a-E interval, and rapid filling wave (RFW) ratio at rest and after exercise.

† C = control tracing, and 1, 2, 4, and 10 represent immediately and 2, 4, and 10 minutes after exercise.

‡ The numbers to the right of the ± sign represent the standard deviation.

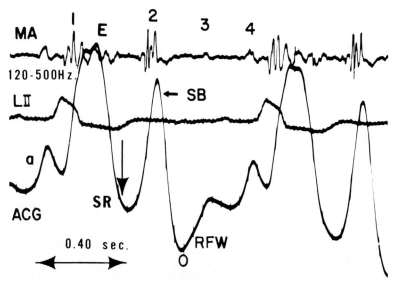

Fig. 8.18. Simultaneously recorded mitral (MA) area phonocardiogram, lead II (LII) of the electrocardiogram, and apexcardiogram (ACG) in a patient with coronary artery disease. Note marked increase in amplitude of the A wave and a prominent systolic retraction (SR) followed by a late systolic bulge (SB). The rapid filling wave (RFW) is also prominent and coincides with the third (3) heart sound. There is a fourth (4) heart sound on the phonocardiogram which coincides with the peak of the A wave on the apexcardiogram.

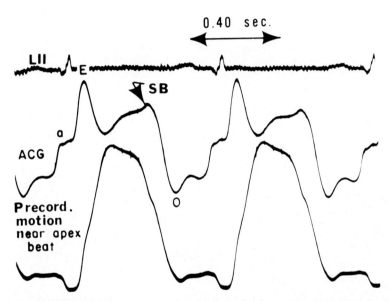

Fig. 8.19. Simultaneously recorded lead II (LII) of the electrocardiogram, apexcardiogram (ACG), and precordial pulsations near the apex beat over an area of left ventricular dyskinesis in a patient with coronary artery disease and a ventricular aneurysm. Note the prominent A wave and late systolic bulge (SB) on the apexcardiogram. The recording of precordial motion over the area of left ventricular dyskinesis shows a late systolic bulge representing paradoxical motion of the apex beat.

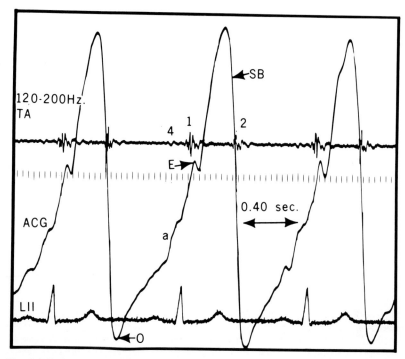

Fig. 8.20. Simultaneously recorded tricuspid (TA) area phonocardiogram, lead II (LII) of the electrocardiogram, and apexcardiogram (ACG) in a 59-year-old patient with coronary artery disease and anterior wall dyskinesis of the left ventricle. The phonocardiogram shows normal first (1) and second (2) heart sounds and a low amplitude fourth (4) heart sound. The apexcardiogram is markedly abnormal showing a late systolic bulge (SB). The E point, well recognized on this tracing, coincides with the first heart sound. The A wave is slightly prominent.

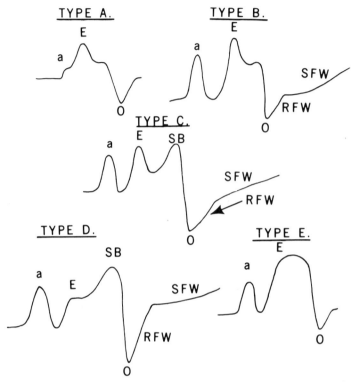

Fig. 8.21. Various types of apexcardiogram abnormalities seen in patients with coronary artery disease. Type A is usually seen in patients with obstructive disease of the coronary arteries who have normal left ventricular functions at rest. Type B is usually seen in patients with elevated left ventricular end-diastolic pressure secondary to associated left ventricular hypertrophy or diminished left ventricular end-diastolic compliance without significant dyskinesis of the anterior wall of the left ventricle. In Type B, one observes a prominent A wave and the systolic component is not significantly altered. Type C, characterized by a prominent A wave and a late systolic bulge (SB) preceded by a systolic retraction, is seen in patients with elevated left ventricular end-diastolic pressure and associated dyskinesis of the left ventricle. Type D is seen in patients with elevated left ventricular end-diastolic pressure and severe hypokinesis or akinesis of the anterior aspect of the left ventricle. The A wave is prominent and is followed by a small systolic retraction and a prominent, late systolic bulge. The peak of the systolic bulge exceeds the E point of the apexcardiogram. In addition, the rapid filling wave (RFW) is quite conspicuous and these patients frequently have a third heart sound in the phonocardiogram. Type E is seen in patients with coronary artery disease and associated hypertensive cardiovascular disease. The A wave is prominent and the systolic wave is round and sustained. The E point is difficult to recognize on these patients. The rapid filling wave is also small. SFW = slow filling wave.

Tables 8.1 and 8.2 show various measurements which can be made on the apexcardiogram in normal subjects and patients with coronary artery disease at rest, after exercise and after administration of sublingual nitroglycerin. If abnormalities are not present in the resting tracing, they

Table 8.2. Mean Values of Percentage Amplitude of "a" Waves of Apex Cardiogram in Normal Subjects and in Patients with Ischemic Heart Disease at Rest, after Exercise, and after Nitroglycerin

		Percentage Amplitude of "a" Wave (Mean)				
		Resting	Imme-diately	2 Minutes	5 Minutes	10 Minutes
Group I: Control group	Exercise (32 cases)	8.0	8.3	8.2	8.1	7.0
Group II: Ischemic group	Exercise (25 cases)	26.5	41.3	35.4	31.3	24.5
	Nitroglycerin (27 cases)	33.3	20.5	15.4	8.3	7.8

may be induced by mild-to-moderate forms of exercise stress testing (figs. 8.12 and 8.13), smoking (fig. 8.22), during Valsalva maneuver, or in the beats following a ventricular premature contraction (fig. 8.23). These changes may be reversed by administration of nitroglycerin (fig. 8.24) or other coronary vasodilators or by application of tourniquets to the extremities (fig. 8.25).

The apexcardiogram is a useful technique to study patients prior to and after aortic coronary bypass surgery. If there is significant improvement in left ventricular function following myocardial revascularization, the A wave decreases in amplitude and there is a decrease in the size of the late systolic bulge. However, ventricular function may be unaltered or actually deteriorate if the patient develops intra-operative myocardial infarction. The apexcardiogram may detect these changes (fig. 8.26). This is particularly true when the left anterior descending artery is the primary vessel involved. The apexcardiogram is also valuable during the recovery phase of acute myocardial infarction, particularly if the infarcted area involves the anterior-apical aspect of the left ventricle. Deterioration of ventricular function eventually leading to cardiogenic shock can be appreciated by a progressive increase in amplitude of the A wave, development of greater systolic retraction, late systolic bulge and prominent rapid filling wave. Improvements in clinical status and ventricular function results in "normalization" of the apexcardiogram. This is evident when the apexcardiogram is recorded simultaneously with the carotid pulse tracing, electrocardiogram and phonocardiogram, so that systolic and diastolic time intervals can be measured in a single recording.

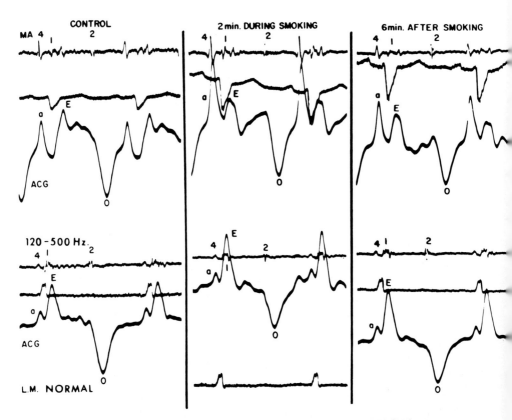

Fig. 8.22. Simultaneously recorded phonocardiogram, lead II (LII) of the electrocardiogram, and apexcardiogram (ACG) in a patient with coronary artery disease and in a normal subject. The apexcardiogram at rest in the patient with coronary artery disease shows a prominent A wave which coincides with a conspicuous fourth (4) heart sound on the phonocardiogram. For 2 minutes during cigarette smoking, there is a significant increase in amplitude of the A wave as well as a fourth (4) heart sound on the phonocardiogram. Six minutes after smoking, the A wave is still slightly prominent. These changes are not observed in the normal subject.

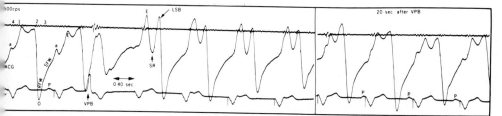

Fig. 8.23. Simultaneously recorded tricuspid (TA) area phonocardiogram, apexcardiogram (ACG), and lead II (LII) of the electrocardiogram in a 62-year-old patient
with coronary artery disease, left ventricular dyskinesis, and a demand pacemaker
implanted in the right ventricle. The third beat is a ventricular premature beat (VPB).
Following the ventricular premature beat a late systolic bulge (LSB) becomes much
more conspicuous and progressively decreases in the subsequent paced beats. This
figure illustrates the importance of recording tracings during cardiac arrhythmias. In
this patient abnormalities of left ventricular contraction became much more prominent in the post-extrasystolic beat. The apexcardiogram and paced beats are abnormal and show a systolic bulge, but not to the degree seen in the post-extrasystolic beats. PI = pacemaker impulse, RFW = rapid filling wave, SFW, slow filling
wave.

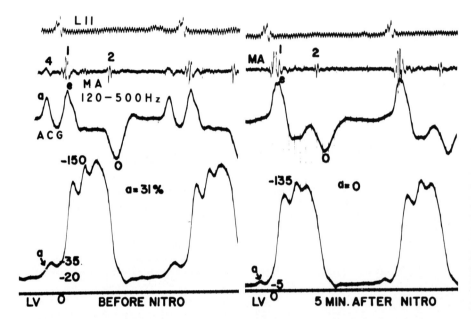

Fig. 8.24. Simultaneously recorded mitral (MA) area phonocardiogram, apexcardiogram (ACG), and left ventricular pressures (LV) before and 5 minutes after sublingual administration of $\frac{1}{150}$ gr nitroglycerin. The prominent fourth (4) heart
sound on the phonocardiogram coincides with the prominent A wave on the apexcardiogram and left ventricular pressure curves. Left ventricular end-diastolic
pressure on the control tracing was elevated to 35 mm Hg. Administration of nitroglycerin results in disappearance of the fourth heart sound and the A wave of the
apexcardiogram, and a marked decrease of the A wave on the left ventricular pressure curve. Left ventricular (LV) end-diastolic pressure, after administration of nitroglycerin, decreased to 7 mm Hg.

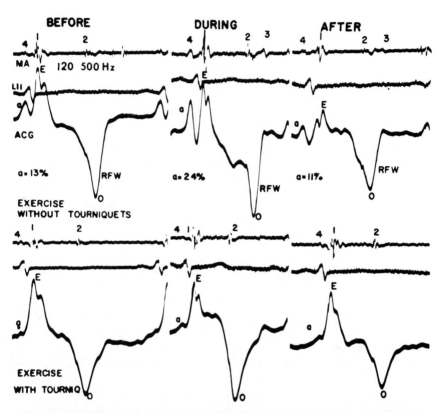

Fig. 8.25. Simultaneously recorded mitral (MA) area phonocardiogram, lead II (LII) of the electrocardiogram, and apexcardiogram (ACG) in a patient with coronary artery disease. The top panel was recorded before, during, and after double Masters two-step exercise test with and without tourniquets applied to the extremities. Exercise without tourniquets resulted in an increase in the A wave ratio to 24%. Application of tourniquets prior to exercise resulted in decreased amplitude of the A wave on the apexcardiogram. Exercise with the tourniquets did not cause any significant increase in amplitude of the A wave. RFW = rapid filling wave.

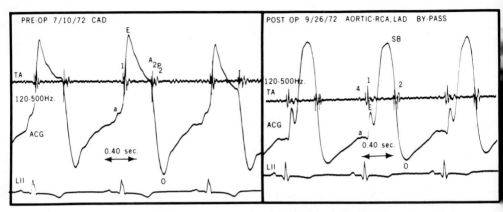

Fig. 8.26. Simultaneously recorded tricuspid (TA) area phonocardiogram, apexcardiogram (ACG), and lead II (LII) of the electrocardiogram in a 41-year-old patient with coronary artery disease. The tracings were recorded before and 3 weeks after aortic coronary saphenous vein bypass to the right coronary and left anterior descending arteries. The pre-operative apexcardiogram shows a small A wave and a normal systolic wave. Following aortic coronary artery bypass the patient developed myocardial infarction. Note the marked changes in the apexcardiogram including the appearance of a very prominent late systolic bulge (SB). The fourth (4) heart sound became conspicuous (see text).

SYSTOLIC TIME INTERVALS

Measurements of systolic time intervals are of some value in evaluating left ventricular function in patients with coronary artery disease. Measurement of the pre-ejection period and corrected ejection time in patients with coronary artery disease without coronary insufficiency is usually normal. Mild prolongation of the time interval between the Q wave of the electrocardiogram and the aortic component of the second heart sound (Q-S$_2$ interval) is shortened slightly in patients with chronic coronary artery disease, but this has not proven to be of clinical value in our large series of patients. It is important to stress that these findings are related to the state of left ventricular function and do not necessarily relate to the degree of severity of obstructive disease of the coronary arteries seen during coronary arteriography. Shortening of ejection time and prolongation of the pre-ejection period may be seen in patients with coronary artery disease, representing decreased stroke volume and ejection fraction. This is usually an indication of marked impairment of left ventricular performance. Following myocardial revascularization using aortic-coronary saphenous vein bypass graft operation or a left internal mammary-left anterior descending artery anastomosis (Green procedure) with resultant improvement in left ventricular performance tends to reverse the pre-ejection period to ejection time ratio toward normal. Great caution should be exercised in relating these measurements to disappearance of angina pectoris following these operations. In our experience, the disappearance or decrease in frequency and intensity of angina pectoris is not necessarily an indicator of graft patency.

During acute myocardial infarction, the pre-ejection period is usually prolonged and ejection time is short. As the patient recovers, there is a tendency toward normalization of these intervals. This has been correlated with various parameters which determine left ventricular performance. With development of congestive heart failure and cardiogenic shock, particularly in patients with extensive anterior wall myocardial infarction, the abnormalities seen in the A and rapid filling waves of the apexcardiogram and systolic time intervals are not as valuable as one would expect. This is probably due to the fact that these patients have a high circulatory level of catecholamines which influences measurement of various intervals of the cardiac cycle.

MANEUVERS, PHARMACOLOGIC AGENTS, CYCLE LENGTH

Exercise stress testing is useful in the diagnosis of patients with coronary artery disease. Through increased use of treadmill exercise testing, correlations have been made between the abnormalities of the ST segments and T waves on the electrocardiogram with the apexcardiogram and systolic time intervals. Earlier studies demonstrated that exercise testing resulted in a significant increase in amplitude of the A and rapid filling waves on the apexcardiogram as shown in figures 8.13 and 8.25. Cigarette smoking also causes an increase in amplitude of the A wave on the apexcardiogram. These changes are probably a reflection of diminished left ventricular compliance with elevated left ventricular end-diastolic pressure (figs. 8.13 and 8.14). Placement of tourniquets on the lower extremities or abdominal binding tends to make these abnormal findings return to normal values as shown in figure 8.25. Many patients subjected to some form of coronary artery surgery develop myocardial infarction and some of these abnormalities may become even more prominent as shown in figure 8.26. Administration of vasopressor agents with increase in the afterload would make these changes more prominent on the apexcardiogram, in the systolic time intervals and/or in the systolic murmur due to papillary muscle dysfunction (fig. 8.37). Administration of vasodilators such as nitroglycerin or amyl nitrite causes a reduction in amplitude of the A wave on the apexcardiogram (fig. 8.24), shortening of the pre-ejection period and prolongation of the systolic time intervals toward normal.

The influence of cycle length on the murmur of papillary muscle dysfunction is shown in figure 8.38. With atrial fibrillation at a rapid ventricular rate, the systolic regurgitant murmur of papillary muscle dysfunction is almost inaudible and unrecordable. However, in the beats preceded by a long diastolic pause, one observes a significant increase in amplitude of the systolic murmur as well as an increase in the amplitude of the carotid pulse tracing.

ECHOCARDIOGRAPHY

Echocardiography has not been definitely established as a valuable diagnostic tool in patients with coronary artery disease. Current work by several investigators has shown that it can be useful under certain circumstances, particularly to evaluate left ventricular function, abnormal patterns of interventricular septal, posterior wall motion and measurement of intracavitary diameters. A good recording of the pulmonic valve helps to determine the presence of elevated right heart pressure in which case the A wave of the pulmonic valve will be diminished or absent. All of these parameters are important for the selection of patients for aortic coronary bypass surgery, in post-operative follow-up and in the assessment of changes in left ventricular function following acute myocardial infarction.

Patients with coronary artery disease may exhibit abnormal motion of the interventricular septum. It may have a diminished, flat (figs. 8.27–8.33) or paradoxical motion during systole. Decreased excursion of the posterior wall of the left ventricle may also be seen (fig. 8.34). Abnormal motion of the anterior leaflet of the mitral valve is seen in patients with elevated left ventricular end-diastolic pressure above 15–20

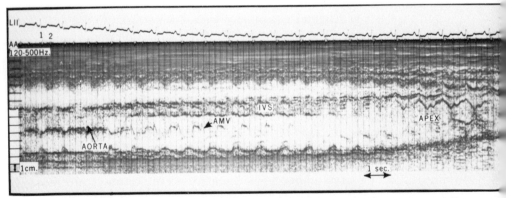

Fig. 8.27. Simultaneously recorded echocardiogram, aortic (AA) area phonocardiogram, and lead II (LII) of the electrocardiogram in a 68-year-old patient with coronary artery disease. On the echocardiographic scan from the aorta to the apex of the left ventricle there is abnormal motion of the interventricular septum (IVS). This structure has markedly diminished excursion. The patient had severe segmental disease of the left anterior descending artery on the coronary arteriograms. AMV = anterior mitral valve.

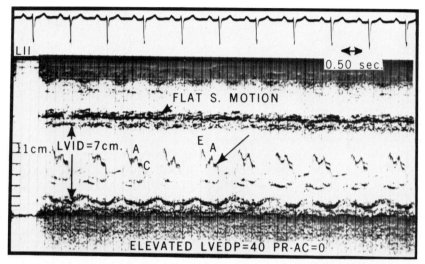

Fig. 8.28. Echocardiogram and lead II (LII) of the electrocardiogram in a 58-year-old patient with coronary artery disease, left ventricular failure and a calcified aortic valve. Note the flat interventricular septal motion. The left ventricular internal diameter (LVID) was increased to 7 cm. Left ventricular end-diastolic pressure was markedly elevated to 40 mm Hg. Measurement of the PR minus A-C interval on the echocardiogram is 0 indicating abnormal left ventricular end-diastolic compliance.

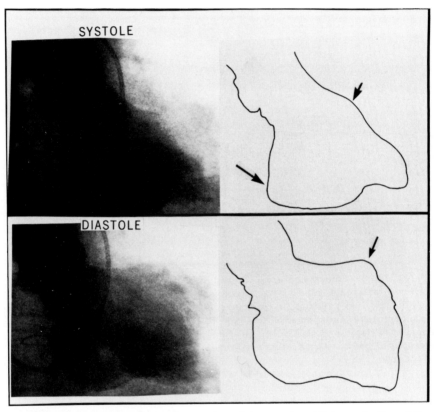

Fig. 8.29. Left ventricular angiogram in a right anterior oblique projection of the patient shown in figure 8.28. Arrows indicate areas of left ventricular dyskinesis during systole and diastole.

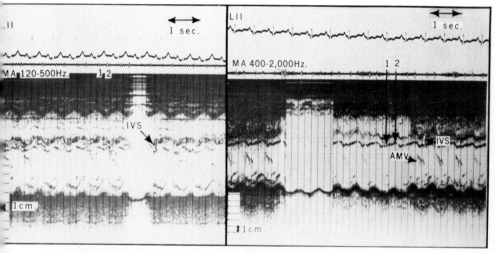

Fig. 8.30. Simultaneously recorded echocardiogram and lead II (LII) of the electrocardiogram in a 58-year-old patient with coronary artery disease. The tracings were recorded before (left panel) and after (right panel) aortic coronary artery bypass surgery. In the pre-operative tracing, there is a marked decrease in the interventricular septal motion (IVS). Following aortic coronary artery bypass surgery there is paradoxical motion of the interventricular septum. AMV = anterior mitral valve.

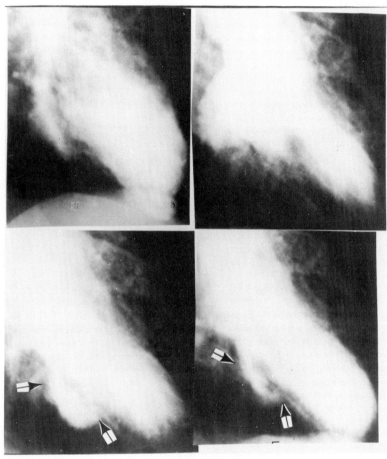

Fig. 8.31. Coronary arteriograms and left ventricular angiograms of the patient shown in figure 8.30. Arrows indicate areas of ventricular dyskinesis and segmental disease in the coronary artery.

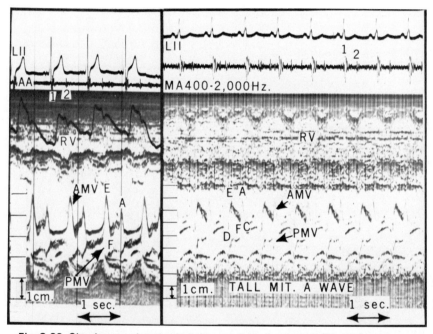

Fig. 8.32. Simultaneously recorded echocardiogram, aortic (AA) area phonocardiogram, and lead II (LII) of the electrocardiogram in a normal subject (left panel) and a
patient with coronary artery disease (right panel), left ventricular aneurysm, and
elevated left ventricular end-diastolic pressure. Note the normal motion of the mitral
valve in the left panel. The A wave is smaller than the E wave in the normal subject. In the patient with coronary artery disease, the A wave exceeds the E point
indicating abnormal left ventricular end-diastolic compliance. RV = right ventricle; AMV = anterior mitral valve; PMV = posterior mitral valve.

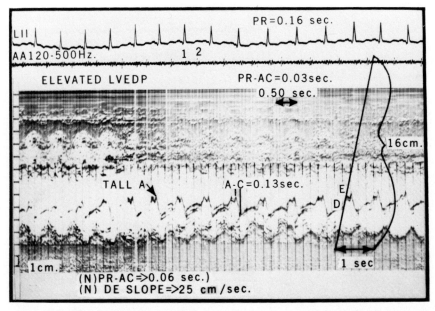

Fig. 8.33. Simultaneously recorded phonocardiogram at the aortic (AA) area, lead II (LII) of the electrocardiogram, and echocardiogram in a 65-year-old patient with severe triple vessel coronary artery disease and elevated left ventricular end-diastolic pressure. The mitral valve motion is abnormal. The PR minus A-C interval and the D-E slope are shortened (N = normal values). There is a tall A wave in the anterior mitral valve motion.

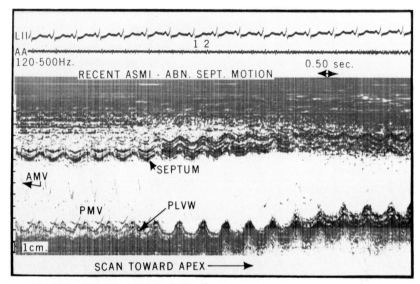

Fig. 8.34. Simultaneously recorded aortic (AA) area phonocardiogram, lead II (LII) of the electrocardiogram, and echocardiogram in a 29-year-old patient with severe coronary artery disease and recent subacute anteroseptal myocardial infarction. Note the abnormal interventricular septal motion and decreased excursion of the posterior wall of the left ventricle (PLVW). AMV = anterior mitral valve, PMV = posterior mitral valve.

mm Hg. In these patients, there is a large excursion of the anterior mitral valve at the time of atrial contraction (A wave) (figs. 8.28, and 8.33). In these recordings, amplitude of the A wave must be higher than the F point (fig. 8.35). The A-C interval is prolonged above the normal range. Measurement of the PR interval on the electrocardiogram minus the A-C interval on the echocardiogram will be shorter in patients with elevated, late left ventricular end-diastolic pressure. Measurement of the slope from the D to the E point is short as shown in figure 8.33.

Echocardiographic studies obtained in patients with acute myocardial infarction have shown abnormalities of the interventricular septum (fig. 8.34) and posterior wall (fig. 8.35) of the left ventricle which undergoes changes that grossly correlate with evolution of the clinical status. Left ventricular internal diameters may be increased in patients with a marked degree of left ventricular dyskinesis. Detection and quantitation of left ventricular aneurysm is difficult to appreciate in most patients but this diagnosis can be suspected if there is abnormal anterior motion of the mitral valve during systole associated with increased motion of the posterior wall of the left ventricle and diminished or paradoxical motion of the interventricular septum (fig. 8.36).

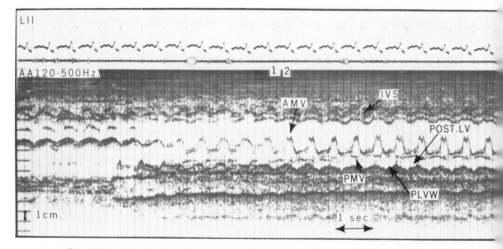

Fig. 8.35. Simultaneously recorded echocardiogram, lead II (LII) of the electro-cardiogram, and aortic (AA) area phonocardiogram in a 62-year-old patient with acute inferior wall myocardial infarction. Note the diminished excursion of the pos-terior wall of the left ventricle and abnormal motion of the anterior mitral valve (see text). AMV = anterior mitral valve, IVS = interventricular septum, POST. LV = posterior left ventricle; PLVW = posterior left ventricular wall.

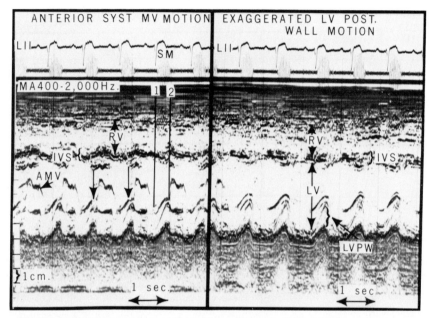

Fig. 8.36. Simultaneously recorded echocardiogram of the mitral valve, mitral area (MA) phonocardiogram, and lead II (LII) of the electrocardiogram in a 74-year-old patient with severe coronary artery disease, left ventricular aneurysm, and mitral insufficiency secondary to papillary muscle dysfunction documented by angiography. Note abnormal, anterior displacement of the mitral valve (left panel) during systole (arrow) and flat motion of the interventricular septum (IVS). The right panel shows exaggerated motion of the left ventricular posterior wall (LVPW). Abnormal systolic, anterior motion of the mitral valve is probably due to left ventricular asymmetry, a vigorously contracting posterior left ventricular wall, and a hypokinetic interventricular septum. AMV = anterior mitral valve, RV = right ventricle, LV = left ventricle.

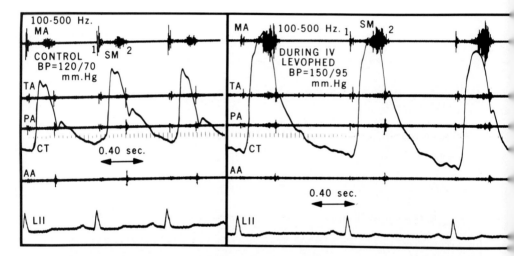

Fig. 8.37. Simultaneously recorded phonocardiogram at the mitral (MA), tricuspid (TA), pulmonic (PA) and aortic (AA) areas, carotid pulse tracing (CT), and lead II (LII) of the electrocardiogram in a 59-year-old patient with coronary artery disease and mitral insufficiency secondary to papillary muscle dysfunction syndrome. The tracings were taken before (left panel) and during (right panel) administration of Levophed. Blood pressure on the control tracing was 120/70 mm Hg. The systolic murmur (SM) has a late systolic peak and is of low amplitude at the mitral area. Administration of Levophed resulted in a marked increase in amplitude of the systolic murmur and an increase in blood pressure to 150/96 mm Hg.

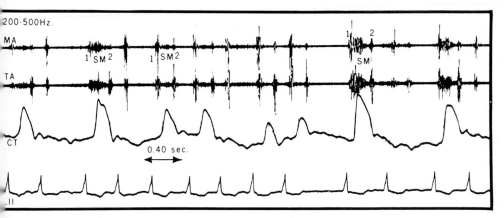

Fig. 8.38. Simultaneously recorded mitral (MA) and tricuspid (TA) area phonocardiogram, carotid pulse tracing (CT), and lead II (LII) of the electrocardiogram in a 66-year-old patient with coronary artery disease and mitral insufficiency secondary to papillary muscle dysfunction. The rhythm is rapid atrial fibrillation with a variable ventricular response. Note the marked decrease in amplitude of the systolic murmur in the beats with a short cycle length. Beats preceded by a long cycle length show a significant increase in amplitude of the systolic murmur (SM). See text.

REFERENCES

1. Abbasi, A. S.: Paradoxical motion of interventricular septum in left bundle branch block. Circulation, *49:* 423, 1972.
2. Abrams, H. L.: Aortocoronary saphenous bypass. N. Engl. J. Med., *282:* 456, 1970.
3. Agress, C. M., and Wegner, S.: The vibrocardiographic exercise test for coronary insufficiency. Am. J. Cardiol., *9:* 541, 1962.
4. Agress, C. M., Wegner, S., Forrester, J. S., Chatterjee, K., Parmley, W. W., and Swan, H. J. C.: An indirect method for evaluation of left ventricular function in acute myocardial infarction. Circulation, *46:* 291, 1972.
5. Anderson, J. W.: Ischemic electrocardiographic changes with reversion after removal of diseased gallbladders. Minn. Med., *55:* 211, 1972.
6. Aranow, W. S., Bowyer, A. F., and Kaplan, M. A.: External isovolumic contraction time and left ventricular ejection time/external isovolumic contraction time ratios at rest and after exercise in coronary artery disease. Circulation, *43:* 59, 1971.
7. Baker, B. M., Scarborough, W. R., Davis, F. W., Jr., Mason, R. E., Singewald, M. L., Walker, S. H., Murphy, E. A., Harrison, W. K., Jr., and Sherwin, R. W.: Predictive considerations and statistical evaluation. Proc. R. Soc. Med., *60:* 1290, 1967.
8. Balcon, R., Bennett, E. D., and Sowton, G. E.: Comparison of pulmonary artery diastolic and left ventricular end-diastolic pressures in patients with ischaemic heart disease. Br. Heart J., *33:* 615, 1971.
9. Bamrah, V. S., Bahler, R. C., and Rakita, L.: Hemodynamic response to supine exercise in patients with chest pain and normal coronary arteriograms. Am. Heart J., *87:* 147, 1974.
10. Baragan, J., Fernandez, F., Coblence, B., Saady, Y., and Lenegre, J.: Left ventricular dynamics in complete right bundle branch block with left axis deviation of QRS. Circulation, *42:* 797, 1970.

11. Baragan, J., Fernandez-Caamano, F., Sozutek, Y., Coblence, B., and Lenegre, J.: Chronic left complete bundle branch block: Phonocardiographic and mechanocardiographic study of 30 cases. Br. Heart J., *30:* 196, 1968.
12. Beilin, L., and Mounsey, P.: The left ventricular impulse in hypertensive heart disease. Br. Heart J., *24:* 409, 1962.
13. Benchimol, A., Asendorf, A., and Dimond, E. G.: The apexcardiogram in coronary artery disease. Heart Bull., *19:* 69, 1970.
14. Benchimol, A., Buxbaum, A., Maroko, P. R., Pedraza, A., and Brener, L.: Chest pain with or without abnormal electrocardiograms in patients with normal coronary arteriograms. Ariz. Med., *26:* 341, 1969.
15. Benchimol, A., Desser, K. B., and Harris, C. L.: Coronary artery spasm—a case report. Ariz. Med., *31:* 356, 1974.
16. Benchimol, A., Desser, K. B., and Massey, B. J.: Coexisting left anterior hemiblock and inferior wall myocardial infarction; vectorcardiographic features. Am. J. Cardiol., *29:* 7, 1972.
17. Benchimol, A., and Dimond, E. G.: The apexcardiogram in ischemic heart disease. Br. Heart J., *24:* 581, 1962.
18. Benchimol, A., and Dimond, E. G.: The apexcardiogram in "normal older" subjects and in patients with arteriosclerotic heart disease; effect of exercise on the "a" wave. Am. Heart J., *65:* 789, 1963.
19. Benchimol, A., Dimond, E. G., and Carson, J. C.: The value of the apexcardiogram as a reference tracing in phonocardiography. Am. Heart J., *61:* 485, 1961.
20. Benchimol, A., and Ellis, J. G.: A study of the period of isovolumic relaxation in normal subjects and in patients with heart disease. Am. J. Cardiol., *19:* 196, 1967.
21. Benchimol, A., Fishenfeld, J., and Desser, K. B.: Influence of atrial systole on first derivative of the apexcardiogram. Chest, *65:* 446, 1974.
22. Benchimol, A., Maia, I. G., and Maroko, P. R.: Selective coronary dye-dilution curves in normal subjects and in patients with coronary disease. Am. J. Cardiol., *22:* 844, 1968.
23. Benchimol, A., and Maroko, P.: The apexcardiogram. The value of the apexcardiogram in coronary artery disease. Dis. Chest., *54:* 378, 1968.
24. Benchimol, A., Marsh, C. A., and Desser, K. B.: Discordant left ventricular pressure and apexcardiographic pulsus alternans. Chest, *67:* 477, 1975.
25. Benchimol, A., Matsuo, S., Desser, K. B., Wang, T. F., and Gartlan, J. L. Jr.: Coronary artery blood flow velocity during ventricular tachycardia in man. Am. J. Med. Sci., *264:* 277, 1972.
26. Benchimol, A., and Tippit, H. C.: The clinical value of the jugular and hepatic pulses. In: Friedberg, C. K. (ed.): *Physical Diagnosis in Cardiovascular Diseases.* Grune & Stratton, New York, 1969.
27. Bennet, E. D.: Significance of atrial sound in acute myocardial infarction. Br. Heart J., *34:* 202, 1972.
28. Bristow, J. D., VanZee, B. E., and Judkins, M. P.: Systolic and diastolic abnormalities of the left ventricle in coronary artery disease; studies in patients with little or no enlargement of ventricular volume. Circulation, *42:* 219, 1970.
29. Burch, G. E., Giles, T. D., and Colcolough, H. L.: Ischemic cardiomyopathy. Am. Heart J., *79:* 291, 1970.
30. Burch, G. E., Giles, T. D., and Martinez, E.: Echocardiographic detection of abnormal motion of the interventricular septum in ischemic cardiomyopathy. Am. J. Med., *57:* 293, 1974.
31. Buyukozturk, K., Kimbiris, D., and Segal, B. L.: Systolic time intervals; relation to severity of coronary artery disease, intercoronary collateralization and left ventricular dyskinesia. Am. J. Cardiol., *28:* 183, 1971.
32. Carlsten, A., Forsberg, S. A., Paulin, S., Varnauskas, E., and Werko, L.: Coronary angiography in the clinical analysis of suspected coronary disease. Am. J. Cardiol., *19:* 509, 1967.
33. Carvalho, F. R., Benchimol, A., and Dimond, E. G.: The usefulness of the apexcardiogram and phonocardiogram and its abnormalities in congenital and

acquired heart diseases. Arq. Bras. Cardiol., *16:* 77, 1963.

34. Caulfield, W. H., Jr., Smith, R. H., and Franklin, R. B.: The second heart sound in coronary artery disease; a phonocardiographic assessment. Am. Heart J., *77:* 187, 1969.
35. Cheng, T. O.: Incidence of ventricular aneurysm in coronary artery disease; an angiographic appraisal. Am. J. Med., *50:* 340, 1971.
36. Cheng, T. O.: Murmurs in coronary artery disease. N. Engl. J. Med., *283:* 1054, 1970.
37. Cohn, P. F., Gorlin, R., Cohn, L. H., and Collins, J. J., Jr.: Left ventricular ejection fraction as a prognostic guide in surgical treatment of coronary and valvular heart disease. Am. J. Cardiol., *34:* 136, 1974.
38. Cohn, P. F., Levine, J. A., Bergeron, G. A., and Gorlin, R.: Reproducibility of the angiographic left ventricular ejection fraction in patients with coronary artery disease. Am. Heart J., *88:* 713, 1974.
39. Collins, M., Obeid, A., Ryan, G. F., Smulyan, H., and Eich, R. H.: Hemodynamic effects of increasing the heart rate in patients with arteriosclerotic heart disease. Am. Heart J., *77:* 466, 1972.
40. Corya, B. C., Feigenbaum, H., Rasmussen, S., and Black, M. J.: Anterior left ventricular wall echoes in coronary artery disease; linear scanning with a single element transducer. Am. J. Cardiol., *34:* 652, 1974.
41. Desser, K. B., and Benchimol, A.: The apexcardiogram in patients with syndrome of midsystolic click and late systolic murmur. Chest, *62:* 739, 1972.
42. Desser, K. B., Benchimol, A., and Schumacher, J. A.: The post-extrasystolic apexcardiogram. Chest, *64:* 747, 1973.
43. Diamond, B., and Killip, T.: Indirect assessment of left ventricular performance in acute myocardial infarction. Circulation, *42:* 579, 1970.
44. Dimond, E. G., and Benchimol, A.: Correlation of intracardiac pressure and precordial movement in ischaemic heart disease. Br. Heart J., *25:* 389, 1963.
45. Dimond, E. G., and Benchimol, A.: The exercise apexcardiogram in angina pectoris; its possible usefulness in diagnosis and therapy. Dis. Chest, *43:* 92, 1963.
46. Dimond, E. G., Duenas, A., and Benchimol, A.: Apexcardiography; a review. Am. Heart J., *72:* 124, 1966.
47. Dimond, E. G., Li, Y. B., and Benchimol, A.: Tourniquets and abdominal binders in ischemic heart disease; effects on the apex cardiogram. J.A.M.A., *187:* 98, 1964.
48. Dowling, J. T., Sloman, G., and Urquhart, C.: Systolic time interval fluctuations produced by acute myocardial infarction. Br. Heart J., *33:* 765, 1971.
49. Eddleman, E. E. Jr.: Kinetocardiographic changes in ischemic heart disease. Circulation, *32:* 650, 1965.
50. Eddleman, E. E. Jr., and Harrison, T. R.: The kinetocardiogram in patients with ischemic heart disease. Prog. Cardiovasc. Dis., *6:* 189, 1963.
51. Eddleman, E. E. Jr., and Langley, J. O.: Paradoxical pulsation of the precordium in myocardial infarction and angina pectoris. Am. Heart J., *63:* 579, 1962.
52. Effler, D. B., Favaloro, R. G., and Groves, L. K.: Coronary artery surgery utilizing saphenous vein graft techniques; clinical experience with 224 operations. J. Thorac. Cardiovasc. Surg., *59:* 147, 1970.
53. Ellestad, M. H., Allen, W., Wan, M. C. K., and Kemp, G. L.: Maximal treadmill stress testing for cardiovascular evaluation. Circulation, *39:* 517, 1969.
54. Fabian, J., Epstein, N., Coulshed, N., and McKendrick, C. S.: Duration of phases of left ventricular systole using indirect methods; II. Acute myocardial infarction. Br. Heart J., *34:* 882, 1972.
55. Frankl, W. S., Deitz, R. D., and Soloff, L.: The Q-T ratio as a guide to the exercise test in the digitalized subject. Dis. Chest, *54:* 119, 1968.
56. Gahl, K., Caspar, P., Pearson, M., Sutton, R., and McDonald, L.: Apical systolic murmurs related to mitral regurgitation at angiography in ischemic heart disease. Br. Heart J., *34:* 965, 1972.
57. Garrard, C. L. Jr., Weissler, A. M., and Dodge, H. T.: The relationship of alterations in systolic time intervals to ejection fraction in patients with cardiac disease. Circulation, *42:* 455, 1970.

58. Greenwald, J., Yap, J. F., Franklin, M., and Lichtman, A. M.: Echocardiographic mitral systolic motion in left ventricular aneurysm. Br. Heart J., *37:* 684, 1975.

59. Hamosh, P., Cohn, J. N., Engleman, K., Broder, M. I., and Freis, E. D.: Systolic time intervals and left ventricular function in acute myocardial infarction. Circulation, *45:* 375, 1972.

60. Harrison, T. R.: Some clinical and physiologic aspects of angina pectoris. Bull. John Hopkins Hosp., *104:* 275, 1959.

61. Harrison, T. R., and Hughes, L.: Precordial systolic bulges during anginal attacks. Trans. Assoc. Am. Physicians, *71:* 174, 1959.

62. Harrison, W. K. Jr., and Talbot, S. A.: Discrimination of the quantitative ultralow-frequency ballistocardiogram in coronary heart disease. Am. Heart J., *74:* 80, 1967.

63. Heikkila, J., Luomanmake, K., and Pyorala, K.: Serial observations on left ventricular dysfunction in acute myocardial infarction. Circulation, *44:* 343, 1971.

64. Hellerstein, H. K., Prozan, G. B., Liebow, I. M., Doan, A. E., and Henderson, J. A.: Two step exercise test as a test of cardiac function in chronic rheumatic heart disease and in arteriosclerotic heart disease with old myocardial infarction. Am. J. Cardiol., *7:* 234, 1961.

65. Hill, J. C., O'Rourke, R. A., Lewis, R. P., and McGranahan, G. M.: The diagnostic value of the atrial gallop in acute myocardial infarction. Am. Heart J., *78:* 194, 1969.

66. Hodges, M., Halpern, B. L., Friesinger, G. C., and Dagenais, G. R.: Left ventricular pre-ejection period and ejection time in patients with acute myocardial infarction. Circulation, *45:* 933, 1972.

67. Hornsten, T. R., and Bruce, R. A.: Computed ST forces of Frank and bipolar exercise electrocardiograms. Am. Heart J., *78:* 346, 1969.

68. Hutchinson, R. G.: The apexcardiogram in the diagnosis of coronary artery disease; a review. Angiology, *25:* 381, 1974.

69. Inoue, K., Smulyan, H., Mookherjee, S., and Eich, R. H.: Ultrasonic measurement of left ventricular wall motion in acute myocardial infarction. Circulation, *43:* 778, 1971.

70. Inoue, K., Young, G. M., Grierson, A. L., Smulyan, H., and Eich, R. H.: Isometric contraction period of the left ventricle in acute myocardial infarction. Circulation, *42:* 79, 1970.

71. Jain, S. R., and Lindahl, J.: Apex cardiogram and systolic time intervals in acute myocardial infarction. Br. Heart J., *33:* 578, 1971.

72. Jeresaty, R. M., and Liss, J. P.: Midsystolic clicks and coronary heart disease. Chest, *63:* 297, 1973.

73. Johnson, W. D., and Lepley, D. Jr.: An aggressive surgical approach to coronary disease. J. Thorac. Cardiovasc. Surg., *59:* 128, 1970.

74. Kattus, A. A. Jr., Hanafee, W. N., Longmire, W. P. Jr., MacAlpin, R. N., and Rivin, A. U.: Diagnosis, medical and surgical management of coronary insufficiency. Ann. Intern. Med., *69:* 115, 1968.

75. Kavanagh-Gray, D.: Left ventricular end-diastolic pressures following selective coronary arteriography. Am. Heart J., *84:* 629, 1972.

76. Kazamias, T. M., Gander, M. P., Ross, J. Jr., and Braunwald, E.: Detection of left-ventricular-wall motion disorders in coronary artery disease by radarkymography. N. Engl. J. Med., *2:* 63, 1971.

77. Khaja, F., Parker, J. O., Ledwich, R. J., West, R. O., and Armstrong, P. W.: Assessment of ventricular function in coronary artery disease by means of atrial pacing and exercise. Am. J. Cardiol., *26:* 107, 1970.

78. Kobayashi, K.: Clinical studies on apexcardiogram; II. Cardiac movement in thyroid dysfunction and coronary heart disease from the point of apexcardiogram. Jap. Circ. J., *35:* 1091, 1971.

79. Kramer, R. J., Goldstein, R., Hirshfeld, I. W., Johnston, G. S., and Epstein, S. E.: Visualization of acute myocardial infarction by radionuclide gallium 67. Circulation, *45:* 20, 1972.

80. Legler, J. F., and Benchimol, A.: The significance of extra systoles in coronary artery disease. Geriatrics, *19:* 468, 1964.

81. Legler, J. F., Benchimol, A., and Dimond, E. G.: The apexcardiogram in the study of 2-OS intervals. Br. Heart J., *25:* 246, 1963.
82. Lewis, R. P., Boudoulas, H., Forester, W. F., and Weissler, A. M.: Shortening of electromechanical systole as a manifestation of excessive adrenergic stimulation in acute myocardial infarction. Circulation, *46:* 856, 1972.
83. Likoff, W.: Myocardial revascularization; a critique. N. Y. State J. Med., *70:* 1983, 1970.
84. Likoff, W., Kasparian, H., Segal, B. L., Forman, H., and Novack, P.: Coronary arteriography; correlation with electrocardiographic response to measured exercise. Am. J. Cardiol., *18:* 160, 1966.
85. Linhart, J. W.: Myocardial function in coronary artery disease determined by atrial pacing. Circulation, *44:* 203, 1971.
86. Lipp, H., Gambetta, M., Schwartz, J., de la Fuente, D., and Resnekov, L.: Intermittent pansystolic murmur and presumed mitral regurgitation after acute myocardial infarction. Am. J. Cardiol., *30:* 690, 1972.
87. Ludbrook, P., Karliner, J. S., London, A., Peterson, K. L., Leopold, G. R., and O'Rourke, R. A.: Posterior wall velocity; an unreliable index of total left ventricular performance in patients with coronary artery disease. Am. J. Cardiol., *33:* 475, 1974.
88. Luisada, A., and Magri, A.: The low frequency tracings of the precordium and epigastrium in normal subjects and cardiac patients. Am. Heart J., *44:* 545, 1952.
89. Lynn, T. N., and Wolf, S.: The prognostic significance of the ballistocardiogram in ischemic heart disease. Am. Heart J., *88:* 277, 1974.
90. McCallister, B. D., Richmond, D. R., Saltups, A., Hallermann, F. J., Wallace, R. B., and Frye, R. L.: Left ventricular hemodynamics before and 1 year after internal mammary artery implantation in patients with coronary artery disease and angina pectoris. Circulation, *42:* 471, 1970.
91. McConahay, D. R., Martin, M. M., and Cheitlin, M. D.: Resting and exercise systolic time intervals; correlations with ventricular performance in patients with coronary artery disease. Circulation, *45:* 529, 1972.
92. McKusick, V. A.: *Cardiovascular Sound in Health and Disease.* Williams & Wilkins Co., Baltimore, 1958.
93. Margolis, C.: Significance of ejection period/tension period as a factor in the assessment of cardiac function and as a possible diagnostic tool for the uncovering of silent coronary heart disease; study of 111 cases. Dis. Chest, *46:* 706, 1964.
94. Martines-Rios, M. A., Bruto da Costa, B. C., Cecena-Seldner, F. A., and Gensini, G. G.: Normal electrocardiogram in the presence of severe coronary artery disease. Am. J. Cardiol., *25:* 320, 1970.
95. Matsuzaki, T.: Calibrated low frequency acceleration vibrocardiography; its hemodynamic determination and clinical application. Jap. Heart J., *13:* 1, 1972.
96. Mielke, J. E.: Functional mitral regurgitation. N. Eng. J. Med., *283:* 1464, 1970.
97. Moss, A. J.: Ischemic heart disease and accelerated cardiovascular aging; a ballistocardiographic study. Circulation, *25:* 369, 1962.
98. Mounsey, P.: Precordial pulsations in relation to cardiac movement and sounds. Br. Heart J., *21:* 457, 1959.
99. Muller, O., and Rorvik, K.: Hemodynamic consequences of coronary heart disease, with observations during anginal pain and on the effect of nitroglycerine. Br. Heart J., *20:* 302, 1958.
100. Nixon, P. G., and Bethell, H. J. N.: Atrial gallop in diagnosis of early coronary heart disease. Br. Heart J., *34:* 202, 1972.
101. Nutter, D. O.. Trujillo, N. P., and Evans, J. M.: The isoenzymes of lactic dehydrogenas; I. Myocardial infarction and coronary insufficiency. Am. Heart J., *72:* 315, 1966.
102. O'Rourke, R. A.: Appearance of atrial sound after reversion of atrial fibrillation. Br. Heart J., *32:* 597, 1970.
103. Pasternac, A., Gorlin, R., Sonnenblick, E. H., Haft, J. I., and Kemp, H. G.: Abnormalities of ventricular motion induced by atrial pacing in coronary artery

disease. Circulation, *45:* 1195, 1972.

104. Piccone, V. A., Leveen, H. H., Potter, R. T., Falk, G., Mandi, A., and Oran, E.: Multiparameter evaluation of internal mammary artery implant function; an experimental study. Ann. Thorac. Surg., *8:* 327, 1969.

105. Piessens, J., VanMieghem, W., Kesteloot, H., and DeGeest, H.: Diagnostic value of clinical history, exercise testing and atrial pacing in patients with chest pain. Am. J. Cardiol., *33:* 351, 1974.

106. Pouget, J. M., Harris, W. S., Mayron, B. R., and Naughton, J. P.: Abnormal responses of the systolic time intervals to exercise in patients with angina pectoris. Circulation, *43:* 289, 1971.

107. Ratchin, R. A., Rackley, C. E., and Russell, R. O.: Serial evaluation of left ventricular volumes and posterior wall movement in the acute phase of myocardial infarction using diagnostic ultrasound. Am. J. Cardiol., *29:* 286, 1972.

108. Rosa, L. M., Constantino, J. P., Karsak, N., Reich, R., and Zezmer, B.: The precordial accelerogram in ischemic heart disease—a study of middle-aged and old patients with angina pectoris; recent and old myocardial infarction. Am. J. Cardiol., *9:* 534, 1962.

109. Rosa, L. M., and Nevzat, K.: Precordial pulsatory mechanism in coronary heart disease. Circulation, *22:* 801, 1960.

110. Ross, R. S., and Friesinger, G. C.: Coronary arteriography. Am. Heart J., *72:* 437, 1966.

111. Rowe, G. G., Thomsen, J. H., Stenlund, R. R., McKenna, D. H., Sialer, S., and Corliss, R. J.: A study of hemodynamics and coronary blood flow in man with coronary artery disease. Circulation, *39:* 139, 1969.

112. Rushmer, R. F.: Initial ventricular impulse; a potential key to cardiac evaluation. Circulation, *29:* 268, 1964.

113. Samson, R.: Changes in systolic time intervals in acute myocardial infarction. Br. Heart J., *32:* 839, 1970.

114. Sangster, J. F., and Oakley, C. M.: Diastolic murmur of coronary artery stenosis. Br. Heart J., *35:* 840, 1973.

115. Sawayama, T., Marumoto, S., Niki, I., and Matsuura, T.: The clinical usefulness of the amyl nitrite inhalation test in the assessment of the third and atrial heart sounds in ischemic heart disease. Am. Heart J., *76:* 746, 1968.

116. Sawayama, T., Ochiai, M., Marumoto, S., Matsuura, T., and Niki, I.: Influence of amyl nitrite inhalation on the systolic time intervals in normal subjects and in patients with ischemic heart disease. Circulation, *40:* 327, 1969.

117. Schweizer, W., Bertrab, R. von, and Reist, P.: Kinetocardiography in coronary artery disease. Br. Heart J., *27:* 263, 1965.

118. Seltzer, C. C.: An evaluation of the effect of smoking on coronary heart disease; I. Epidemiological evidence. J.A.M.A., *203:* 193, 1968.

119. Shelburne, J. C., Rubinstein, D., and Gorlin, R.: A reappraisal of papillary muscle dysfunction; correlative clinical and angiographic study. Am. J. Med., *46:* 862, 1969.

120. Skinner, N. S. Jr., Leibeskind, R. S., Phillips, H. L., and Harrison, T. R.: Angina pectoris; effect of exertion and of nitrites on the precordial movements. Am. Heart J., *61:* 250, 1961.

121. Sonnenblick, E. H.: Non-Invasive evaluation of regional ventricular dysfunction. N. Engl. J. Med. *285:* 114, 1971.

122. Spodick, D. H.: Coronary bypass operations. N. Engl. J. Med., *285:* 55, 1971.

123. Spodick, D. H.: Coronary surgery. Am. Heart J., *7:* 579, 1970.

124. Suh, S. K., and Eddleman, E. E. Jr.: Kinetocardiographic findings of myocardial infarction. Circulation, *19:* 531, 1959.

125. Tippit, H. C., and Benchimol, A.: The apex cardiogram J.A.M.A., *201:* 24, 1967.

126. Toutouzas, P., Gupta, D., Samson, R., and Shillingford, J.: Q-second sound interval in acute myocardial infarction. Br. Heart J., *31:* 462, 1969.

127. Turner, P. P., and Hunter, J.: The atrial sound in ischaemic heart disease. Br. Heart J., *35:* 657, 1973.

128. Urschel, H. C. Jr., Razzuk, M. A., Nathan, M. J., Miller, E. R., Nicholson, D. M., and

Paulson, D. L.: Combined gas (CO_2) endarterectomy and vein bypass graft for patients with coronary artery disease. Ann. Thorac. Surg., *10:* 119, 1970.

129. Walston, A., Hackel, D. B., Estes, E. H., and Durham, N. C.: Acute coronary occlusion and the "power failure" syndrome. Am. Heart J., *79:* 613, 1970.

130. Weissler, A. M., and Garrard, C. L. Jr.: Systolic time intervals in cardiac disease. Mod. Concepts Cardiovasc. Dis., *40:* 1, 1970.

131. Weissler, A. M., Peeler, R. G., and Toehill, W. H.: Relationships between left ventricular ejection time, stroke volume, and heart rate in normal individuals and patients with cardiovascular disease. Am. Heart J., *62:* 367, 1961.

132. Whitsett, T. L., and Naughton, J.: The effect of exercise on systolic time intervals in sedentary and active individuals and rehabilitated patients with heart disease. Am. J. Cardiol., *27:* 352, 1971.

133. Wolferth, C., and Margolies, A.: *Stroud's Diagnosis and Treatment of Cardiovascular Disease.* F. A. Davis Co., Philadelphia, 1945.

134. Wood, P.: *Disease of the Heart and Circulation.* J. B. Lippincott Co., Philadelphia, 1956.

135. Yurchak, C. M., and Gorlin, R.: Paradoxical splitting of the second heart sound in coronary disease. N. Engl. J. Med., *269:* 741, 1963.

chapter 9

Congenital Heart Disease

ATRIAL SEPTAL DEFECTS

Atrial septal defects are commonly of two varieties, ostium secundum and ostium primum. Ostium primum septal defects belong to a group of congenital abnormalities called endocardial cushion defects. In patients with ostium primum defects, associated congenital malformations of either the mitral and/or tricuspid valve resulting in valvular insufficiency are seen.

SECUNDUM DEFECTS

Heart Sounds and Murmurs

The first heart sound is split and the tricuspid component is accentuated. In about 25% of cases a systolic ejection click due to dilatation of the pulmonary artery or abnormal pulmonary valve motion is present (fig. 9.1). The incidence of ejection clicks increases in patients with pulmonary hypertension and this sound is inscribed very early in systole (0.02–0.04 sec) after the initial vibration of the first heart sound. In some patients it is inscribed with the first heart sound and therefore becomes inaudible. The second heart sound is widely split, and fixed with the A2-P2 interval ranging from 0.04 to 0.08 sec (figs. 9.1–9.5). The pulmonic component of the second heart sound is of normal intensity in the absence of pulmonary hypertension and is transmitted well to the mitral area. This is probably related to dilatation of the right ventricle with anterior rotation of this chamber which then forms the "apex" of the heart. The A2-P2 interval is "fixed" during both phases of the respiratory cycle or it may decrease slightly during expiration. Splitting of the second heart sound has been attributed to the presence of complete or incomplete right bundle branch block which is frequently seen in this condition. It may also be due to increased, fixed pulmonary flow and abnormal pulmonary compliance.

A tricuspid opening snap is rare and seen only in patients with large left-to-right shunts (fig 9.4). Prominent third heart sounds are frequently heard and recorded best at the tricuspid area (fig. 9.5). Fourth

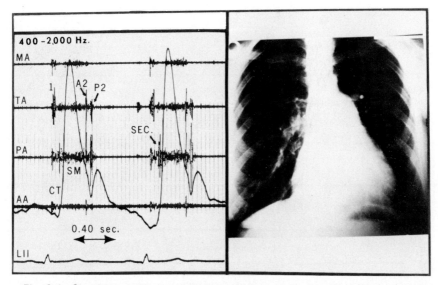

Fig. 9.1. Simultaneously recorded phonocardiogram at the mitral (MA), tricuspid (TA), pulmonic (PA), and aortic areas (AA), carotid pulse tracing (CT) and lead II (LII) of the electrocardiogram in a 21-year-old patient with a secundum type atrial septal defect (left panel). The first heart sound is normal. The second heart sound shows fixed splitting and the A2-P2 interval is 0.05 sec. Both components have normal amplitude. A systolic ejection click (SEC) follows the first heart sound and coincides with the beginning of the upstroke of the carotid pulse tracing. A high frequency, high amplitude systolic ejection murmur (SM) begins with the ejection click and terminates with the aortic closure sound. There are no diastolic murmurs. The carotid pulse tracing is normal. The chest x-ray (right panel) shows a large cardiac silhouette due to enlargement of the right ventricle, a prominent main pulmonary artery and increased pulmonary blood flow. The right atrium is dilated.

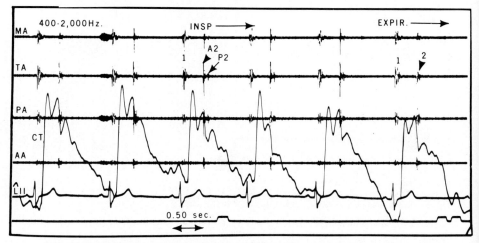

Fig. 9.2. Simultaneously recorded phonocardiogram at the mitral (MA), tricuspid (TA), pulmonic (PA) and aortic (AA) areas, carotid pulse tracing (CT), and lead II (LII) of the electrocardiogram in a 23-year-old patient with an atrial septal defect. During inspiration the second heart sound is split and the A2-P2 interval is approximately 0.05 sec. During expiration the second heart sound remains split but the A2-P2 interval shortens to 0.03 sec. The carotid pulse tracing is normal.

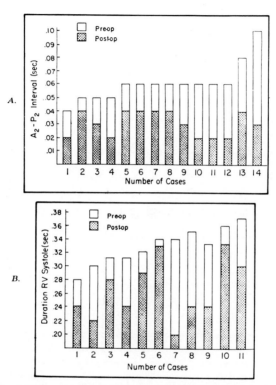

Fig. 9.3. (Panel A) Pre- and post-operative changes in the duration of splitting of the second heart sound in a group of patients with secundum type atrial septal defects. (Panel B) Pre- and post-operative changes in the duration of right ventricular systole in the same group of patients. There is a significant decrease in duration of the A2-P2 interval and a decrease in duration of right ventricular systole following closure of the atrial septal defect. However, in many of these patients the second heart sound continues to be split in the post-operative tracings.

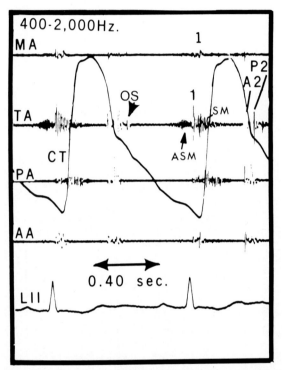

Fig. 9.4. Simultaneously recorded phonocardiogram at the mitral (MA), tricuspid (TA), pulmonic (PA) and aortic (AA) areas, carotid pulse tracing (CT), and lead II (LII) of the electrocardiogram in a 48-year-old patient with a secundum type atrial septal defect. The tracing was recorded during expiration. The first heart sound is normal. The second heart sound is widely split and the pulmonic component is slightly accentuated. The prominent, high frequency vibration in early diastole is the opening snap of the tricuspid valve (TOS). A high frequency, medium amplitude systolic ejection murmur (SM) is best recorded at the pulmonic area. A medium frequency, high amplitude atriosystolic murmur (ASM) follows the P wave of the electrocardiogram. The carotid pulse tracing is normal. Cardiac catheterization revealed the presence of a large left-to-right shunt at the atrial level, mild elevation of pulmonary artery pressures and dilated pulmonary arteries.

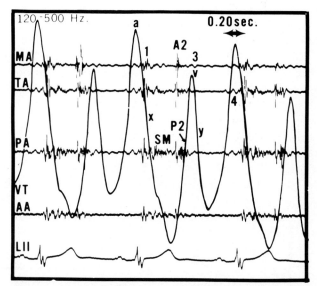

Fig. 9.5. Simultaneously recorded phonocardiogram at the mitral (MA), tricuspid (TA), pulmonic (PA) and aortic (AA) areas, jugular venous tracing (VT), and lead II (LII) of the electrocardiogram in a 23-year-old patient with a secundum type atrial septal defect. The first heart sound is normal. The second heart sound is widely split and is recorded best at the pulmonic area. There are low amplitude third and fourth heart sounds. A high frequency, low amplitude systolic ejection murmur (SM) is best recorded at the pulmonic area. The jugular venous tracing shows prominent A and V waves and normal x and y descents.

heart sounds in patients below age 30 are rare, but are frequently heard in patients with pulmonary hypertension (fig. 9.6).

A systolic ejection murmur in patients with secundum type atrial septal defects is the result of increased flow across the outflow tract of the right ventricle and pulmonic valve. This murmur of varying intensity is best recorded at the pulmonic and tricuspid areas (figs. 9.1, 9.2, 9.4, and 9.5). Atrial ventricular diastolic murmurs and atrial systolic murmurs (fig. 9.4) may be heard providing that magnitude of the left-to-right shunt is large with pulmonary blood flow to systemic flow ratio exceeding 2:1. This murmur is probably the result of increased turbulent flow across the tricuspid valve. Flow through the atrial septal defect which occurs during systole and diastole does not cause any significant audible heart murmur despite the fact that a small fraction of a left-to-right shunt does occur during atrial contraction, as demonstrated with use of phasic measurement of flow velocities in the right atrium using the Doppler flowmeter catheter technique. In the presence of pulmonary hypertension with mean pulmonary artery pressure exceeding 50 mm Hg, there is a progressive disappearance of the right ventricular third heart sound and atrial ventricular diastolic murmur

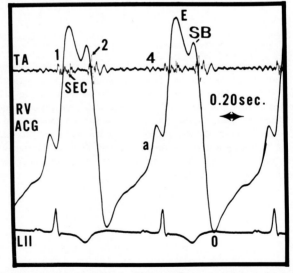

Fig. 9.6. Simultaneously recorded phonocardiogram at the tricuspid area (TA), right ventricular apexcardiogram, and lead II (LII) of the electrocardiogram in a patient with an atrial septal defect and pulmonary hypertension. The normal first heart sound is followed by a systolic ejection click (SEC). The second heart sound is single and accentuated. The fourth heart sound coincides with the peak of a prominent A wave in the right ventricular apexcardiogram (RV ACG) which also shows a late systolic bulge (SB) prior to inscription of the second heart sound. These findings are usually seen in patients with right ventricular hypertrophy.

because of decreased magnitude of the left-to-right shunt. In addition, the systolic ejection murmur decreases in amplitude and the A2-P2 interval becomes very short. Pulmonic insufficiency murmurs are seen in patients with marked dilatation of the pulmonary artery or in cases with severe pulmonary hypertension. The systolic regurgitant murmur representing tricuspid insufficiency is usually indicative of a large left-to-right shunt or severe pulmonary hypertension and is seen in patients with marked dilatation of the right ventricle. Successful closure of the atrial septal defect causes a decrease in amplitude of the systolic murmur and the A2-P2 interval, and disappearance of the atrioventricular diastolic murmur as shown in figure 9.6.

Carotid Pulse Tracing

The carotid pulse tracing is of no diagnostic value in secundum type atrial septal defect.

Jugular Venous Pulse Tracing

The jugular venous pulse tracing is abnormal, showing prominent A and V waves (fig. 9.5). The relative increase in these waves is recognized by their increase in relation to the C wave. These waves reflect the left-to-right shunt which occurs during atrial contraction and early ventricular diastole. When pulmonary artery pressure begins to rise the V wave becomes progressively smaller and the A wave progressively larger. Tricuspid insufficiency occurs in the late natural history of this disease and the abnormalities of the venous pulse essentially are those described for tricuspid insufficiency (see Chapter 6).

Apexcardiogram

The apexcardiogram of the left ventricle is of no value in the diagnosis of secundum type atrial septal defects. However, right ventricular precordial motion can be recorded with a transducer placed over the tricuspid or subxyphoid area. It shows a prominent systolic retraction followed by a late systolic bulge and a conspicuous rapid filling wave. In patients with severe right ventricular hypertrophy, the systolic wave is sustained, round and the A wave becomes larger.

Systolic Time Intervals

Systolic time intervals are of no value in the diagnosis of atrial septal defects, however, when patients develop severe pulmonary hypertension the left ventricular ejection time decreases.

Echocardiography

Echocardiography is a useful non-invasive technique in the diagnosis of secundum type atrial septal defects. The most common findings include: (1) increase in right ventricular internal diameter due to increased diastolic volume loading. This particular finding is seen in patients with a large left-to-right shunt. (2) Abnormal motion of the interventricular septum. Two abnormalities of septal motion may be seen in patients with right ventricular volume loading. In type A (paradoxical septal motion), the septum moves anteriorly in systole and posteriorly in diastole (fig 9.7). Paradoxical septal motion, which is commonly seen in patients with atrial septal defects, is usually the result of increased diastolic volume loading of the right ventricle and usually regresses after successful closure of the atrial septal defect. Type B is recognized by flat septal motion throughout systole and a brief small posterior deflection noted in early diastole. This abnormality is rarely seen in patients with atrial septal defects. If present, it is usually indicative of a marked increase in the right ventricular intracavitary diameter. Caution should be exercised in the interpretation of these findings since normal septal motion has been seen in patients with atrial septal defect. Therefore, absence of abnormal septal motion does not exclude this diagnosis. A technically good echocardiographic scan is important in these patients and the interventricular septum should be analyzed in the recording showing mid-left ventricular cavitary structures.

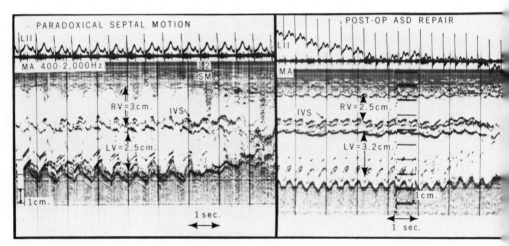

Fig. 9.7. Simultaneously recorded echocardiogram, mitral area (MA) phonocardiogram, and lead II (LII) of the electrocardiogram in a 5-year-old patient before and after closure of an atrial septal defect. In the pre-operative tracing (left panel) note the increase in right ventricular internal diameter to 3 cm and paradoxical motion of the interventricular septum. In the right panel, approximately 1 month after closure of the atrial septal defect, there is a decrease in right ventricular (RV) cavity size to 2.5 cm and flat motion of the interventricular septum (IVS). Left ventricular (LV) internal diameter pre-operatively was 2.5 cm and post-operatively, 3.2 cm.

A decrease in the D-E slope of the anterior and posterior mitral leaflets has been noted in some patients with atrial septal defect. Abnormalities of mitral valve motion simulating idiopathic hypertrophic subaortic stenosis have also been described, with systolic anterior motion. This is present in approximately 35–40% of patients with secundum type atrial septal defects. Approximately 30–40% of patients with this type of congenital lesion show findings which simulate the ones seen in prolapse of the posterior mitral valve (see Chapter 4).

ENDOCARDIAL CUSHION DEFECTS

Endocardial cushion defects include a variety of cardiac lesions which should be considered in generic terms. Most lesions are due to a lack of fusion of the endocardial cushions, therefore, a variety of combined malformations may be seen. The simplest form is a low placed atrial septal defect with associated cleft of the mitral valve, also called an ostium primum atrial septal defect. Total absence of fusion of the cushion may result in both atrial and ventricular septal defects and associated mitral and/or tricuspid insufficiencies. In addition, some patients may have a left ventricular right atrial shunt. Due to the variety of anatomical defects seen in these patients, the auscultatory, phonocardiographic, pulse wave and echocardiographic abnormalities may not be identical.

Heart Sounds and Murmurs

The first heart sound is normal in patients with endocardial cushion defects. If a severe degree of mitral insufficiency is present, the first heart sound is diminished. The second heart sound is usually widely split and fixed (figs. 9.8 and 9.9). A third heart sound is frequently heard at the mitral and tricuspid areas and is secondary to increased early right ventricular filling. Fourth heart sounds and systolic ejection clicks are not generally heard unless there is associated pulmonary hypertension.

The typical murmurs associated with ostium primum defects are mitral and/or tricuspid insufficiency due to congenital deformities of these valves (figs. 9.8 and 9.9). The pansystolic regurgitant murmur starts with the first heart sound, therefore, during the period of isovolumic contraction. It reaches a plateau throughout systole and terminates with the aortic or pulmonary valve closure sound. Low frequency atrioventricular diastolic murmurs representing increased flow across the mitral or tricuspid valves are seen in patients with large left-to-right shunts. This murmur is usually preceded by a prominent third heart sound and terminates prior to atrial contraction. Systolic ejection murmurs are frequently present due to increased flow across the pulmonary valve. Rare diastolic murmurs of pulmonary insufficiency are associated with a very large left-to-right shunt and/or severe pulmonary hypertension.

Carotid Pulse Tracing

The carotid pulse tracing is of no diagnostic value in patients with ostium primum atrial septal defects.

Jugular Venous Pulse Tracing

The jugular venous pulse tracing usually shows an abnormal contour similar to the findings described for secundum type atrial septal defects, namely prominent A and V waves (fig 9.9).

Systolic Time Intervals

Systolic time intervals are of no diagnostic value in patients with endocardial cushion defects; however, in the presence of mitral insufficiency with a large left-to-right shunt, left ventricular ejection time decreases secondary to decrease in left ventricular forward stroke volume.

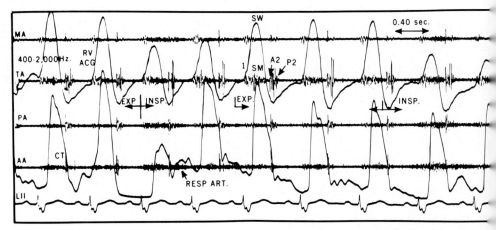

Fig. 9.8. Simultaneously recorded phonocardiogram at the mitral (MA), tricuspid (TA), pulmonic (PA) and aortic areas (AA), carotid pulse tracing (CT), right ventricular apexcardiogram (RV ACG), and lead II (LII) of the electrocardiogram in a 12-year-old patient with an endocardial cushion defect and a large left-to-right shunt. A high frequency, high amplitude systolic regurgitant murmur (SM) best recorded at the tricuspid and mitral areas is secondary to mitral insufficiency. The first heart sound is diminished. The second heart sound is widely split (0.07 sec) and fixed. The pulmonic component is slightly accentuated. The tracings were recorded during inspiration (INSP) and expiration (EXP) to demonstrate fixed splitting of the second heart sound. The right ventricular apexcardiogram shows a sustained systolic wave (SW) and an inconspicuous E point. The electrocardiogram shows complete right bundle branch block. The carotid pulse tracing is normal.

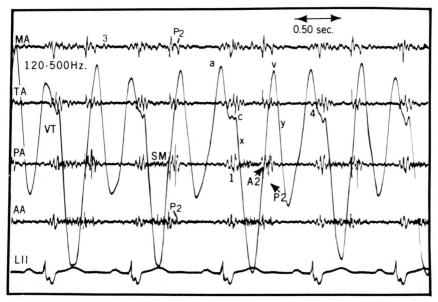

Fig. 9.9. Simultaneously recorded phonocardiogram at the mitral (MA), tricuspid (TA), pulmonic (PA) and aortic areas (AA), jugular venous tracing (VT), and lead II (LII) of the electrocardiogram in a 12-year-old patient with an endocardial cushion defect and mitral insufficiency. The first and second heart sounds are normal. There is a high frequency, low amplitude systolic regurgitant murmur (SM) recorded at the mitral and pulmonic areas due to mitral insufficiency. The second heart sound has fixed splitting and the pulmonic component is well transmitted to the mitral and aortic areas. The jugular venous tracing shows prominent A and V waves and normal x and y descents.

Echocardiography

The echocardiogram in patients with endocardial cushion defects varies depending upon the types of lesions associated with the disease. The most common type of ostium primum septal defect is usually associated with the right ventricular volume overloading. The echocardiogram may show multiple mitral valve echoes during systole and diastole with normal posterior left atrial wall motion. In addition, there is exaggeration of the anterior mitral valve excursion which protrudes through the interventricular septum and decreased excursion of the tricuspid leaflet.

Paradoxical septal motion is frequently seen and right ventricular internal diameter may be increased (fig 9.10). The various anatomical landmarks for mitral valve motion, such as recording of the E-F slope, are difficult to record. The D-E slope can usually be recorded and is abnormal. In advanced forms of endocardial cushion defects such as

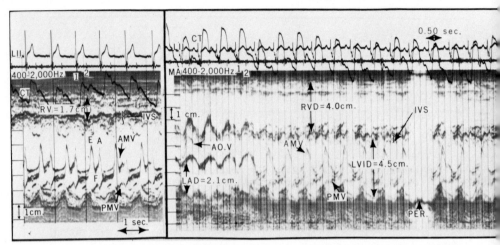

Fig. 9.10. Echocardiogram of a normal subject (left panel) showing normal motion of the mitral valve and interventricular septum (IVS). The right panel shows an echocardiogram of a 5-year-old patient with an ostium primum type atrial septal defect with paradoxical motion of the interventricular septum and a greatly increased right ventricular dimension (RVD) of 4 cm. Left ventricular internal diameter (LVID) is slightly increased for the age group at 4.5 cm. The aortic root measurement of 2.0 cm and left atrial dimension (LAD) of 2.1 cm are in the normal range. AMV = anterior mitral valve, PMV = posterior mitral valve, PER = pericardium, AO V = aortic valve.

artrioventricular canal, patients will exhibit an unusual atrioventricular valve motion pattern. In these instances the mitral and tricuspid leaflet seem to join together at the level of the aortic root during the systolic phase of the cardiac cycle. During diastole the mitral valve moves posteriorly and the tricuspid valve moves anteriorly. The interventricular septum is absent in patients with common atrioventricular canal.

TOTAL ANOMALOUS PULMONARY VENOUS RETURN

Anomalous pulmonary venous return can be partial or total. Most frequently in this type of congenital heart disease, the pulmonary veins will drain into the right atrium, superior vena cava, or coronary sinus.

The phonocardiographic and pulse wave abnormalities are somewhat similar to the ones described in patients with secundum type atrial septal defects (see above under "Secundum Defects"). A high amplitude, high frequency atrioventricular diastolic murmur may be present as seen in figure 9.11, representing marked increase in flow across the tricuspid valve.

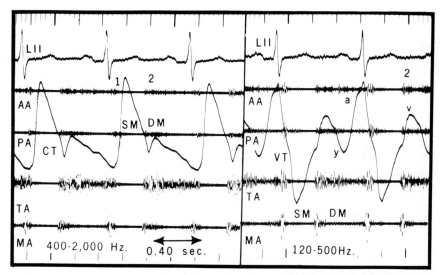

Fig. 9.11. Simultaneously recorded phonocardiogram at the aortic (AA), pulmonic (PA), tricuspid (TA) and mitral areas (MA), lead II (LII) of the electrocardiogram, and carotid pulse tracing (CT) (left panel) and with a jugular venous tracing (VT) (right panel), in a 2-year-old patient with total anomalous pulmonary venous return to the coronary sinus and associated atrial septal defect. The first heart sound is normal. The second heart sound is slightly accentuated. A high frequency, low amplitude systolic ejection murmur (SM) is recorded best at the aortic area. The most important feature on the phonocardiogram is the high frequency, high amplitude diastolic murmur (DM) which begins with the second heart sound, continues through middiastole and terminates with atrial contraction. It most likely represents a marked increase in flow across the tricuspid valve due to a large left-to-right shunt. The carotid pulse tracing is normal. The jugular venous tracing shows a slightly prominent A wave and normal x and y descents. (From C. Harris, Baylor University Medical Center, Dallas, Texas, with permission.)

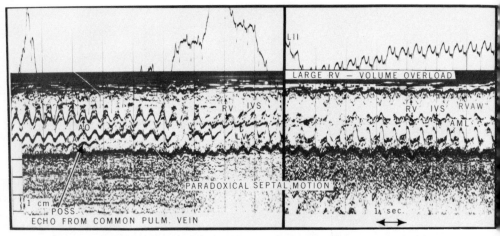

Fig. 9.12. Echocardiogram of a 7-day-old infant with total anomalous pulmonary venous drainage into a left superior vena cava. On the scan (left panel) from the aorta (AO) to the left ventricle (LV), echoes possibly derived from the common pulmonary vein are indicated by an arrow. The recording in the right panel shows an increase in right ventricular dimension to 1.5 cm and paradoxical motion of the interventricular septum (IVS) which is frequently seen in this condition. It is probably due to large diastolic volume loading of the right ventricle (RV). LA = left atrium, RVAW = right ventricular anterior wall, AML = anterior mitral leaflet.

Echocardiogram

No definite echocardiographic pattern has been established in patients with total anomalous pulmonary venous return. Some reports have indicated a decrease in left atrial internal diameter. Paradoxical septal motion has been described in a few isolated cases but this has not been demonstrated by all investigators. The right ventricular dimensions are increased (fig 9.12).

VENTRICULAR SEPTAL DEFECT

Non-invasive techniques are valuable in evaluating patients with ventricular septal defects.

Heart Sounds and Murmurs

The first heart sound is normal. The second heart sound is single or shows a narrow split. The splitting of the second heart sound in this condition is not as wide as it is in patients with atrial septal defects or pulmonary valvular stenosis and has little variation, if any, during the two phases of the respiratory cycle. With progressive increase in pulmonary artery pressure and resistance, decrease in magnitude of the left-to-right shunt, or with development of a bidirectional shunt, pulmonary blood flow decreases. As a result of the decreased flow, the pulmonary valve closes early and the second heart sound becomes single and accentuated (figs. 9.15–9.19). In some patients with a marked degree of pulmonary hypertension (Eisenmenger complex), right ventricular systole becomes so short the pulmonic valve closes very early and pulmonic paradoxical splitting of the second heart sound may be seen (P2 precedes A2). This type of splitting can also be seen in patients with congenital or acquired heart disease associated with severe pulmonary hypertension.

Third heart sounds are frequently present in patients with large ventricular septal defects, particularly if the pulmonary systemic flow ratio exceeds 2:1. This sound is probably due to an increase in rapid filling of the left ventricle secondary to increased flow across the mitral valve.

Fourth heart sounds are rare in patients without pulmonary hypertension, particularly in younger age groups. Systolic ejection clicks occur more frequently in patients when the mean pulmonary artery pressure exceeds 60 mm Hg, and are usually due to dilatation of the pulmonary artery or abnormal motion of the pulmonic valve in early systole.

The systolic murmur is the most striking finding in patients with ventricular septal defects. This murmur has the combined characteristics of a systolic regurgitant and ejection murmur (fig. 9.13). The regurgitant feature is due to the fact that the murmur starts with the first heart sound, during the period of isovolumic contraction, at which time the left-to-right shunt is already present. The ejection feature is due to turbulent flow across a relatively small orifice, resulting in a diamond shape murmur with a maximal peak during mid-systole. This murmur terminates with aortic valve closure. It is best recorded at the tricuspid area although it is transmitted well to most precordial areas. As pulmonary hypertension develops and the magnitude of the left-to-right shunt decreases there is a progressive diminution of intensity and duration of the systolic murmur (figs. 9.14–9.16). When right ventricular systolic pressure equalizes the left ventricular systolic pressure, the systolic murmur may not be present.

A low amplitude, low frequency atrioventricular diastolic murmur (fig. 9.15) recorded in patients with large left-to-right shunts probably represents increased flow across the mitral valve. Atrial-systolic murmurs also have been described in this condition and are usually associated with large ventricular septal defects with large left-to-right shunts. As pulmonary artery pressure increases the diastolic murmur becomes shorter and may disappear completely. Murmurs of pulmonic insufficiency are present in approximately 20–30% of patients with severe pulmonary hypertension. This murmur is usually due to dilatation of the pulmonary valve (figs. 9.14 and 9.15).

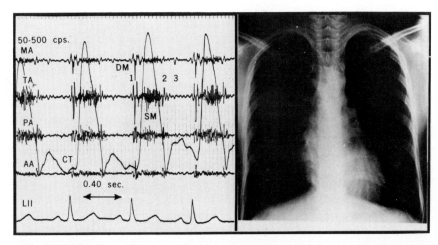

Fig. 9.13. Simultaneously recorded phonocardiogram at the mitral (MA), tricuspid (TA), pulmonic (PA) and aortic areas (AA) carotid pulse tracing (CT), and lead II (LII) of the electrocardiogram in a 12-year-old patient with a ventricular septal defect (left panel). The first and second heart sounds are normal. There is a low frequency third heart sound followed by a low frequency atrial ventricular diastolic murmur (DM) and a high frequency, high amplitude systolic regurgitant murmur (SM) which is recorded best at the tricuspid and pulmonic areas. The carotid pulse tracing is normal. The chest x-ray (right panel) shows a normal cardiac silhouette and slightly increased pulmonary vascular markings. At cardiac catheterization the patient had a large left-to-right shunt and normal pulmonary artery pressures.

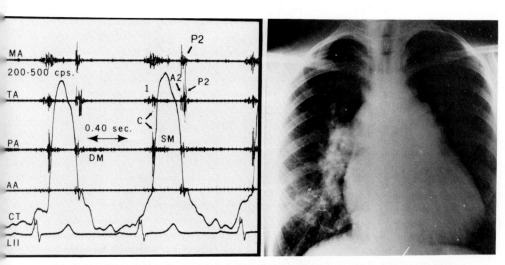

Fig. 9.14. Simultaneously recorded phonocardiogram at the mitral (MA), tricuspid (TA), pulmonic (PA) and aortic areas (AA), carotid pulse tracing (CT), and lead II (LII) of the electrocardiogram in a 23-year-old patient with a ventricular septal defect, small right-to-left shunt and severe pulmonary hypertension (left panel). The first heart sound is normal. The second heart sound has narrow splitting (A2-P2 interval, 0.03 sec) and the pulmonic component is markedly accentuated. The pulmonary valve closure sound is well recorded at the pulmonic and mitral areas which is usual in patients with a dilated right ventricle with or without associated pulmonary hypertension. A systolic ejection click (C) is followed by a short, high frequency, low amplitude systolic murmur (SM) recorded best at the pulmonic area. The carotid pulse tracing is normal. The chest x-ray (right panel) shows cardiomegaly with enlargement of the pulmonary artery and right atrium and decreased pulmonary blood flow.

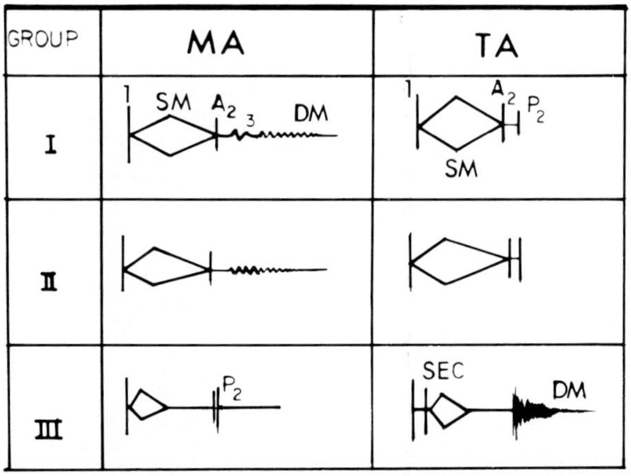

Fig. 9.15. Graphic representation of the phonocardiographic findings in patients with ventricular septal defect. (Group I) Phonocardiographic findings in patients with pulmonary artery pressures between 20 and 40% of systemic arterial pressure. In this group the systolic murmur occupies the entire duration of systole at the mitral (MA) and tricuspid areas (TA). A third heart sound at the mitral area is followed by a low frequency atrioventricular diastolic murmur (DM). The second heart sound is split by approximately 0.03 to 0.05 sec at the tricuspid area. (Group II) Phonocardiographic findings in patients with pulmonary artery pressures between 40 and 70% of the systemic arterial pressure. The systolic murmur (SM) at the mitral area has smaller amplitude. The third heart sound is absent and the atrioventricular diastolic murmur has decreased amplitude, and shorter duration. The splitting of the second heart sound is shorter at the tricuspid area. (Group III) Phonocardiographic findings in patients with pulmonary artery pressures exceeding 70% of the systemic arterial pressure. The pulmonic component of the second heart sound is well recorded at the mitral area. The third heart sound and atrioventricular diastolic murmur are absent. At the tricuspid area a systolic ejection click is recorded and an arterial diastolic murmur of pulmonary insufficiency is present.

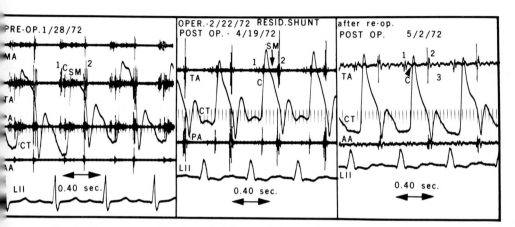

Fig. 9.16. Pre-operative phonocardiogram (left panel) recorded at the mitral (MA), tricuspid (TA), pulmonic (PA) and aortic areas (AA), carotid pulse tracing (CT), and lead II (LII) of the electrocardiogram in an 18-year-old patient with a ventricular septal defect and severe pulmonary hypertension. The normal first heart sound is followed by a systolic ejection click (C). After the click there is a high frequency, low amplitude systolic murmur (SM) which terminates during midsystole. The second heart sound is single and accentuated. Following closure of the ventricular septal defect (middle panel) the systolic ejection click is still recordable and the second heart sound is accentuated. The systolic murmur is not as prominent as it was in the pre-operative tracing. Post-operative cardiac catheterization revealed the presence of a residual left-to-right shunt at the ventricular level. The patient was re-operated and the second post-operative tracing (right panel) shows disappearance of the systolic murmur. The systolic ejection click and third heart sound are still present. The contour of the carotid pulse tracing is normal in all three recordings.

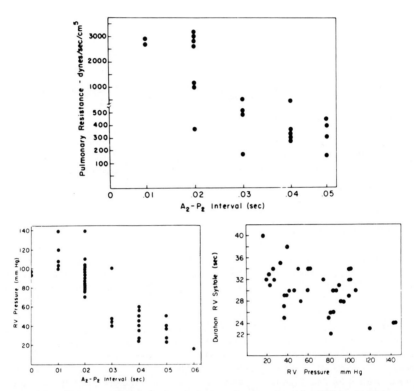

Fig. 9.17. (Top panel) Correlation between the duration of splitting of the second heart sound (A2-P2 interval) and pulmonary vascular resistance. With increased pulmonary vascular resistance the A2-P2 interval becomes quite short. (Lower left panel) Correlation of right ventricular pressure and splitting of the second heart sound. With the increase in right ventricular pressure the A2-P2 interval becomes quite short. (Lower right panel) Correlation of the duration of right ventricular systole with right ventricular pressure. As right ventricular pressure increases, right ventricular systole becomes shorter due to early closure of the pulmonic valve.

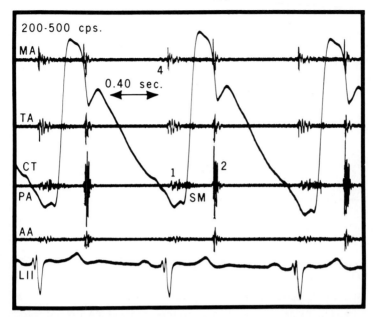

Fig. 9.18. Simultaneously recorded phonocardiogram at the mitral (MA), tricuspid (TA), pulmonic (PA) and aortic areas (AA), carotid pulse tracing (CT), and lead II (LII) of the electrocardiogram in a 39-year-old patient with a ventricular septal defect and severe pulmonary hypertension. The first heart sound is normal. The second heart sound is single and accentuated. A short, high frequency, early systolic murmur (SM) terminates during mid-systole. There is a faint fourth heart sound at the mitral area. The carotid pulse tracing shows a short ejection time due to decreased left ventricular stroke volume.

Carotid Pulse Tracing

The carotid pulse tracing has a normal contour in ventricular septal defects.

Jugular Venous Pulse Tracing

The jugular venous tracing is useful in identifying the degree of elevation of pulmonary artery pressure and resistance. If pulmonary artery pressure is normal, the jugular venous tracing is normal. With progressive increase in pulmonary pressure and resistance, the A wave becomes progressively larger. Giant A waves are seen only when the mean pulmonary artery pressure exceeds 80–100 mm Hg (fig. 9.19). They are due to abnormal, late right ventricular end-diastolic compliance requiring a forceful atrial contraction.

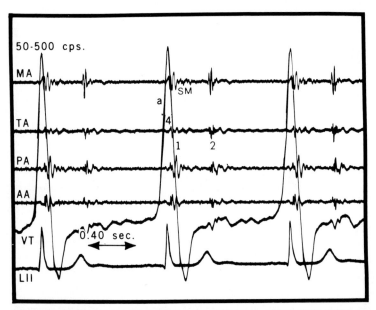

Fig. 9.19. Simultaneously recorded phonocardiogram at the mitral (MA), tricuspid (TA), pulmonic (PA) and aortic areas (AA), jugular venous tracing (VT), and lead II (LII) of the electrocardiogram in a 38-year-old patient who had a ventricular septal defect with a bidirectional shunt at the ventricular level and severe pulmonary hypertension. The first heart sound is normal. The second heart sound is single. A prominent fourth heart sound coincides with a very prominent A wave on the jugular venous tracing. There is also a faint third heart sound. A high frequency, low amplitude systolic murmur (SM) is recorded best at the mitral area.

Apexcardiogram

The apexcardiogram of the left ventricle may show slight exaggeration of the rapid filling wave with the peak coinciding with the third heart sound, but this may be a normal finding in young subjects with small left-to-right shunts (Roger type of ventricular septal defect) representing a normal physiologic third heart sound. The right ventricular apexcardiogram, recorded at the right sternal border near the fourth, left intercostal space or subxyphoid area is valuable in patients with large left-to-right shunts. It may show exaggeration of the A wave, a sustained systolic wave, and a diminished rapid filling wave if the left-to-right shunt is large and the patient has right ventricular hypertrophy.

Systolic Time Intervals

Systolic time intervals are not valuable in evaluating ventricular septal defects because definite abnormalities have not been described for the pre-ejection period or pre-ejection period-left ventricular ejection time ratio (PEP/LVET) in these patients.

Echocardiogram

Echocardiography has not been completely established as a diagnostic tool in evaluating patients with ventricular septal defect. In patients with normal pulmonary artery pressure and small left-to-right shunts, the pulmonic valve motion is normal and the A dip has normal amplitude in the range of 2–8 mm. In patients with moderate to severe pulmonary hypertension the pulmonic valve exhibits abnormal motion with a progressive decrease in amplitude of the A dip (fig. 9.20) or the A dip is absent. Abnormal systolic notching of the valve and a flat E–F slope are commonly seen. If a good recording of the tricuspid valve is obtained, one may detect a prolonged A-C interval. This technique is also useful to demonstrate an increase in left atrial and left ventricular internal diameters, particularly in patients with large left-to-right shunts. Left ventricular and right ventricular wall thickness are usually normal and interventricular septal motion is normal.

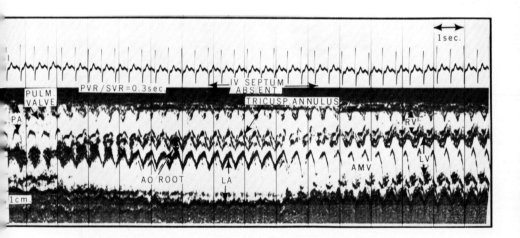

Fig. 9.20. Simultaneously recorded lead II (LII) of the electrocardiogram and echocardiographic scan from the pulmonary artery (PA) to the left ventricle (LV) in a 14-month-old patient with a large ventricular septal defect and pulmonary hypertension. Cardiac catheterization revealed a large left-to-right shunt at the interventricular level with pulmonary blood flow to systemic ratio of 4:1. Pulmonary vascular/systemic vascular resistance (PVR/SVR) was 0.3. The structure on the left of this illustration is a large pulmonary artery. The pulmonic valve has a small A dip. The left atrium (LA) is enlarged to 2.6 cm. The right ventricle (RV) is enlarged to 1.6 cm. Left ventricular internal dimension is increased to 3.4 cm. AMV = anterior mitral valve, LV = left ventricle, AO = aorta.

PRIMARY IDIOPATHIC PULMONARY HYPERTENSION

Primary or idiopathic pulmonary hypertension is a condition associated with marked increase in pulmonary artery pressure and resistance
with associated dilatation of the pulmonary artery. The etiology of this
condition is unknown. The phonocardiographic (fig. 9.21), auscultatory
features, pulse wave abnormalities, and echocardiographic features (fig.
9.22) in this condition are quite similar to the ones described in patients
with ventricular septal defects and pulmonary hypertension with Eise-
menger's syndrome (see "Ventricular Septal Defects").

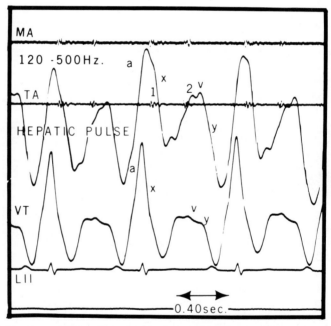

Fig. 9.21. Simultaneously recorded phonocardiogram at the mitral (MA), and
tricuspid areas (TA), hepatic pulse tracing, jugular venous pulse tracing (VT), and
lead II (LII) of the electrocardiogram in a 29-year-old patient with severe pulmonary
hypertension and tricuspid insufficiency. Note the prominent A waves in the jugular
venous and hepatic pulse tracings. In both pulse wave recordings the x descents are
small and prominent v waves are followed by rapid y descents. At cardiac catheterization the pulmonary artery pressures were identical to aortic pressures.

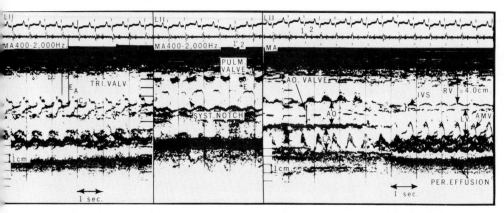

Fig. 9.22. Simultaneously recorded mitral area (MA) phonocardiogram, lead II (LII) of the electrocardiogram, and echocardiographic recording of the tricuspid and pulmonic valves with a scan from the aorta (AO) to the left ventricle (LV) in a 30-year-old patient with idiopathic pulmonary hypertension and marked elevation of right ventricular end-diastolic pressure to 18 mm Hg. The tricuspid (TRI) valve recording (left panel) demonstrates abnormal motion of the anterior tricuspid valve with prolongation of the A-C interval. Time of inscription of the first and second heart sounds is indicated. The pulmonic (PULM) valve recording (middle panel) shows abnormal motion which is indicated by the presence of a systolic (SYST) notch (flying W), flat E-F slope and an absent A dip. The scan from the aorta to the left ventricle (right panel) shows an increase in right ventricular (RV) dimension to 4 cm. A clear echo free space between the epicardium and posterior pericardium indicates the presence of pericardial effusion since this patient was in congestive heart failure. The aortic root and left atrium (LA) measure 2.6 cm. AMV = anterior mitral valve, IVS = interventricular septum.

PATENT DUCTUS ARTERIOSUS

Heart Sounds and Murmurs

The first heart sound is normal. The second heart sound is normal providing the patient has normal pulmonary artery pressure. If the second heart sound is split and there is associated pulmonary hypertension, the pulmonary component is accentuated and well transmitted to the aortic and mitral areas. Multiple high frequency systolic sounds are heard in mid- and/or late systole representing turbulent flow across the ductus arteriosus. This has been attributed to turbulent currents through the ductus. A third heart sound is present at the mitral area in patients with large left-to-right shunts with pulmonary systemic flow ratio exceeding 2:1.

Fourth heart sounds are rarely recorded. Systolic ejection clicks are present only in patients with severe pulmonary hypertension with or without reversal of the shunt. These patients have marked dilatation of the pulmonary arteries.

The auscultatory and phonocardiographic findings in patients with patent ductus arteriosus include the presence of a continuous machinery murmur throughout systole and diastole. This high frequency murmur starts immediately after the first heart sound, reaches maximal intensity at the time of the second heart sound, continues throughout diastole, and terminates at the time of atrial contraction (fig. 9.23). The murmur is heard best at the pulmonic or left infraclavicular area and is well transmitted to the spine. It is difficult to differentiate this murmur from those caused by arteriovenous fistula and aortic-pulmonary window, since they may also be continuous murmurs. The murmur of aortic pulmonary window, however, is usually loudest at the tricuspid area. In patients with patent ductus arteriosus and large left-to-right shunts, a low frequency, mid-diastolic rumbling murmur is heard at the mitral area corresponding to increased flow across the mitral valve. The murmur is usually preceded by a prominent third heart sound. As pulmonary artery pressure increases, there is a progressive diminution of the diastolic component of the machinery murmur and disappearance of the diastolic rumble and the third heart sound. Further increase in the pulmonary artery pressures and resistance may cause disappearance of the systolic ejection murmur (silent patent ductus arteriosus). The murmur of pulmonic insufficiency is seen in only a few cases in the late stage of the natural history of this disease and is due to dilatation of the pulmonary valve.

Carotid Pulse Tracing

The carotid pulse tracing may show the same features described in patients with aortic insufficiency, consisting of a rapid upstroke time, midsystolic retraction followed by a late systolic bulge and sharp downward displacement of the dicrotic notch. A large, early diastolic wave may be present (dicrotic pulse).

Jugular Venous Pulse Tracing

The jugular venous pulse tracing is normal in patients with normal pulmonary artery pressures. With elevated pulmonary and right ventricular pressures, the A wave becomes quite prominent.

Apexcardiogram

The apexcardiogram shows a normal E point and normal systolic wave. In the presence of left ventricular hypertrophy, seen in patients with large left-to-right shunts, the systolic wave is round and sustained throughout systole. The rapid filling wave is prominent when the

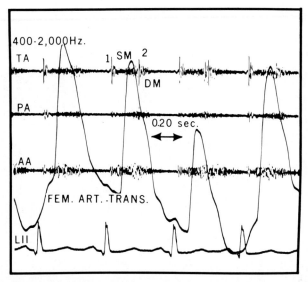

Fig. 9.23. Simultaneously recorded phonocardiogram at the tricuspid (TA), pulmonic (PA) and aortic areas (AA), transcutaneous femoral artery tracing, and lead II (LII) of the electrocardiogram in an 8-month-old patient with patent ductus arteriosus and a large left-to-right shunt. A high frequency, high amplitude, continuous machinery murmur seen in all precordial areas is recorded best at the pulmonic and aortic areas. This murmur starts shortly after the first heart sound, reaches a maximal peak at the level of the second heart sound, continues through diastole and terminates prior to atrial systole. DM = diastolic murmur, SM = systolic murmur.

pulmonic to systemic flow ratio exceeds 2:1 reflecting left ventricular diastolic overloading. The A wave is normal.

Systolic Time Intervals

The systolic time intervals are of no diagnostic value in patients with patent ductus arteriosus.

Echocardiogram

Echocardiography has not been established as a diagnostic tool in patients with patent ductus arteriosus. However, in these infants and children one usually detects an increase in left atrial internal dimension as compared with the aortic root (fig. 9.24). This is usually seen in patients with large left-to-right shunts. Reports have indicated that serial echocardiograms obtained in these patients may demonstrate a progressive increase in left atrial size which appears to be related to progressive increase in the left-to-right shunt through the ductus.

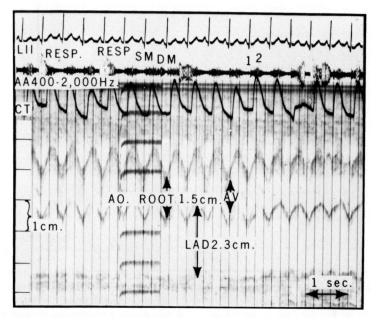

Fig. 9.24. Simultaneously recorded echocardiogram, aortic area (AA) phonocardiogram, carotid pulse tracing (CT), and lead II (LII) of the electrocardiogram in an 8-month-old patient with patent ductus arteriosus with a pulmonary systemic flow ratio exceeding 2:1. The tracing shows an enlarged left atrium (2.3 cm) and a normal aortic root (1.5 cm). Respiratory (RESP) artifacts on the phonocardiogram are indicated. Systolic (SM) and diastolic (DM) murmurs are recorded on the phonocardiogram. LAD = left atrial diameter, AV = aortic valve, AO = aorta.

However, caution must be exercised in the interpretation of these findings since an increase in the left atrial diameter can be seen in patients with respiratory distress syndrome. Spontaneous or surgical closure of the ductus will result in a decrease in left atrial size. Since the echocardiographic findings are non-specific for this particular lesion, it is important that an increase in left atrial size be correlated with all of the previously described non-invasive techniques to study the disease state.

COARCTATION OF THE AORTA

Heart Sounds and Murmurs

The first heart sound is normal. The second heart sound may be single or split. Paradoxical splitting of the second heart sound is seen in about 10% of paients with coarctation of the aorta due to delayed emptying of the left ventricle. The aortic component of the second heart sound is accentuated due to an increase in aortic pressures.

A systolic ejection murmur with maximal intensity in mid-systole is often heard best at the level of the thoracic spine and the left upper chest at the sternal area. The murmur may extend through the aortic component of the second heart sound terminating in early diastole. This murmur represents turbulent flow across the coarctation segment of the aorta (fig. 9.25). Patients with severe coarctation of the aorta and a marked degree of collateral circulation through the intercostal arteries may exhibit a continuous high frequency machinery type murmur with maximum intensity at the time of the second heart sound. This murmur is due to increased flow through dilated collateral circulation. Arterial diastolic murmurs of aortic insufficiency heard in approximately 35% of patients with coarctation of the aorta are related to the presence of an insufficient bicuspid aortic valve.

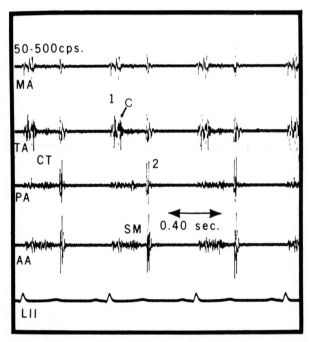

Fig. 9.25. Simultaneously recorded phonocardiogram at the mitral (MA), tricuspid (TA), pulmonic (PA) and aortic areas (AA), and lead II (LII) of the electrocardiogram in a 10-year-old patient with coarctation of the aorta. The first heart sound is normal. The second heart sound is single and accentuated due to increased amplitude of the aortic valve closure sound. A systolic ejection click (C) is followed by a high frequency, low amplitude systolic ejection murmur (SM) which terminates prior to the second heart sound.

Carotid Pulse Tracing

The carotid pulse tracing is not diagnostic in patients with coarctation of the aorta except to rule out the possibility of associated aortic valve disease. Recording of the peripheral arterial pulses, especially the femoral artery pulse tracing compared with the carotid pulse tracing, shows a delay in the upstroke time of the transcutaneous femoral pulse tracing, which exceeds the normal delay of 0.09 sec. The contour of the femoral artery pulse tracing is essentially identical to the one described in patients with aortic valvular stenosis (see Chapter 5).

Jugular Venous Pulse Tracing

The jugular venous pulse tracing is non-diagnostic in this condition.

Apexcardiogram

The apexcardiogram frequently shows a prominent A wave usually exceeding 15% of the total amplitude of the apexcardiogram (E through

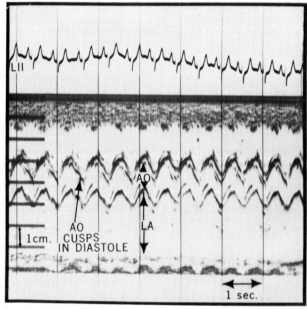

Fig. 9.26. Simultaneously recorded lead II (LII) of the electrocardiogram and echocardiogram in a 14-month-old patient with coarctation of the aorta, patent ductus arteriosus, and associated bicuspid aortic (AO) valve. Note the eccentrically located diastolic aortic valve echoes, probably related to the presence of bicuspid aortic valve. The aorta measures 1.4 cm. The enlarged left atrium (3.5 cm) supports the diagnosis of a significant left-to-right shunt through the patent ductus arteriosus. The aortic valve measures 1 cm which is within normal limits.

O amplitude). A sustained systolic wave representing left ventricular hypertrophy may be seen in patients with severe coarctation of the aorta.

Systolic Time Intervals

Systolic time intervals have no value in the diagnosis of patients with coarctation of the aorta.

Echocardiogram

No definite abnormalities have been described usng echocardiography in patients with coarctation of the aorta unless the patient has an associated bicuspid aortic valve (fig 9.26) or aortic insufficiency, in which case the findings are identical to the ones seen in those conditions.

PULMONARY VALVULAR STENOSIS

Heart Sounds and Murmurs

The first heart sound is normal and is usually followed by a systolic ejection click which grossly correlates with post-stenotic dilatation of the pulmonary artery and the distorted structure of the pulmonary valve. The time inverval between the first heart sound and the systolic ejection click is a gross indicator of the gradient across the pulmonic valve. The shorter the first sound-click interval, the higher the gradient across the pulmonic valve. An ejection click is present in only 10–15% of patients with pulmonary infundibular stenosis, and this finding may be useful to differentiate valvular from infundibular stenosis (see "Tetralogy of Fallot").

The second heart sound is important in assessing the presence and degree of severity of pulmonary valvular stenosis. This sound is widely split and fixed; the pulmonic component is diminished in proportion to the degree of stenosis and may be absent in approximately 20% of patients with gradients exceeding 80–100 mm Hg (figs. 9.27–9.29). The aortic valve closure sound is normal. The time interval between the aortic closure sound-pulmonary closure sound (A2-P2 interval) is grossly proportional to the gradient across the stenotic pulmonic valve. The longer the A2-P2 interval, the greater the gradient across the valve, as shown in figure 9.28. Third heart sounds are rare. Fourth heart sounds are part of the auscultatory and phonocardiographic findings in this condition and they do not always correlate with the degree of severity of the stenotic lesion.

The murmur of pulmonary valvular stenosis is characteristically a high frequency, noisy systolic ejection murmur having maximal intensity in mid- or late systole. This murmur is best heard at the pulmonic and tricuspid areas. Timing of the peak of this murmur is grossly proportional to the gradient across the valve. With gradients exceeding 80 mm

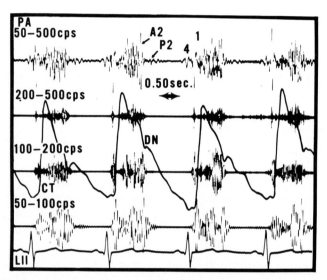

Fig. 9.27. Simultaneously recorded phonocardiogram at the pulmonic (PA) area with a wide band filter at 50–500 cycles per second (CPS). The output of that amplifier was connected into the input of three additional phonocardiographic amplifiers to record tracings at 200–500, 100–200, and 50–100 cps. The tracings were recorded with a carotid pulse tracing (CT) and lead II (LII) of the electrocardiogram. The first heart sound is normal. There is a prominent fourth heart sound and a high frequency, high amplitude systolic ejection murmur with a late systolic peak which terminates at the time of aortic valve closure. The A2-P2 interval is markedly prolonged to 0.08 sec and the pulmonic component of the second heart sound is markedly diminished. The high frequency characteristics of the murmur are best appreciated in the recording at 200–500 cps. The carotid pulse tracing is normal. DN = dicrotic notch.

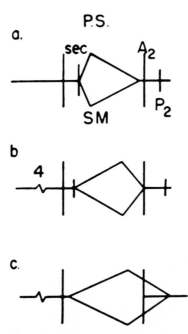

Fig. 9.28. Diagrammatic representation of a group of patients with pulmonary valvular stenosis. (a) Phonocardiographic findings in patients with a mild degree of pulmonary valvular stenosis. The first heart sound is normal and is followed by a systolic ejection click (sec). After the click there is a high amplitude systolic ejection murmur (SM) with an early to mid-systolic peak which terminates prior to aortic valve closure. The second heart sound is split and the pulmonic component is diminished. In this group the gradient across the pulmonic valve is in the range of 20–50 mm Hg. (b) Patients with a moderate degree of pulmonary valvular stenosis with a gradient across the pulmonary valve between 60 and 80 mm Hg. A fourth heart sound is present. The systolic ejection click is inscribed close to the first heart sound. The systolic murmur has a late systolic peak and terminates with the aortic valve closure sound. The A2-P2 interval is increased as compared with group a. (c) Patients with severe pulmonary valvular stenosis with gradients exceeding 80 mm Hg. A fourth heart sound is present. The systolic ejection click may be absent or was recorded simultaneously with the first heart sound. The murmur has a late systolic peak and continues through the aortic component of the second heart sound. The pulmonic component of the second heart sound is usually absent.

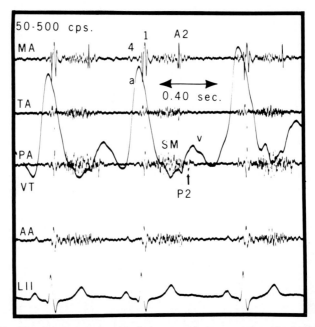

Fig. 9.29. Simultaneously recorded phonocardiogram at the mitral (MA), tricuspid (TA), pulmonic (PA) and aortic areas (AA), jugular venous pulse tracing (VT), and lead II (LII) of the electrocardiogram in a 7-year-old patient with severe pulmonary valvular stenosis. The first heart sound is normal. The second heart sound is widely split. The aortic valve closure sound is normal. The pulmonic valve closure sound is markedly diminished and the A2-P2 interval is prolonged to 0.05 sec. There is a high frequency, high amplitude systolic ejection murmur (SM) with maximal intensity near the second heart sound. The jugular venous tracing shows a marked increase in amplitude of the A wave. The X and Y descents are normal.

Hg the murmur has late systolic accentuation continuing through the aortic valve closure sound and terminating with P2. This murmur, at times, is well transmitted to the carotid arteries. Diastolic murmurs are not heard in this condition.

Carotid Pulse Tracing

The carotid pulse contour is normal. However, recording of the pulse wave is useful as a reference tracing to identify the component of the splitting of the second heart sound.

Jugular Venous Pulse Tracing

The jugular venous pulse tracing is of important diagnostic value in pulmonary stenosis. The A wave increases in amplitude in proportion to the increased pressures in the right ventricle. In very severe forms of pulmonary valvular stenosis, the A wave becomes extremely prominent with A/V ratio exceeding 3 (normal 1.5:1). In mild forms of pulmonary valvular stenosis, the jugular venous tracing may be normal.

Apexcardiogram

The apexcardiogram of the left ventricle is of no value in the diagnosis of pulmonary valvular stenosis. However, in many patients the right ventricular impulse can be recorded. In mild forms of pulmonary valvular stenosis, the right ventricular impulse recorded near the tricuspid area may show a normal systolic retraction and a small A wave. However, in patients with severe pulmonary stenosis and associated right ventricular hypertrophy, the A wave of the right ventricular apexcardiogram becomes quite prominent, the systolic retraction is absent, and there is a sustained systolic wave. The rapid filling wave of the right ventricular apexcardiogram becomes inconspicuous or absent, indicating decreased left ventricular early diastolic compliance.

Systolic Time intervals

Systolic time intervals are of no value in the diagnosis of pulmonary valvular stenosis.

Maneuvers and Pharmacologic Agents

Inhalation of amyl nitrite usually causes an increase in amplitude of the systolic ejection murmur. This is probably related to an increase in venous return resulting in an increased right ventricular stroke volume and increased gradient across the stenotic pulmonary valve. This pharmacologic test is useful in the differential diagnosis between isolated pulmonary stenosis and tetralogy of Fallot. In the latter condition, the systolic murmur decreases in intensity during inhalation of this agent. The systolic murmur decreases during Valsalva maneuver as shown in figure 9.30.

Echocardiogram

Echocardiography is of some value in the diagnosis of pulmonary valvular stenosis. Two of the three cusps of the pulmonic valve are usually recorded in infants but are sometimes difficult to record in children. Definite diagnostic criteria for pulmonary valvular stenosis by echocardiography has not been established. Anatomical fusion of the pulmonic cusps results in a doming effect of the valve (figs. 9.31 and 9.32) and the separation of the cusps cannot be used as diagnostic criteria for determination of the severity of pulmonary valvular stenosis. A forceful atrial contraction against a non-distensible right ventricle and rigid

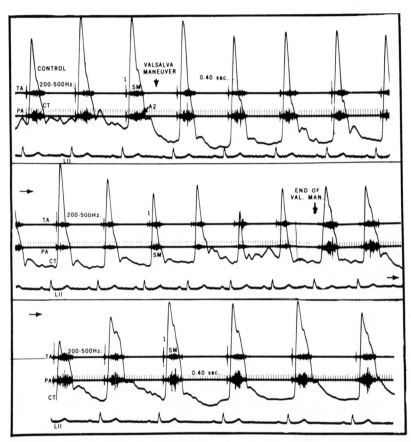

Fig. 9.30. Simultaneously recorded phonocardiogram at the tricuspid (TA) and pulmonic areas (PA) before (upper panel), during (middle panel) and after Valsalva maneuver (VAL. MAN), carotid pulse tracing (CT), and lead II (LII) of the electrocardiogram in a 34-year-old patient with pulmonary valvular stenosis. In the control tracing, note the presence of a high frequency, high amplitude systolic ejection murmur (SM) recorded in both precordial areas. The murmur decreases significantly during the Valsalva maneuver and increases in amplitude immediately afterward. The contour of the carotid pulse tracing is normal. The tracings were recorded continuously prior to, during and after the maneuver.

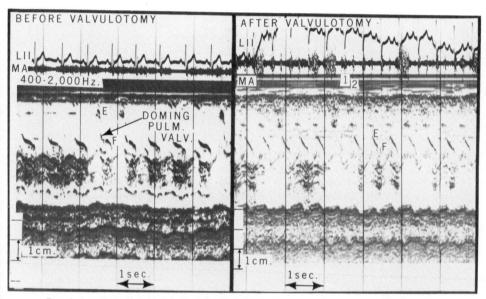

Fig. 9.31. Simultaneously recorded echocardiogram, mitral area (MA) phonocardiogram, and lead II (LII) of the electrocardiogram in a 5-year-old patient with pulmonary valvular stenosis. The recording prior to pulmonary valvulotomy (left panel) shows abnormal doming of the pulmonic valve. After valvulotomy (right panel) doming of the pulmonic valve is no longer present.

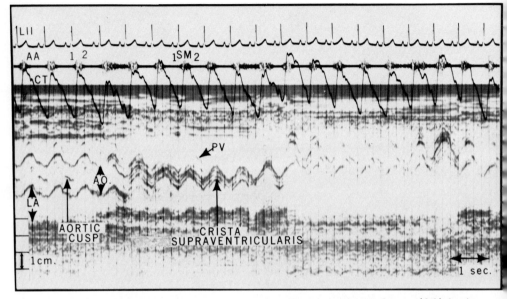

Fig. 9.32. Simultaneously recorded phonocardiogram at the aortic area (AA), lead II (LII) of the electrocardiogram, carotid pulse tracing (CT), and echocardiographic scan from the left atrium (LA) to the pulmonary valve (PV) in a 5-year-old patient with severe pulmonary valvular stenosis. The pulmonary valve structure has a doming appearance. The crista supraventricularis has increased thickness. The aortic root dimension is 1.65 cm, left atrial internal dimension (LA) is 2 cm, and the aortic valve opening (AO) is 1.3 cm. These measurements are all normal.

pulmonic valve may cause the stenotic pulmonic valve to move. This presystolic excursion of the valve called A dip or A motion usually exceeds the normal 2–8 mm of deflection. When this occurs, the gradient across the pulmonic valve is usually above 40–60 mm Hg. The more severe the stenosis, the greater the excursion of the A dip. Great caution must be exercised in interpreting this finding because some patients with moderately severe pulmonary stenosis may show normal excursion of the pulmonic valve at the time of the atrial contraction.

PULMONARY ARTERY STENOSIS

In patients with peripheral pulmonary artery stenosis, the stenotic lesion can be single or multiple and can involve either the right or left pulmonary artery, or both. The phonocardiographic and pulse wave abnormalities are somewhat similar to the ones described in patients with pulmonary valvular stenosis with a few exceptions. The first heart sound is normal. Systolic ejection clicks are rare and the second heart sound is normal. If it is split both components are of normal amplitude. Systolic ejection murmurs are best heard at the second or third intercostal space close to the anterior axillary line, either on the right or left depending on the anatomical location of the stenosis. This murmur has a tendency to radiate toward the spine. The carotid pulse tracing, apexcardiogram, and systolic time intervals are of no value in this condition. The jugular venous tracing may show an exaggerated A wave if right ventricular pressure is elevated.

Echocardiogram

No definite echocardiographic features have been described for this condition, although one might expect normal motion of the pulmonic valve instead of the abnormal features described for patients with pulmonary valvular stenosis.

TETRALOGY OF FALLOT

Heart Sounds and Murmurs

The first heart sound is normal. The second heart sound is single and accentuated due to aortic valve closure. The pulmonary valve closure sound is usually absent (figs. 9.33 and 9.34). Accentuation of the aortic valve closure sound is due to a large aortic stroke volume secondary to the right-to-left shunt. Systolic ejection clicks are rare in this condition but are heard in about 5–10% of cases particularly in patients with dilated ascending aortas. Third heart sounds are also rare. Fourth heart sounds, part of the normal auscultatory findings, are of no diagnostic value in assessing the severity of the stenotic lesion. In tetralogy of Fallot, the obstructive disease is located in the infundibular tract of the right ventricle in about 85% of patients. Combinations of infundibular and pulmonary valvular stenosis may cause auscultatory findings similar to those described in patients with pulmonary valvular stenosis.

Systolic, high frequency ejection murmurs are heard best at the level of the third left intercostal space (figs. 9.33–9.35). The murmur starts shortly after the first heart sound, has a maximal peak in early systole and terminates in the last third of systole. The murmur is due to turbulent flow across the infundibular stenosis and not through the ventricular septal defect. Diastolic murmurs are not present unless the patient has prominent bronchial artery collateral circulation therefore causing a continuous murmur which is heard at multiple areas over the precordium or has been subjected to operative correction (figs. 9.35–9.38).

Carotid Pulse Tracing

The carotid pulse tracing is normal in patients with tetralogy of Fallot.

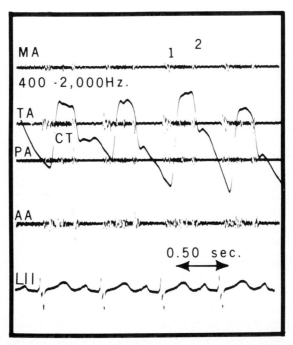

Fig. 9.33. Simultaneously recorded phonocardiogram at the mitral (MA), tricuspid (TA), pulmonic (PA) and aortic areas (AA), carotid pulse tracing (CT), and lead II (LII) of the electrocardiogram in a 5-year-old patient with tetralogy of Fallot. The first heart sound is normal. The second heart sound is single and accentuated and is due to aortic valve closure. A high frequency, medium amplitude systolic murmur begins with the first heart sound and terminates prior to the second heart sound. The murmur is recorded well in all precordial areas but is most prominent at the pulmonic and aortic areas. The carotid pulse tracing is normal.

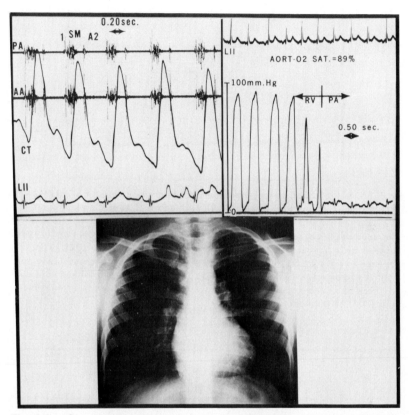

Fig. 9.34. Simultaneously recorded phonocardiogram at the pulmonic (PA) and aortic areas (AA), carotid pulse tracing (CT), and lead II (LII) of the electrocardiogram (upper left panel) in a 6-year-old patient with tetralogy of Fallot. The first heart sound is normal. The second heart sound is single and accentuated and is due to aortic valve closure. A high frequency, short, high amplitude systolic murmur (SM) with maximal intensity in early systole terminates in the middle third of systole. The carotid pulse tracing is normal. The continuous recording of pressure curves from the right ventricle (RV) to the pulmonary artery (PA) (upper right panel) demonstrates a gradient between the inflow tract and outflow tract of the right ventricle and a gradient between the outflow tract and the pulmonary artery indicating the presence of infundibular and pulmonary valvular stenosis. Aortic oxygen saturation was 89%, due to a right-to-left shunt at the ventricular level. The chest x-ray (lower panel) shows right ventricular prominence and decreased pulmonary vascular markings.

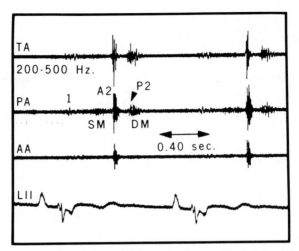

Fig. 9.35. Simultaneously recorded phonocardiogram at the mitral (MA), tricuspid (TA), pulmonic (PA) and aortic areas (AA), and lead II (LII) of the electrocardiogram in a 42-year-old patient who was subjected to total correction of tetralogy of Fallot and has mild degree of residual pulmonary insufficiency. The normal first heart sound is followed by a high frequency, low amplitude systolic murmur (SM). The second heart sound is widely split by 0.12 sec. The aortic component is accentuated and the pulmonic component is markedly diminished. Following the pulmonary valve closure sound there is a high frequency, medium amplitude decrescendo arterial diastolic murmur (DM) of pulmonary insufficiency.

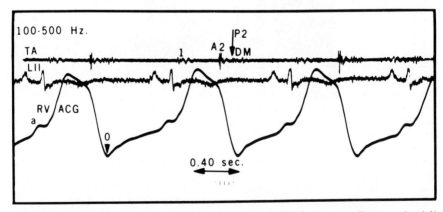

Fig. 9.36. Simultaneously recorded tricuspid area (TA) phonocardiogram, lead II (LII) of the electrocardiogram, and right ventricular apexcardiogram (RV ACG) in a 42-year-old patient after surgical correction of tetralogy of Fallot. The patient had a mild degree of pulmonic insufficiency. A diastolic murmur (DM) of pulmonic insufficiency is well delineated. The right ventricular apexcardiogram shows a small A wave and a sustained systolic wave, and small rapid filling wave of the type seen in patients with right ventricular hypertrophy.

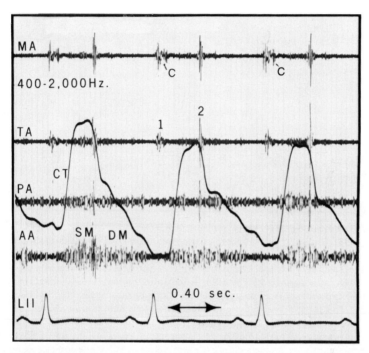

Fig. 9.37. Simultaneously recorded phonocardiogram at the mitral (MA), tricuspid (TA), pulmonic (PA) and aortic areas (AA), carotid pulse tracing (CT), and lead II (LII) of the electrocardiogram in a 21-year-old patient with tetralogy of Fallot who was subjected to a Blalock shunt procedure (right subclavian artery to pulmonary artery anastomosis). The normal first heart sound is followed by a systolic ejection click (C) which is best recorded at the mitral area. A high frequency, high amplitude continuous murmur recorded best at the aortic area represents systolic and diastolic flow from the Blalock shunt procedure. The carotid pulse tracing is normal. SM = systolic murmur, DM = diastolic murmur.

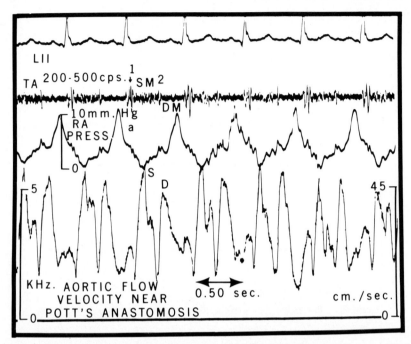

Fig. 9.38. Simultaneously recorded tricuspid area (TA) phonocardiogram, lead II (LII) of the electrocardiogram, right atrial pressure curve (RA PRESS), and aortic flow velocity measured with the Doppler flowmeter catheter technique in a 22-year-old patient with tetralogy of Fallot and Pott's (aorta-pulmonary artery) anastomosis. The flowmeter catheter tip was located near the Pott's anastomosis. The first heart sound is normal. The second heart sound is single. There is a high frequency, low amplitude systolic murmur (SM) and a high frequency decrescendo diastolic murmur (DM). The right atrial pressure curve demonstrates a prominent A wave. The aortic flow velocity curve demonstrates a major systolic (S) and diastolic (D) wave indicative of a large shunt through the anastomosis during systole and diastole.

Jugular Venous Pulse Tracing

The jugular venous pulse usually shows a prominent A wave but not to the extent seen in patients with moderate to severe isolated pulmonary valvular stenosis.

Apexcardiogram

The apexcardiogram of the right ventricle may show a sustained systolic wave with diminished rapid filling wave and a slightly prominent A wave due to right ventricular hypertrophy.

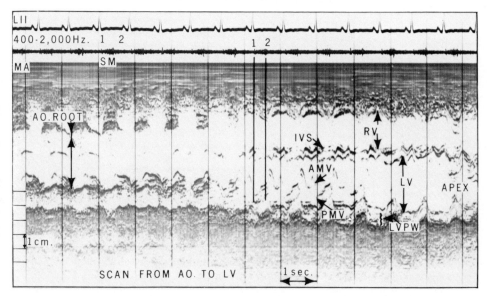

Fig. 9.39. Simultaneously recorded echocardiogram, mitral area (MA) phonocardiogram, and lead II (LII) of the electrocardiogram in a 25-year-old patient with tetralogy of Fallot. The echocardiographic scan from the aorta (AO) to the left ventricle (LV) shows the aortic root overriding the interventricular septum (IVS). The right ventricular (RV) dimension is increased to 3.5 cm, the aortic root is dilated and measures 4 cm. The left atrium has a normal dimension of 1.7 cm and left ventricular (LV) dimension is also normal at 4 cm. The interventricular septum and posterior wall of the left ventricle (LVPW) are normal, measuring 0.9 cm. AMV = anterior mitral valve, PMV = posterior mitral valve.

Echocardiogram

Echocardiographic features in tetralogy of Fallot include demonstration of the anatomical discontinuity of the interventricular septum (figs. 9.39 and 9.40) in relation to the anterior aortic wall. This corresponds to what is usually described as overriding of the aorta. There is a continuity between the mitral annulus and the posterior aortic wall. Because of the increase in right ventricular pressure and subsequent right ventricular hypertrophy which are present in this condition, the recording may demonstrate an increase in thickness of the right ventricular anterior wall, and the outflow tract of the right ventricle may be small. Recording of the pulmonic valve is technically difficult. When obtained, it helps in the differential diagnosis between tetralogy of Fallot and truncus arteriosus.

Some of the echocardiographic features described above for patients with tetralogy of Fallot are also seen in patients with truncus arteriosus (see below under "Truncus Arteriosus"). Additional echocardiographic

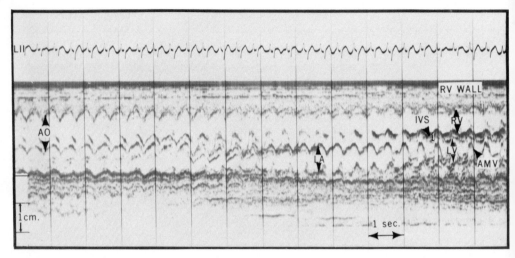

Fig. 9.40. Simultaneously recorded lead II (LII) of the electrocardiogram and echocardiographic scan from the aorta (AO) to the left ventricle (LV) in a 5-day-old infant with pseudo truncus arteriosus (tetralogy of Fallot with pulmonary atresia). The echocardiographic findings include absence of the pulmonic valve and discontinuity of the interventricular septum (IVS) and anterior aortic wall. The right ventricle (RV) is enlarged to 1.3 cm. Note that the posterior wall of the aorta is in continuity with the anterior mitral valve (AMV) leaflet. The aortic root measures 1 cm and the left atrial (LA) internal dimension is 0.9 cm.

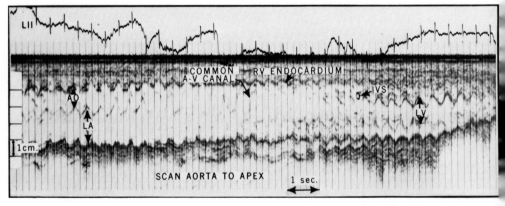

Fig. 9.41. Simultaneously recorded echocardiogram and lead II (LII) of the electrocardiogram in a 1-week-old infant with tetralogy of Fallot and associated atrioventricular (A-V) canal. The common atrioventricular canal is seen on the scan from the aorta (AO) to the apex of the left ventricle (LV). The common atrioventricular valve has a wide excursion and protrudes through the interventricular septum (IVS). At the level of the apex of the heart the motion of the interventricular septum is normal. The aortic root and aortic valve opening have normal values of 1.5 and 1.1 cm respectively. The left atrium (LA) is enlarged to 2 cm.

features in patients with tetralogy of Fallot include an enlarged aorta, a thickened right ventricular septum and right ventricular anterior wall and occasionally dilatation of the right ventricle. In severe forms of tetralogy of Fallot with marked decrease in size of the pulmonary artery, also called pseudo truncus, one may not identify the small segments of the pulmonic valve which is almost atretic in this condition. Patients with tetralogy of Fallot may also present with associated atrioventricular canal as shown in figure 9.41. Patients with tetralogy of Fallot can be subjected to a number of operative procedures which include creation of a right subclavian artery-pulmonary artery anastomosis (Blalock procedure), aortic-pulmonary artery anastomosis (Potts procedure), or total correction of the lesion. The palliative shunt procedure at times can cause large left-to-right shunts and some of these patients may develop heart failure. Echocardiography is useful to detect progressive enlargement of the left atrium in these patients.

TRILOGY OF FALLOT

Trilogy of Fallot consists of pulmonary stenosis with an atrial septal defect and a right-to-left shunt at the atrial level. The auscultatory, phonocardiographic and pulse wave abnormalities are essentially identical to those described in patients with pulmonary valvular stenosis.

TRUNCUS ARTERIOSUS

This congenital disease consists of an arterial trunk which receives blood from the right and left ventricles. A ventricular septal defect is almost always associated with this condition. The pulmonary arteries arise from this common trunk.

Heart Sounds and Murmurs

The first heart sound is single or slightly accentuated. The second heart sound is also single because of the presence of a single truncal valve. The third heart sound is usually present and probably due to a large volume diastolic loading of the ventricles. A systolic ejection click is present in approximately 15% of patients with a common trunk.

Patients with truncus arteriosus usually present with a systolic ejection murmur which is probably secondary to a high turbulent flow across the large truncus, and an arterial diastolic murmur representing truncal valve insufficiency. Continuous machinery murmurs are rare but have been found in patients with large pulmonary blood flow.

Carotid Pulse Tracing

The carotid pulse tracing is of no value in the diagnosis of this condition.

Jugular Venous Pulse Tracing

The jugular venous tracing usually shows an increase in the amplitude of the A wave.

Apexcardiogram

The apexcardiogram on these infants is difficult to record. If a tracing is obtained, one usually sees a sustained systolic wave and a prominent rapid filling wave.

Systolic Time Intervals

The systolic time intervals are of no value in the diagnosis of this condition.

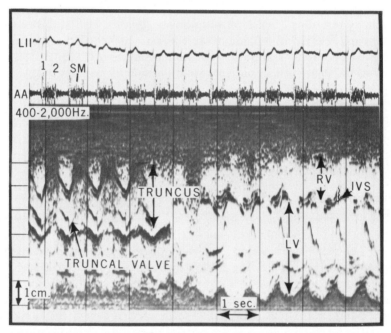

Fig. 9.42. Simultaneously recorded aortic area (AA) phonocardiogram, lead II (LII) of the electrocardiogram, and echocardiogram in a 5-year-old patient with truncus arteriosus. Note the large truncus and the truncal valve. The anterior wall of the truncus overrides the interventricular septum (IVS). The aortic root measures 1.9 cm; aortic valve 1.3 cm; left atrial internal dimension, 2.5 cm; left ventricular (LV) internal dimension, 3.7 cm. On the phonocardiogram the first heart sound is normal. The second heart sound is single and accentuated. There is a high frequency, high amplitude systolic regurgitant murmur (SM). RV = right ventricle.

Echocardiogram

The echocardiographic features of patients with truncus arteriosus are somewhat similar to the ones seen in patients with tetralogy of Fallot (fig. 9.42). Discontinuity of the anterior truncus wall and the interventricular septum is frequently present. The pulmonic valve is not recorded and there is an increase in right ventricular wall thickness. This condition may be difficult to differentiate from patients with tetralogy of Fallot.

TRANSPOSITION OF GREAT VESSELS (SITUS SOLITUS)

Transposition of the great vessels is a condition in which the pulmonary artery and aorta have abnormal origins and positions. The pulmonary artery arises from the left ventricle and is posteriorly located and the aorta is anterior and arises from the right ventricle. The auscultatory and phonocardiographic findings are not specific and they reflect the associated malformations such as ventricular septal defect, atrial septal defect, etc. As a result, the abnormalities of the heart sounds, murmurs, and pulse waves are somewhat similar to the ones described in those conditions. The first heart sound is normal. The second heart sound is split and the pulmonic component is accentuated. A high frequency, medium amplitude systolic murmur with maximal intensity in early or mid-systole is commonly seen (fig. 9.43). Atrioventricular diastolic murmurs representing increased rate of flow across the mitral valve are also frequently present.

Echocardiogram

In this congenital heart disease, the aortic valve is located to the right, the pulmonary valve leftward and inferiorly. However, echocardiograms of this condition must be recorded with caution and transducer angulation is very important. The transducer should be placed at the fourth left intercostal space, and directed posteriorly in an attempt to record both aortic and pulmonic valves simultaneously. Recording of both semilunar valves with this transducer location is difficult in normal individuals but occurs in most cases of D-transposition. Continuity of the posterior semilunar valve and the posterior wall vessel is not always helpful in the diagnosis of this congenital malformation, since this finding can be seen in normal patients. The posterior semilunar valve opens earlier in patients with transposition of the great vessels; therefore, simultaneous timing of the opening of the two valves is important in the diagnosis of this disease since the pulmonary valve almost always opens earlier and closes later than the aortic valve when pulmonary resistance is normal. Additional echocardiographic findings in this condition are an increase in right ventricular wall thickness and an increase in intracavitary diameter

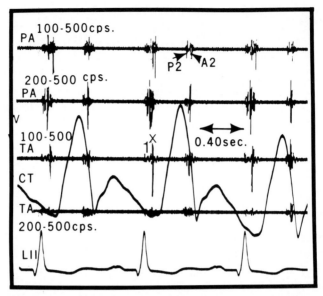

Fig. 9.43. Simultaneously recorded phonocardiogram at the pulmonic (PA) and tricuspid areas (TA) at bandpass filter settings of 100–500 cycles per second (cps) and 200–500 cps, carotid pulse tracing (CT) and lead II (LII) of the electrocariodgram in a 22-year-old patient with transposition of the great vessels. The first heart sound is normal. The second heart sound has paradoxical splitting and both components precede the dicrotic notch of the carotid pulse tracing. A high frequency vibration which occurs shortly after the first heart sound probably represents a systolic ejection click. The contour of the carotid pulse tracing is normal.

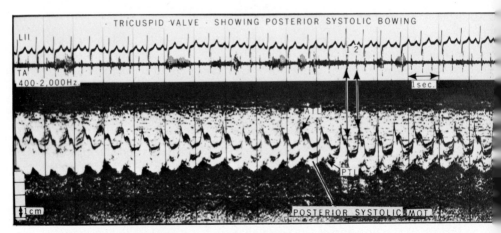

Fig. 9.44. Simultaneously recorded tricuspid area (TA) phonocardiogram, lead II (LII) of the electrocardiogram, and echocardiogram in a 6-year-old patient who was subjected to a Mustard procedure (intra-atrial baffle) for correction of transposition of the great vessels. Note abnormal motion of the tricuspid valve which exhibits posterior systolic bowing. ATL = anterior tricuspid leaflet, PTL = posterior tricuspid leaflet.

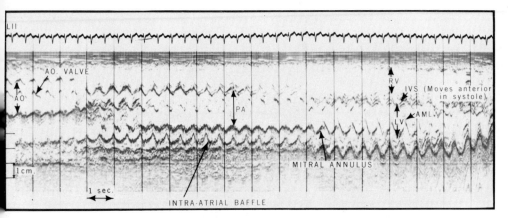

Fig. 9.45. Simultaneously recorded lead II (LII) of the electrocardiogram and echocardiographic scan from the aortic valve to the mitral valve in a 3-year-old patient with transposition of the great vessels who was subjected to a Mustard procedure. The scan shows increased right ventricular (RV) diameter of 2.2 cm and a dilated pulmonary artery (PA) to 2.5 cm. The multiple echoes at the atrial level are intra-atrial baffle echoes. The mitral annulus is well recorded. The interventricular septum (IVS) has paradoxical motion. Left ventricular (LV) internal dimension is approximately 3 cm and the aorta (AO) measures 2 cm.

of the left atrium and left ventricle secondary to a large left-to-right shunt. When these patients are subjected to palliative procedures for correction of this condition, they may present with abnormal echocardiograms as shown in figures 9.44 and 9.45.

CORRECTED TRANSPOSITION OF GREAT VESSELS

In patients with corrected transposition of the great vessels, the aorta originates from the anatomical right ventricle and the pulmonary artery from the anatomical left ventricle. There are multiple combinations of this type of congenital heart disease. From a physiologic standpoint, this anomaly is functionally correct since the systemic ventricle (morphologically the right ventricle) ejects arterial blood into the aorta and the right sided ventricle (anatomically the left ventricle) ejects non-oxygenated blood into the pulmonary artery.

The auscultatory and phonocardiographic findings in this condition are not specific. Phonocardiographic and pulse wave abnormalities, with the exception of splitting of the second heart sound which is frequently present in this anomaly, are best noted at the aortic area. Patients with this type of congenital heart disease may also exhibit a systolic regurgitant murmur usually due to insufficiency of the left-sided atrioventricular valve (fig. 9.46). They may also present with associated atrial septal defects and/or pulmonary stenosis. In this situation the

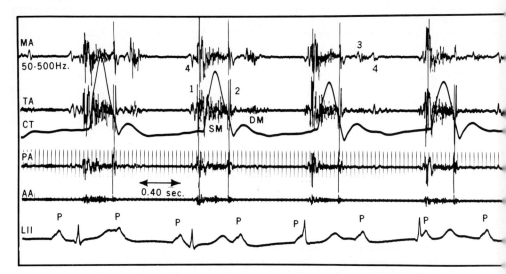

Fig. 9.46. Simultaneously recorded phonocardiogram at the mitral (MA), tricuspid (TA), pulmonic (PA) and aortic areas (AA), carotid pulse tracing (CT), and lead II (LII) of the electrocardiogram in a 22-year-old patient with corrected transposition of the great vessels and complete heart block. The first and second heart sounds are normal. Time of inscription of the P wave on the electrocardiogram is indicated. A fourth heart sound is inscribed following the P wave of the electrocardiogram (wandering fourth heart sound). There is a prominent third heart sound. A high frequency, low amplitude systolic regurgitant murmur (SM) due to left sided atrioventricular valve insufficiency is best recorded at the mitral and tricuspid areas. A short atrioventricular diastolic murmur (DM) which follows the third heart sound is due to increased flow across that valve. The carotid pulse tracing shows a normal contour.

phonocardiographic findings are essentially identical to the ones defined in those conditions (fig. 9.47).

The carotid pulse, jugular venous tracings, and apexcardiogram are of no value in the diagnosis of this condition. There are no definite echocardiographic features for this congenital heart disease.

TRICUSPID ATRESIA

Tricuspid atresia is a condition characterized by a hypoplastic or atretic tricuspid valve, dilatation of the left ventricular cavity, and a variable degree of hypoplasia of the right ventricle. The presence of a left-to-right shunt is essential for survival, and these shunts may occur through atrial, or ventricular septal defects or through a patent ductus arteriosus.

Auscultation and phonocardiography usually shows a single second heart sound due to aortic valve closure. The murmur which may be

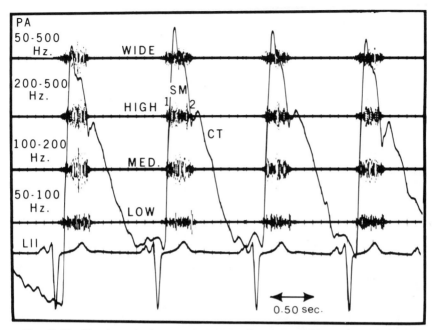

Fig. 9.47. Simultaneously recorded pulmonic area (PA) phonocardiogram at bandpass filter settings of 50–500, 200–500, 100–200, and 50–100 Hz, carotid pulse tracing (CT), and lead II (LII) of the electrocardiogram in a 10-year-old patient with corrected transposition of the great vessels, ventricular septal defect and pulmonary valvular stenosis. The first heart sound is normal. The second heart sound is single and has diminished amplitude. A high frequency, high amplitude systolic ejection murmur (SM) recorded in all frequency ranges was most prominent at 200–500 Hz and is probably due to pulmonary valvular stenosis. The carotid pulse tracing is normal. The electrocardiogram shows a short P-R interval, and pre-excitation syndrome.

present in tricuspid atresia is usually pansystolic and due to the ventricular septal defect.

The jugular venous pulse tracing usually shows prominent A waves. The carotid pulse and apexcardiogram are of no diagnostic value in this condition.

Echocardiogram

Echocardiography can be used in this condition to demonstrate the absence of the tricuspid valve, increased intracavitary left ventricular diameter, small right ventricular cavity, and increased left atrial internal dimension (figs. 9.48–9.50).

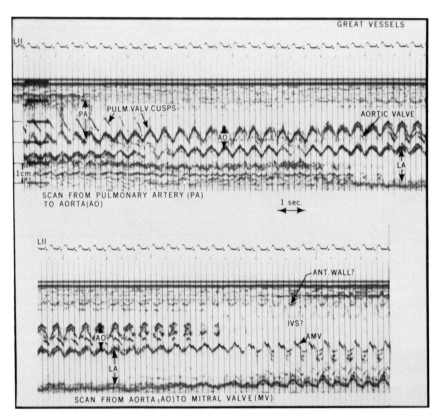

Fig. 9.48. Simultaneously recorded lead II (LII) of the electrocardiogram and echocardiographic scan from the pulmonary artery (PA) to the aorta (AO) and from the aorta to the mitral valve (MV). This 3-week-old infant had tricuspid atresia, normally related great vessels and increased pulmonary blood flow. The left atrial size is increased at 1.7 cm as compared with the aortic root which measures 0.8 cm. There is a questionable recording of the interventricular septum (IVS?) which appears late on the scan, possibly due to the presence of a ventricular septal defect. The tricuspid valve was not recorded in its usual position. The aortic valve measures 0.55 cm and the pulmonary artery appears to be almost twice the size of the aortic root. LA = left atrium, AMV = anterior mitral valve.

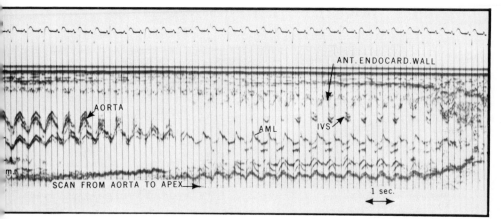

Fig. 9.49. Simultaneously recorded lead II (LII) of the electrocardiogram and echocardiographic scan from the aorta to the apex in a 3-week-old infant with tricuspid atresia and a ventricular septal defect. Small echoes recorded from the interventricular septum (IVS) are not detected until mid-cavity due to the presence of a large ventricular septal defect. The interventricular septum is well seen at the level where mitral valve motion is recorded. AML = anterior mitral leaflet.

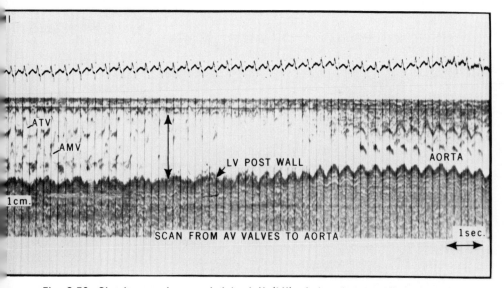

Fig. 9.50. Simultaneously recorded lead II (LII) of the electrocardiogram and echocardiographic scan from the mitral valve to the aorta in a two-week-old infant with a single ventricle (double inlet left ventricle). The tracing records both the anterior tricuspid valve (ATV) and anterior mitral valve (AMV) motion. There is a large, single intracavitary ventricular chamber and absence of the interventricular septum. The aorta measures 2.5 cm and the left ventricular internal diameter is increased to 6 cm.

DOUBLE OUTLET RIGHT VENTRICLE

This relatively uncommon form of congenital heart disease is characterized by an anatomical displacement of the aorta and associated
ventricular septal defect (Taussig-Bing syndrome). Both the pulmonary
artery and aorta originate from the right ventricle, therefore the mitral
valve and aortic or pulmonic valve continuity is interrupted since the
ventricular septal defect is located between the valves.

Heart Sounds and Murmurs

The auscultatory and phonocardiographic findings in this condition,
usually due to the presence of an intracardiac shunt through the
ventricular septal defect, include a high frequency, high amplitude
systolic regurgitant murmur, best recorded at the level of the left third or
fourth intercostal space (fig. 9.51). The first heart sound is usually
normal. The second heart sound may be single and/or accentuated due to

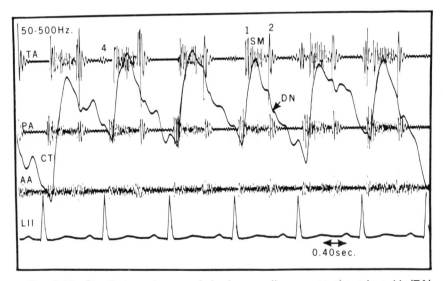

Fig. 9.51. Simultaneously recorded phonocardiogram at the tricuspid (TA),
pulmonic (PA), and aortic areas (AA), carotid pulse tracing (CT), and lead II (LII) of
the electrocardiogram in a 2-year-old patient with double outlet right ventricle,
ventricular septal defect and associated pulmonary valvular stenosis. The first heart
sound is normal. The second heart sound is single. A high frequency, medium
amplitude systolic murmur (SM) starts with the first heart sound and terminates at
the second heart sound. This murmur probably represents flow across the ventricular
septal defect and the pulmonary valvular stenosis. The carotid pulse tracing is
normal. DN = dicrotic notch.

an increase in pulmonary artery pressure. Atrial ventricular diastolic murmurs are uncommon in this condition.

Echocardiogram

The echocardiogram in patients with double outlet right ventricle may show discontinuity of the mitral valve in relation to the aortic annulus. This is best appreciated on a scan from the mitral to the aortic valve. Caution should be exercised in diagnosing this condition since patients without double outlet right ventricle may show discontinuity of the basic structures due to transducer angulation.

This congenital heart disease is frequently associated with a large left-to-right shunt, and patients may have increased left atrial and left ventricular internal diameters. The pulmonary and aortic valve may exhibit slight anterior displacement in relation to the septum, but this finding is not of definite diagnostic value. Echocardiographic findings in patients with this condition are shown in figures 9.52 and 9.53.

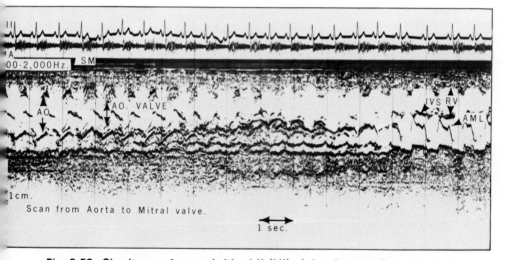

Fig. 9.52. Simultaneously recorded lead II (LII) of the electrocardiogram, mitral area (MA) phonocardiogram, and echocardiographic scan from the aorta (AO) to the mitral valve in a 5-year-old patient with double outlet right ventricle. Note the discontinuity of the mitral valve with the posterior aorta and of the interventricular septum (IVS) and anterior aorta. The aortic root is enlarged to 3 cm, the aortic valve measures 2 cm, and the left atrium measures 1.5 cm. Right ventricular (RV) internal dimension appears to be large. AML = anterior mitral leaflet.

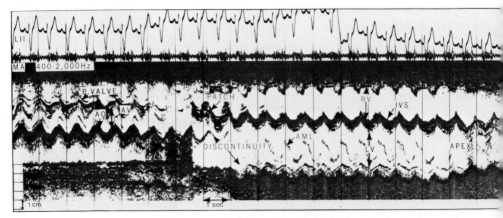

Fig. 9.53. Simultaneously recorded mitral area (MA) phonocardiogram, lead II (LII) of the electrocardiogram and echocardiographic scan from the aorta (AO) to the apex in a 13-year-old patient with double outlet right ventricle, residual ventricular septal defect, pulmonary insufficiency and pulmonary valvular stenosis. Note discontinuity of the posterior aorta with the anterior mitral valve. Right ventricular (RV) internal diameter is increased to approximately 4.5 cm, and left ventricular (LV) internal diameter to 4.4 cm. The interventricular septum (IVS) measures 1 cm and moves paradoxically. The aortic root measures 2.7 cm and the left atrial diameter is increased to 3 cm. A patch placed at the interventricular septum is well seen between the anterior aortic root and the septum. AML = anterior mitral leaflet, AV = aortic valve.

RUPTURE OF SINUS OF VALSALVA

Patients with ruptured sinus of Valsalva into the left ventricle exhibit the typical features described in patients with aortic insufficiency (see Chapter 5). The arterial insufficiency murmur is very prominent and usually has musical characteristics. However, when the sinus rupture is into the right ventricle, right atrium, or pulmonary artery, it results in phonocardiographic and auscultatory findings similar to the ones described for patients with patent ductus arteriosus and arteriovenous fistula.

EBSTEIN'S ANOMALY

This congenital heart disease is characterized by abnormal displacement of the leaflets of the tricuspid valve. In most patients, excessive valvular tissue is present and the tricuspid leaflets have varying depths of connection with the papillary muscles of the right ventricle or the right side of the interventricular septum. The most common form is characterized by posterior and downward displacement of the posterior leaflet of the tricuspid valve. Because the valve is located downward in the right ventricular cavity, segments of the right ventricular muscle become part of the anatomical right atrium.

Clinically, we see varying degrees of severity in this congenital anatomical defect ranging from mild to very severe forms. Patients with marked enlargement of the right atrium exhibit the typical findings associated with tricuspid insufficiency. Ebstein's anomaly of the mitral valve has been described in association with other congenital malformations but this anomaly is very rare as compared with the ones seen in the tricuspid valve.

Heart Sounds and Murmurs

The first heart sound usually has normal amplitude, is widely split and may be slightly diminished. It has a delayed inscription and the time interval from the Q wave of the electrocardiogram to the first heart sound is prolonged. This sound frequently has two components with the first component occurring approximately 0.04–0.07 sec after the Q wave of the electrocardiogram. The second component, which may be due to tricuspid valve closure, is recorded in the range of 0.07–0.16 sec after the Q wave of the electrocardiogram. A third transient may be present in some patients and is recorded quite late during ventricular systole in the range of 0.12–0.22 sec after the Q wave of the electrocardiogram. The second heart sound is single and is usually due to the aortic valve closure sound. Splitting of the second heart sound is seen only in the presence of right or left bundle branch block. Right bundle branch block is the most common conduction defect seen in this condition and its presence results in wide and fixed splitting of the second heart sound. The duration of splitting of the second heart sound ranges from 0.03 to 0.10 sec with little variation during the respiratory cycle. Reverse splitting of the second heart sound is rare in this condition but it is seen in patients with associated Wolff-Parkinson-White syndrome. Patients with Ebstein's malformation of the tricuspid valve may have associated atrioventricular conduction abnormalities such as pre-excitation syndrome and the most common is type B which electrocardiographically is similar to the pattern seen in the patients with left bundle branch block. One of the most important phonocardiographic features in this condition is the presence of a prominent third heart sound (figs. 9.54 and 9.55). The sound has special auscultatory and phonocardiographic characteristics. It usually occurs in the range of 0.04–0.12 sec after the aortic valve closure sound and has a high frequency characteristic resembling the opening snap of the tricuspid or mitral valve. Rarely, one may record a fourth heart sound. The high frequency, low amplitude systolic regurgitant murmur of tricuspid insufficiency is found in the majority of these patients. Atrioventricular

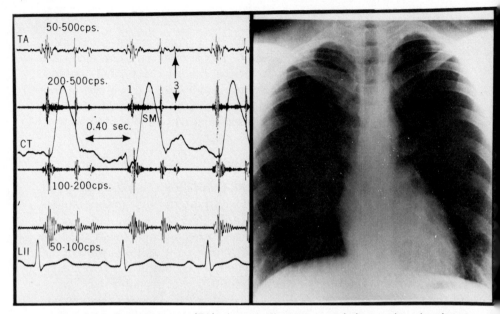

Fig. 9.54. Tricuspid area (TA) phonocardiogram recorded at various bandpass filter settings, carotid pulse tracing (CT), and lead II (LII) of the electrocardiogram (left panel) in a 20-year-old patient with Ebstein's anomaly of the tricuspid valve of a mild degree of severity. The first and second heart sounds are normal. A high frequency third heart sound is recorded 0.12 sec after the second heart sound. A high frequency, low amplitude systolic murmur (SM) starts with the first heart sound and terminates in mid-systole. The carotid pulse tracing is normal. The chest x-ray (right panel) shows normal heart size.

diastolic murmurs due to increased flow across the tricuspid valve may be present in approximately 25% of patients and are usually due to increased diastolic flow across the deformed tricuspid valve. Atrial systolic murmurs are rare.

Jugular Venous Pulse Tracing

The jugular venous tracing may show the typical features described for patients with tricuspid insufficiency. A prominent A wave may be present.

Echocardiogram

One of the most important echocardiographic features in patients with Ebstein's anomaly is a delayed tricuspid valve closure in relation to mitral valve closure. Unfortunately, this is difficult to demonstrate since it requires simultaneous recording of both valves on the echocardiogram with a good quality phonocardiogram showing delayed tricuspid valve closure and abnormally wide splitting of the first heart sound. In addition,

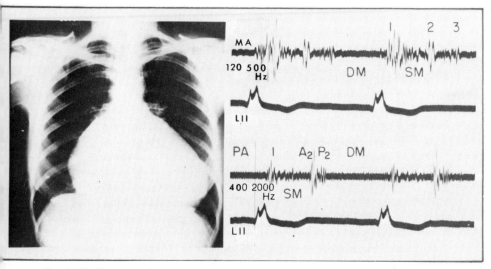

Fig. 9.55. (Left panel) Chest x-ray of a patient with Ebstein's disease, an anomaly of the tricuspid valve, showing marked enlargement of the cardiac silhouette and right atrium. (Top right panel) Mitral area (MA) phonocardiogram and lead II (LII) of the electrocardiogram. (Lower right panel) Pulmonic area (PA) phonocardiogram and lead II of the electrocardiogram. Note the presence of a short, high frequency, low amplitude systolic murmur (SM) which begins with the first heart sound and terminates before the second heart sound. The second heart sound is split at the pulmonic area and the pulmonic component is diminished. A low amplitude diastolic murmur (DM) is recorded best at the pulmonic area. There are high frequency, early diastolic vibrations at the mitral area inscribed 0.12–0.16 sec after the second heart sound.

one may find a decrease in the E-F slope of the anterior tricuspid valve. This valve may have an abnormal anterior position during the diastolic phase of the cardiac cycle and increased excursion as compared with the mitral valve (fig. 9.56). Abnormal motion of the interventricular septum has been described in this condition. The most common one is type B or flat motion of the septum. Type A, paradoxical septal motion, can be seen in this condition and occasionally one may find normal septal motion. In addition, if a good recording of the pulmonary valve is obtained, it shows a normal configuration which helps to differentiate from patients with severe pulmonary valvular stenosis or pulmonic atresia which may mimic this condition (see above under "Pulmonary Valvular Stenosis"). In the adult, great care must be exercised in the diagnosis of this condition because the markedly enlarged right atrium makes the pulmonic valve recording difficult to obtain. Patients with this anomaly may have abnormal displacement of the tricuspid valve which is located more to the left as compared with normal subjects.

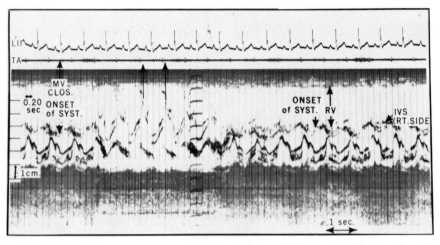

Fig. 9.56. Simultaneously recorded tricuspid area (TA) phonocardiogram, lead II (LII) of the electrocardiogram, and echocardiogram in a 7-year-old patient with Ebstein's anomaly of the tricuspid valve. The echocardiogram demonstrates markedly increased excursion of the tricuspid valve as compared with the mitral valve (MV). The tricuspid valve closes late as compared with closure of the mitral valve. Right ventricular (RV) internal dimension increases to 3.7 cm and left ventricular internal dimension measures 2.7 cm. IVS = interventricular septum.

CORONARY ARTERIOVENOUS FISTULA

Congenital coronary arteriovenous fistula is a rare anomaly. The more common coronary artery-chamber fistulas result from persistence of the embryonic myocardial trabeculae, which usually develop into sinusoids. In contrast, coronary artery-pulmonary artery communications are thought to represent abnormal origin of a coronary artery from the pulmonary trunk. The accessory artery communicates with branches of the normal coronary artery. Flow goes from the high pressure aortic area to the low pressure pulmonary artery.

The phonocardiographic and auscultatory features of the condition are similar to those described in patients with patent ductus arteriosus. However, a continuous murmur is uniformly present in these patients. Since continuous murmurs may be caused by a number of cardiovascular disorders, it is important to attempt to establish a definite diagnosis of the etiology of the continuous murmur. A clue to the presence of coronary arteriovenous fistula is that although the murmur is continuous, the systolic component starts earlier in systole and has ejection type characteristics as shown in figures 9.57 and 9.58.

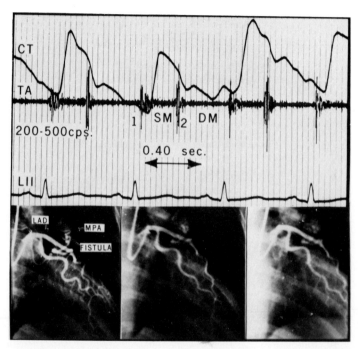

Fig. 9.57. Simultaneously recorded tricuspid area (TA) phonocardiogram, carotid pulse tracing (CT), and lead II (LII) of the electrocardiogram in a 41-year-old patient with left anterior descending coronary artery and pulmonary arteriovenous fistula. The first and seoncd heart sounds are normal. There is a high frequency, low amplitude systolic murmur (SM) and a diastolic murmur (DM) which starts with the second heart sound. However, this murmur is not continuous as usually seen in patients with patent ductus arteriosus. Selective left coronary arteriograms (bottom) show opacification of the left anterior descending (LAD) and left circumflex arteries. The left anterior descending artery-pulmonary arteriovenous fistula is indicated by an arrow with an early opacification of the main pulmonary artery (MPA).

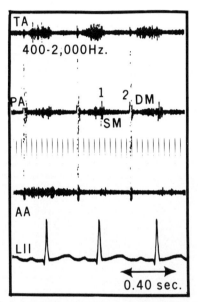

Fig. 9.58. Simultaneously recorded phonocardiogram at the tricuspid (TA), pulmonic (PA) and aortic areas (AA), and lead II (LII) of the electrocardiogram in a 1-year-old patient with left anterior descending artery fistula into the right ventricle. A high frequency, high amplitude systolic murmur (SM) recorded best at the pulmonic area terminates prior to the second heart sound. There is also a high frequency, high amplitude arterial diastolic murmur (DM) with maximal accentuation during mid-diastole, at the time of atrial contraction. At the tricuspid area the systolic murmur had maximal accentuation at the time of the second heart sound and the diastolic murmur begins with the second heart sound, resembling the continuous murmur seen in patients with patent ductus arteriosus.

REFERENCES

1. Abbasi, A. S., MacAlpin, R. N., Eber, L. M., and Pearce, M. L.: Echocardiographic diagnosis of idiopathic hypertrophic cardiomyopathy without outflow obstruction. Circulation, *46:* 897, 1972.
2. Abbasi, A. S., MacAlpin, R. N., Eber, L. M., and Pearce, M. L.: Left ventricular hypertrophy diagnosed by echocardiography. N. Engl. J. Med., *289:* 118, 1973.
3. Abraganseb, A. M., Grendahl, H., and Muller, C.: Hemodynamic effects of methoxamine in patients with left-to-right shunts. Acta Med. Scand., *191:* 283, 1972.
4. Alderman, E. L., Rytand, D. A., Crow, R. S., Finegan, R. E., and Harrison, D. C.: Normal and prosthetic atrioventricular valve motion in atrial flutter; correlation of ultrasound, vectorcardiographic, and phonocardiographic findings. Circulation, *45:* 1206, 1972.
5. Allen, H. D., and Goldberg, S. J.: Echocardiography in congenital heart disease. Ariz. Med., *31:* 571, 1974.
6. Baritt, D. W., Davies, D. H., and Jacob, G.: Heart sounds and pressures in atrial septal defect. Br. Heart J., *27:* 90, 1965.
7. Belenkie, I., Nutter, D., Clark, D., McCraw, B., and Raizner, A. E.: Assessment of left ventricular dimensions and function by echocardiography. Am. J. Cardiol., *31:* 755, 1973.
8. Beller, B. M., and Dexter, L.: Clinical and hemodynamic stability in a patient with a large atrial septal defect; a 17-year follow-up. J.A.M.A., *195:* 588, 1966.
9. Benchimol, A., Barreto, E. C., and Gartlan, J. L.: Right atrial flow velocity in patients with atrial septal defect. Am. J. Cardiol., *25:* 381, 1970.
10. Benchimol, A., and Desser, K. B.: Diagnostic value of arterial and venous wave forms. Cardiovasc. Clin., *6:* 73, 1975.
11. Benchimol, A., and Dimond, E. G.: Phonocardiography in ventricular septal defect; correlation between hemodynamics and phonocardiographic findings. Am. J. Med., *28:* 347, 1960.
12. Benchimol, A., and Lucena, E. G.: Vectorcardiography in congenital heart disease with the use of the Frank system. Br. Heart J., *27:* 236, 1965.
13. Benchimol, A., Wu, T. L., and Dimond, E. G.: Apexcardiogram in the diagnosis of congenital heart disease. Am. J. Cardiol., *17:* 63, 1966.
14. Benchimol, A., Tio, S., and Sundararajan, V.: Congenital corrected transposition of the great vessels in a 58-year-old man. Chest, *59:* 634, 1971.
15. Benchimol, A., and Tippit, H. C.: The clinical value of the jugular and hepatic pulses. Prog. Cardiovasc. Dis., *10:* 159, 1967.
16. Betriu, A., Wigle, E. D., Felderhof, D. H., and McLouglin, M. J.: Prolapse of the posterior leaflet of the mitral valve associated with secundum atrial septal defect. Am. J. Cardiol., *33:* 126, 1974.
17. Bialostozky, D., Horwitz, S., and Espino-Vela, J.: Ebstein's malformation of the tricuspid valve; a review of 65 cases. Am. J. Cardiol., *29:* 826, 1972.
18. Bonner, A. J. Jr., and Tavel, M. E.: The relationship of the jugular "C" wave to changing diastolic intervals. Am. Heart J., *84:* 441, 1972.
19. Bousvaros, G. A.: Diagnostic auscultatory complex in coarctation of the aorta. Br. Heart J., *29:* 443, 1967.
20. Brammell, H. L., Vogel, J. H. K., Pryor, R., and Blount, S. G. Jr.: The Eisenmenger syndrome; a clinical and physiologic reappraisal. Am. J. Cardiol., *28:* 679, 1971.
21. Brown, O. R., Harrison, D. C., and Popp, R. L.: Echocardiographic study of right ventricular hypertension producing asymmetric septal hypertrophy. Circulation, *48* (Suppl. IV): 47, 1973.
22. Castle, R. F.: Transmission patterns of cardiac murmurs. J.A.M.A., *199:* 838, 1967.
23. Chang, J. H., and Burrington, J. D.: Coarctation of the aorta in infants and children. J. Pediatr. Surg., *7:* 127, 1972.
24. Chesler, E., Joffe, H. S., Beck, W., and Schrire, V.: Echocardiographic recognition of mitral-semilunar valve discontinuity. Circulation, *43:* 725, 1971.
25. Chesler, E., Joffe, H. S., Beck, W., and Schrire, V.: Echocardiography in the diagnosis of congenital heart disease. Pediatr. Clin. North Am., *18:* 1163, 1971.

26. Chesler, E., Joffe, H. S., Vecht, R., Beck, W., and Schrire, V.: Ultrasound cardiography in single ventricle and the hypoplastic left and right heart syndromes. Circulation, *42:* 123, 1970.

27. Christ, M. L., Silber, E., Shaffer, A. B., Pick, A., and Levin, B.: Eisenmenger complex. Am. Heart J., *82:* 236, 1971.

28. Chung, K., Alexson, C. G., Manning, J. A., and Gramiak, R.: Echocardiography in truncus arteriosus; the value of pulmonic valve detection. Circulation, *48:* 281, 1973.

29. Clark, C. E., Henry, W. L., and Epstein, S. E.: The sensitivity and specificity of echocardiography in diagnosing IHSS by detection of asymmetrical septal hypertrophy. Circulation, *46:* (Suppl. II): 139, 1972.

30. Clarkson, P. M., and Orgill, A. A.: Continuous murmurs in infants of low birth weight. J. Pediatr., *84:* 208, 1974.

31. Cohen, L. S., and Roberts, W. C.: Tetralogy of Fallot; its unusual variants and its simulators. Chest, *57:* 266, 1970.

32. Colman, A. L.: *Clinical Examination of the Jugular Venous Pulse.* Springfield, Ill.: Charles C Thomas, 1966.

33. Craig, R. J., and Selzer, A.: Natural history and prognosis of atrial septal defect. Circulation, *37:* 805, 1968.

34. Crews, T. L., Pridie, R. B., Benham, R., and Leatham, A.: Auscultatory and phonocardiographic findings in Ebstein's anomaly; correlation of first heart sound with ultrasonic records of tricuspid valve movement. Br. Heart J., *34:* 681, 1972.

35. Davis, R. H., Feigenbaum, H., Chang, S., Konecke, L. L., and Dillon, J. C.: Echocardiographic manifestations of discrete subaortic stenosis. Am. J. Cardiol., *33:* 277, 1974.

36. DeMonchy, C.: Phonocardiograhy and external pulsation tracings in infants with congenital heart disease. Cardiologia, *52:* 160, 1968.

37. Diamond, M. A., Dillon, J. C., Haine, C. L., Chang, S., and Feigenbaum, H.: Echocardiographic features of atrial septal defect. Circulation, *43:* 129, 1971.

38. Dillon, J. C., Chang, S., and Feigenbaum, H.: Echocardiographic manifestations of left bundle branch block. Circulation, *49:* 876, 1974.

39. Dillon, J. C., Feigenbaum, H., Konecke, L. L., Keutel, J., Hurwitz, R. A., Davis, R. H., and Chang, S.: Echocardiographic manifestations of d-transposition of the great vessels. Am. J. Cardiol., *32:* 74, 1973.

40. Dimond, E. G., and Benchimol, A.: Phonocardiography in atrial septal defect; correlation between hemodynamics and phonocardiographic findings. Am. Heart J., *58:* 343, 1959.

41. Dimond, E. G., and Benchimol, A.: Phonocardiography in pulmonary stenosis; correlation between hemodynamics and phonocardiographic findings. Ann. Intern. Med., *52:* 145, 1960.

42. Dippel, W. F., and Kerber, R. E.: Mechanism of the echocardiographic abnormality of interventricular septum motion in right ventricular volume overload. Circulation, *46* (Suppl. II): 36, 1972.

43. Duchak, J., Chang, S., and Feigenbaum, H.: The posterior mitral valve echo and the echocardiographic diagnosis of mitral stenosis. Am. J. Cardiol., *29:* 628, 1972.

44. Dugan, W. T., Char, F., Gerald, B. E., and Campbell, G. S.: Pseudocoarctation of the aorta in childhood. Am. J. Dis. Child., *119:* 401, 1970.

45. Edler, I.: The diagnostic use of ultrasound in heart disease. Acta Med. Scand., *308:* 32, 1955.

46. Edler, I.: Ultrasound cardiography in mitral valve stenosis. Am. J. Cardiol., *19:* 18, 1967.

47. Eshaghpour, E., Turnoff, H. B., Kingsley, B., and Linhart, J. W.: Echocardiographic features of endocardial cushion defect. Am. J. Cardiol., *33:* 135, 1974.

48. Feigenbaum, H.: *Echocardiography.*, Philadelphia: Lea & Febiger, 1972.

49. Feigenbaum, H., Popp, R. L., Chip, J. N., and Haine, C. L.: Left ventricular wall thickness measured by ultrasound. Arch. Intern. Med., *121:* 391, 1968.

50. Feigenbaum, H., Popp, R. L., Wolfe, S. B., Troy, B. L., Pombo, J. F., Haine, C. L., and Dodge, H. T.: Ultrasound measurements of the left ventricle; a correlative study with angiocardiography. Arch. Intern. Med., *129:* 461, 1972.

51. Feigenbaum, H., Stone, J. M., Lee, D. A., Nasser, W. K., and Chang, S.: Identification of ultrasound echoes from the left ventricle by use of intracardiac injections of indocyanine green. Circulation, *51:* 615, 1970.
52. Fisher, E., and Paul, M. H.: Transposition of the great arteries; recognition and management. Cardiovasc. Clin., *2:* 211, 1970.
53. Fixler, D. E.: Congenital corrected transposition with atrial inversion and normal hemodynamics. Am. Heart J., *8:* 387, 1971.
54. Fontana, M. E., and Wooley, C. F.: Sail sound in Ebstein's anomaly of the tricuspid valve. Circulation, *46:* 155, 1972.
55. Fortuin, N. J., and Craige, E.: On the mechanism of Austin Flint murmur. Circulation, *45:* 558, 1972.
56. Fortuin, N. J., Hood, W. P. Jr., Sherman, M. E., and Craige, E.: Determination of left ventricular volumes by ultrasound. Circulation, *44:* 575, 1971.
57. Friedman, S., Harris, T. N., Atac, M. S., and Peker, H.: Some characteristics of diastolic flow murmurs in congenital and acquired heart disease. J. Pediatr., *71:* 52, 1967.
58. Friedman, W. F., Mehrizi, A., and Pusch, A. L.: Multiple muscular ventricular septal defects. Circulation, *32:* 35, 1965.
59. Furuta, S.: Evaluation of phonocardiography in congenital heart diseases; with special reference to the influence of the double stenosis of the right ventricular outflow tract on the systolic murmurs in tetralogy of Fallot. Jap. Circ. J., *30:* 1541, 1966.
60. Fyler, D. C., Gallaher, M. E., and Nadas, A. S.: Auscultation in the evaluation of children with heart disease. Prog. Cardiovasc. Dis., *10:* 363, 1968.
61. Genton, E., and Blount, S. G.: The spectrum of Ebstein's anomaly. Am. Heart J., *73:* 395, 1967.
62. Gibson, D. G., and Brown, D.: Measurement of instantaneous left ventricular volumes and filling rate in man by echocardiography. Br. Heart J., *35:* 559, 1973.
63. Glaser, J., Bharati, S., Whitman, V., and Liebman, J.: Echocardiographic findings in patients with anomalous origin of the left coronary artery. Circulation, *48:* (Suppl. IV): 63, 1973.
64. Glaser, J., Whitman, V., and Liebman, J.: The differential diagnosis of total anomalous pulmonary venous drainage in infancy by echocardiography. Circulation, *46:* (Suppl. II): 38, 1972.
65. Glasser, S. P., Cheitlin, M. D., McCarty, R. J., Haas, J. H., Hall, R. J., and Mullins, C. E.: Thirty-two cases of interventricular septal defect and aortic insufficiency. Am. J. Med., *53:* 473, 1972.
66. Godman, M. J., Tham, P., and Kidd, B. S. L.: Echocardiography in the evaluation of the cyanotic newborn infant. Br. Heart J., *36:* 154, 1974.
67. Goldberg, B. B.: Suprasternal ultrasonography. J.A.M.A., *15:* 245, 1971.
68. Goldberg, B. B., Ostrum, B. J., and Isard, H. J.: Ultrasonic determination of pericardial effusion. J.A.M.A., *202:* 927, 1967.
69. Goldberg, S. J., Allen, H. D., and Sahn, D. J.: *Pediatric and Adolescent Echocardiography, A Handbook.* Chicago: Year Book Medical Publishers, Inc., 1975.
70. Goldblatt, E.: Diseases of the heart and blood-vessels. Innocent systolic murmurs in childhood. Br. Med. J., *5505:* 95, 1966.
71. Gould, L., Reddy, C. V., and Gomprecht, R. F.: Atypical ausculatory findings in patent ductus arteriosus and stenosis of the pulmonary artery branch. Angiology, *25:* 504, 1974.
72. Gramiak, R., Chung, K. J., Nanda, N., and Manning, J.: Echocardiographic diagnosis of transposition of the great vessels. Radiology, *106:* 187, 1973.
73. Gramiak, R., Nanda, N. C., and Shah, P. M.: Echocardiographic detection of the pulmonary valve. Radiology, *102:* 153, 1972.
74. Gramiak, R., and Shah, P. M.: Cardiac ultasonography; a review of current applications. Radiol. Clin. North Am., *9:* 469, 1971.
75. Gramiak, R., and Shah, P. M.: Echocardiography of the normal and diseased aortic valve. Radiology, *96:* 1, 1970.
76. Grossman, W., McLaurin, L. P., Moos, S. P., Stefadouros, M., and Young, D. T.: Wall thickness and diastolic properties of the left ventricle. Circulation, *49:* 129, 1974.

77. Guller, B., and Bozie, C.: Right-to-left shunting through a patent ductus arteriosus in a newborn with myocardial infarction. Cardiology, *57:* 348, 1972.
78. Gustafson, A.: Correlation between ultrasound cardiography, hemodynamics and surgical findings in mitral stenosis. Am. J. Cardiol., *19:* 32, 1967.
79. Hagan, A., Francis, G., Sahn, D., Karliner, J., Friedman, W., and O'Rourke, R.: Systolic anterior septal motion: an unreliable echocardiographic finding. Circulation, *48:* (Suppl. IV): 173, 1973.
80. Hansen, J. F., and Wennevold, A.: The diagnosis of Ebstein's disease of the heart. Acta Med. Scand., *189:* 515, 1971.
81. Hartmann, A. F. Jr., Goldring, D., and Carlsson, E.: Development of right ventricular obstruction by aberrant muscular bands. Circulation, *30:* 679, 1964.
82. Henry, W. L., Clark, C. E., and Epstein, S. E.: Asymmetric septal hypertrophy. Circulation, *47:* 225, 1973.
83. Henry, W. L., Clark, C. E., and Epstein, S. E.: Asymmetric septal hypertrophy (ASH), the unifying link in the IHSS disease spectrum; observations regarding its pathogenesis, pathophysiology, and course. Circulation *47:* 827, 1973.
84. Henry, W. L., Clark, C. E., Glancy, D. L., and Epstein,S. E.: Echocardiographic measurement of the left ventricular outflow gradient in idiopathic hypertrophic subaortic stenosis. N. Engl. J. Med., *288:* 989, 1973.
85. Henry, W. L., Maron, B. J., Griffith, J. M., and Epstein, S. E.: The differential diagnosis of anomalies of the great vessels by real-time, two-dimensional echocardiography. Am. J. Cardiol., *33:* 143, 1974.
86. Hipona, F. A., and Arthachinta, S.: Ebstein's anomaly of the tricuspid valve; a report of 16 cases and review of the literature. Prog. Cardiovasc. Dis., *7:* 434, 1965.
87. Hirata, T., Wolfe, S. B., Popp, R. L., Helmen, C. H., and Feigenbaum, H.: estimation of left atrial size using ultrasound. Am. Heart J., *78:* 43, 1969.
88. Hirschfeld, S., Meyer, R. A., and Kaplan, S.: Non-invasive right and left systolic time intervals by echocardiography. Pediatr. Res., *8:* 350, 1974.
89. Hoffman, J. I.: Natural history of congenital heart disease. Problems in its assessment with special reference to ventricular septal defects. Circulation, *37:* 97, 1968.
90. Johnson, M. L., Paton, B. C., and Holmes, J. H.: Ultrasonic evaluation of prosthetic valve motion. Circulation, *41:* (Suppl. II): 3, 1970.
91. Johnson, S. L., Baker, D. W., Lute, R. A., and Kawabori, I.: Detection of left-to-right shunts and right ventricular outflow tract obstruction by Doppler echocardiography. Circulation, *48:* (Suppl. IV): 82, 1973.
92. Johnson, S. L., Baker, D. W., Lute, R. A., and Murray, J. A.: Detection of mitral regurgitation by Doppler echocardiography. Am. J. Cardiol., *33:* 147, 1974.
93. Joyner, C. R., Dyrda, I., and Reid, J. M.: Behavior of the anterior leaflet of the mitral valve in patients with the Austin Flint murmur. Clin. Res., *14:* 251, 1966.
94. Joyner, C. R., Hey, E. D., Johnson, J., and Reid, J. M.: Reflected ultrasound in the diagnosis of tricuspid stenosis. Am. J. Cardiol., *19:* 66, 1967.
95. Kamigaki, M., and Goldschlager, N.: Echocardiographic analysis of mitral valve motion in atrial septal defect. Am. J. Cardiol., *30:* 343, 1972.
96. Keith, J. D., Rowe, R. D., and Vlad, P.: *Heart Disease in Infancy and Childhood.* New York, The Macmillan Co., 1967.
97. Kerber, R. E., Greene, R. A., Cohn, L. H., Wexler, L., Kriss, J. P., and Harrison, D. C.: Multiple left ventricular outflow obstructions; aortic valvular and supravalvular stenosis and coarctation of the aorta. J. Thorac. Cardiovasc. Surg., *63:* 374, 1972.
98. King, D. L., Steeg, C. N., and Ellis, K.: Demonstrations of transposition of the great arteries by cardiac ultrasonography. Radiology, *107:* 181, 1973.
99. King, D. L., Steeg, C., and Ellis, K.: Visualization of ventricular septal defects by cardiac ultrasonography. Circulation, *48:* 1215, 1973.
100. King, S. M., Vogel, J. H. K., and Blount, S. G.: Idiopathic muscular subvalvular aortic stenosis with associated congenital cardiovascular lesions. Am. J. Cardiol., *15:* 837, 1965.
101. Kingsley, B.: Stroke volume and cardiac output by echocardiography. J. Audio Eng. Soc., *18:* 692, 1970.

CONGENITAL HEART DISEASE353

102. Kloster, F. E., Roelandt, J., Cate, F. J. T., Bom, N., and Hugenholtz, P. G.: Multiscan echocardiography; II. Technique and initial clinical results. Circulation, *48:* 1075, 1973.
103. Kotler, M. N.: Tricuspid valve in Ebstein's anomaly. Circulation, *47:* 597, 1973.
104. Kraus, Y., Yahini, J. H., Shem-Tov, A., and Neufeld, H. N.: Precordial pulsations in corrected transposition of the great vessels. Diagnostic value of the electromechanical interval. Am. J. Cardiol., *23:* 684, 1969.
105. Kusukawa, R.: Reliability of phonocardiogram in the diagnosis of heart disease. Jap. Circ. J., *30:* 1556, 1966.
106. Lambert, E. C., Timgelstad, J. B., and Hohn, A. R.: Diagnosis and management of congenital heart disease in the first week of life. Pediatr. Clin. North Am., *13:* 943, 1966.
107. Lester, R. G., Osteen, R T., and Robinson, A. E.: Infundibular obstruction secondary to pulmonary valvular stenosis. Am. J. Roentgenol. Radium Ther. Nucl. Med., *94:* 78, 1965.
108. Levy, A. M., Leaman, D. M., and Hanson, J. S.: Effects of digoxin on systolic time intervals of neonates and infants. Circulation, *46:* 816, 1972.
109. Linhart, J. W., and Razi, B.: Late systolic murmur: a clue to the diagnosis of aneurysm of the membranous ventricular septum. Chest, *60:* 283, 1971.
110. Lucena, E. G., Benchimol, A., and Dimond, E. G.: Auscultation and phonocardiography in atrial and ventricular septal defects and pulmonary stenosis. Arq. Bras. Cardiol., *16:* 349, 1963.
111. Luisada, A. A., and Feigen, L. P.: Technical progress in phonocardiography and pulse tracings. Acta Cardiol., *28:* 392, 1972.
112. Lundstrom, N. R.: Echocardiography in the diagnosis of Ebstein's anomaly of the tricuspid valve. Circulation, *47:* 597, 1973.
113. Lundstrom, N. R., and Edler, I.: Ultrasound cardiography in infants and children. Acta Paediatr. Scand., *60:* 117, 1971.
114. Lundstrom, N. R., and Mortensson, W.: Clinical applications of echocardiography in infants and children; II. Estimation of aortic root diameter and left atrial size, a comparison between echocardiography and angiocardiography. Acta Paediatr. Scand., *63:* 33, 1974.
115. Lundstrom, N. R.: Ultrasoundcardiographic studies of the mitral valve region in young infants with mitral atresia, mitral stenosis, hypoplasia of the left ventricle, and cor triatriatum. Circulation, *45:* 324, 1972.
116. Macartney, F., Deverall, P., and Scott, O.: Significance of continuous murmurs in cyanotic congenital heart disease. Br. Heart J., *34:* 205, 1972.
117. Martin, C. E., Reddy, P. S., Leon, D. F., and Shaver, J. A.: Genesis, frequency, and diagnostic significance of ejection sound in adults with tetralogy of Fallot. Br. Heart J., *35:* 402, 1973.
118. Martinez, E. C., Giles, T. D., and Burch, G. E.: Echocardiographic diagnosis of left atrial myxoma. Am. J. Cardiol., *33:* 281, 1974.
119. McCann, W. D., Harbold, N. B., and Giuliani, E. R.: The echocardiogram in right ventricular overload. J.A.M.A., *221:* 1243, 1972.
120. McDonald, I. G.: Echocardiographic demonstration of abnormal motion of the interventricular septum in left bundle branch block. Circulation, *48:* 272, 1973.
121. McDonald, I. G., Feigenbaum, H., and Chang, S.: Analysis of left ventricular wall motion by reflected ultrasound. Circulation, *46:* 14, 1972.
122. Meyer, R. A., and Kaplan, S.: Echocardiography in the diagnosis of hypoplasia of the left or right ventricles in the neonate. Circulation, *46:* 55, 1972.
123. Meyer, R., Schwartz, D. C., Benzing, G., and Kaplan, S.: Ventricular septum in right ventricular volume overload. Am. J. Cardiol., *30:* 349, 1972.
124. Meyer, R. A., Schwartz, D. C., Covitz, W., and Kaplan, S.: Echocardiographic assessment of cardiac malposition. Am. J. Cardiol., *33:* 896, 1974.
125. Meyer, R. A., Stockert, J., and Kaplan, S.: Echographic determination of left ventricular volumes. Pediatr. Res., *7:* 300, 1973.
126. Michaelsson, M.: Aspects on the clinical diagnosis of congenital heart disease in

infancy. Acta Paediatr. Scand., *206* (Suppl.): 15, 1970.

127. Millward, D. K., McLaurin, L. P., and Craige, E.: Echocardiographic studies of the mitral valve in patients with congestive cardiomyopathy and mitral regurgitation. Circulation, *46* (Suppl. II): 42, 1972.

128. Millward, D. K., McLaurin, L. P., and Craige, E.: Echocardiographic studies to explain opening snaps in presence of nonstenotic mitral valves. Am. J. Cardiol., *31:* 64, 1973.

129. Moreyra, E., Klein, J. J., Shimada, H., and Segal, B. L.: Idiopathic hypertrophic subaortic stenosis diagnosed by ultrasound. Am. J. Cardiol., *23:* 32, 1969.

130. Moss, A. J., and Adams, F. H. (Eds.): *Heart Disease in Infants, Children and Adolescents*. Baltimore: The Williams & Wilkins Co., 1968.

131. Moss, A. J., Hutter, A. M., Jr., Lipchik, E. O., and Gallagher, R. E.: Congenital corrected transposition of the great vessels without cardiac anomalies. Am. J. Med., *47:* 986, 1969.

132. Moss, A. J., and Siassi, B.: Natural history of ventricular septal defect. Cardiol. Clin., *2:* 139, 1970.

133. Myler, R. K., and Sanders, C. A.: Normal splitting of the second heart sound in atrial septal defect. Am. J. Cardiol., *19:* 874, 1967.

134. Nagle, R. E., and Tamara, F. A.: Left parasternal impulse in pulmonary stenosis and atrial septal defect. Br. Heart J., *29:* 735, 1967.

135. Nanda, N. C., Gramiak, R., Manning, J., Lipchik, E. O., Mahoney, E. B., and DeWeese, J. A.: Echocardiographic recognition of congenital bicuspid aortic valve. Am. J. Cardiol., *33:* 159, 1974.

136. Nanda, N. C., Gramiak, R., Manning, J., Mahoney, E. B., Lipchik, E. O., and DeWeese, J. A.: Echocardiographic recognition of the congenital bicuspid aortic valve. Circulation, *49:* 870, 1974.

137. Neufeld, H. N., Lucas, R. V. Jr., Lester, R. G., Adams, P. Jr., Anderson, R. C., and Edwards, J. E.: Origin of both great vessels from the right ventricle without pulmonary stenosis. Br. Heart J., *24:* 393, 1962.

138. Nimura, Y., Matsumoto, M., Beppu, S., Matsuo, H., Sakakibara, H., and Hoe, H.: Noninvasive preoperative diagnosis of cor triatriatum with ultrasonocardiotomogram and conventional echocardiogram. Am. Heart J., *88:* 240, 1974.

139. Perasalo, O., Halonen, P. I., and Siltanen, P.: Endocardial cushion defect; clinical and surgical considerations. Acta Chir. Scand., *128:* 592, 1964.

140. Perloff, J. K.: Diagnostic inferences drawn from observation and palpation of the precordium with special reference to congenital heart disease. Adv. Cardiopulm. Dis., *4:* 13, 1969.

141. Perloff, J. K., Caulfield, W. H., and DeLeon, A. C.: Peripheral pulmonary artery murmur of atrial septal defect. Br. Heart J., *29:* 411, 1967.

142. Perry, L. W., Wells, C. R., and Voci, G.: The transmission of systolic murmurs from the pulmonary artery into the left atrium. Am. Heart J., *68:* 443, 1964.

143. Pestana, C., Weidman, W. H., Swan, H. J. C., and McGoon, D. C.: Accuracy of preoperative diagnosis in congenital heart disease. Am. Heart J., *72:* 446, 1966.

144. Pieroni, D. R., Bell, B. B., Krovetz, L. J., Varghese, P. J., and Rowe, R. D.: Auscultatory recognition of aneurysm of the membranous ventricular septum associated with small ventricular septal defect. Circulation, *44:* 733, 1971.

145. Pieroni, D. R., Freedom, R. M., and Homey, E.: Echocardiography in atrio-ventricular canal defects; a clinical spectrum. Excerpta Medica, International Congress Series, Second World Congress on Ultrasonics in Medicine, #277, abstract 28, p. 12. Rotterdam, June 4–8, 1973.

146. Pombo, J. F., Troy, B. L., and Russell, R. O.: Left ventricular volumes and ejection fraction by echocardiography. Circulation, *43:* 480, 1971.

147. Popp, R. L., Brown, O. R., and Harrison, D. C.: Diagnostic accuracy of an ultrasonic multitransducer cardiac imaging system. Circulation, *48:* (Suppl. IV): 125, 1973.

148. Popp, R. L., and Harrison, D. C.: Ultrasonic cardiac echography for determing stroke volume and valvular regurgitation. Circulation, *41:* 493, 1970.

149. Popp, R. L., Silverman, J. F., French, J. W., Stinson, E. B., and Harrison, D. C.:

Echocardiographic findings in discrete subvalvular aortic stenosis. Circulation, *49:* 226, 1974.

150. Popp, R. L., Wolfe, S. B., Hirata, T., and Feigenbaum, H.: Estimation of right and left ventricular size by ultrasound. Am. J. Cardiol., *24:* 523, 1969.

151. Pridie, R. B., Behnam, R., and Wild, J.: Ultrasound in cardiac diagnosis. Clin. Radiol., *23:* 160, 1972.

152. Pridie, R. B., and Oakley, C. M.: Mitral valve movement in hypertrophic obstructive cardiomyopathy. Br. Heart J., *31:* 390, 1969.

153. Rashkind, W. J.: Transposition of the great arteries. Pediatr. Clin. North Am., *18:* 1075, 1971.

154. Rao, B. N., and Edwards, J. E.: Conditions simulating the tetralogy of Fallot. Circulation, *49:* 173, 1974.

155. Ravin, A., and Frame, F. K.: *International Bibliography of Cardiovasular Ausculta- tion and Phonocardiography.* New York: The American Heart Association, Inc., 1971.

156. Rosenthal, T., and Kariv, I.: A pathognomonic murmur of "atypical" patent ductus arteriosus. Dis. Chest, *56:* 350, 1969.

157. Rossen, R. M., Goodman, D. J., Ingham, R. E., and Popp, R. L.: Ventricular systolic septal thickening and excursion in idiopathic hypertrophic subaortic stenosis. N. Engl. J. Med., *291:* 1317, 1974.

158. Sahn, D. J., Deeley, W. J., Hagan, A. D., and Friedman, W. F.: Echocardiographic assessment of left ventricular performance in normal newborns. Circulation, *49:* 232, 1974.

159. Sahn, D. J., Terry, R., O'Rourke, R., and Friedman, W. F.: Multiple crystal cross-sectional echocardiography in the diagnosis of cyanotic congenital heart disease. Circulation, *50:* 230, 1974.

160. Sanchez, J., Rodriguez-Torres, R., Jer-Shoung, L., Goldstein, S., and Kavety, V.: Diagnostic value of the first heart sound in children with atrial septal defect. Am. Heart J., *78:* 467, 1969.

161. Sato, F.: Symposium on limitation of diagnostic value of electrocardiography and phonocardiography; I. Electrocardiogram and phonocardiogram in relation to opera- tive findings, electrocardiogram of congenital heart disease in relation to their operative findings. Jap. Circ. J., *30:* 1537, 1966.

162. Segal, B. L. (Guest Ed.): Symposium on echocardiography. Diagnostic ultrasound. Am. J. Cardiol., *19:* 1, 1967.

163. Shah, P. M., Gramiak, R., Adelman, A. G., and Wigle, E. D.: Role of echocardiogra- phy in diagnostic and hemodynamic assessment of hypertrophic subaortic stenosis. Circulation, *44:* 891, 1971.

164. Shah, P. M., Gramiak, R., and Kramer, D. H.: Ultrasound localization of left ventricular outflow obstruction in hypertrophic obstructive cardiomyopathy. Circula- tion, *40:* 3, 1969.

165. Shepherd, R. L., Glancy, D. L., Jaffe, R. B., Perloff, J. K., and Epstein, S. E.: Acquired subvalvular right ventricular outflow obstruction in patients with ventricu- lar septal defect. Am. J. Med., *53:* 446, 1972.

166. Shibuya, M.: Auscultatory findings of heart sounds and murmurs in congenital heart anomalies and acquired valvular disease; special reference to the determination of the severity of the condition on the basis of phonocardiography. Jap. J. Thorac. Surg., *18:* 1008, 1965.

167. Solinger, R., Elbl, F., and Minhas, K.: Echocardiographic features of the hypoplastic atrioventricular valve. Circulation, *46* (Suppl. II): 224, 1972.

168. Solinger, R., Elbl, F., and Minhas, K.: Echocardiography in congenital heart disease. Lancet, *2:* 1093, 1971.

169. Steinbrunn, W., Cohn, K. E., and Selzer, A.: The Lutembacher syndrome revisited; atrial septal defect associated with mitral stenosis. Am. J. Med., *48:* 295, 1970.

170. Steinfeld, L.: Clinical diagnosis of isolated subpulmonic (supracristal) ventricular septal defect. Am. J. Cardiol., *30:* 19, 1972.

171. Storstein, O., Rokseth, R., and Sorland, S.: Congenital heart disease in a clinical material; an analysis of 1,000 consecutive cases. Acta Med. Scand., *176:* 195, 1964.

172. Sweet, R. L., Russell, R. O. Jr., Moraski, R. E., and Rackley, C. E.: Comparison of left ventricular volumes obtained by biplane angiography and echocardiography in patients with abnormally contracting segments. Circulation, *48:* (Suppl. IV): 116, 1973.

173. Tajik, A. J., Gau, G. T., Giuliani, E. R., Ritter, D. G., and Schattenberg, T. T.: Echocardiogram in Ebstein's anomaly with Wolff-Parkinson-White preexcitation syndrome, type B. Circulation, *47:* 813, 1973.

174. Tajik, A. J., Gau, G. T., Ritter, D. G., and Schattenberg, T. T.: Echocardiogram in tetralogy of Fallot. Chest, *64:* 107, 1973.

175. Tajik, A. J., Gau, G. T., Ritter, D. G., and Schattenberg, T. T.: Echocardiographic pattern of right ventricular diastolic volume overload in children. Circulation, *46:* 36, 1972.

176. Tajik, A. J., Gau, G. T., Ritter, D. G., and Schattenberg, T. T.: Illustrative echocardiogram; echocardiogram in tetralogy of Fallot. Chest, *64:* 107, 1973.

177. Tajik, A. J., Gau, G. T., Ritter, D. G., and Schattenberg, T. T.: The echocardiographic pattern of right ventricular volume overload in children. Circulation, *46* (Suppl. II): 228, 1972.

178. Tajik, A. J., Gau, G. T., and Schattenberg, T. T.: Echocardiogram in atrial septal defect. Chest, *62:* 213, 1972.

179. Tajik, A. J., Gau, G. T., and Schattenberg, T. T.: Echocardiogram in atrial septal defect with small left-to-right shunt. Chest, *63:* 95, 1973.

180. Tajik, A. J., Gau, G. T., and Schattenberg, T. T.: Echocardiogram in total anomalous pulmonary venous drainage; report of a case. Mayo Clin. Proc., *47:* 247, 1972.

181. Tajik, A. J., Gau, G. T., and Schattenberg, T. T.: Echocardiographic "pseudo-IHSS" pattern in atrial septal defect. Chest, *62:* 324, 1972.

182. Tajik, A. J., Gau, G. T., Schattenberg, T. T., and Ritter, D. G.: Normal ventricular septal motion in atrial septal defect. Mayo Clin. Proc., *47:* 635, 1972.

183. Tatsuno, K., Konno, S., Ando, M., and Sakakibara, S.: Pathogenetic mechanisms of prolapsing aortic valve and aortic regurgitation associated with ventricular septal defect; anatomical, angiographic, and surgical considerations. Circulation, *48:* 1028, 1973.

184. Tavel, M. E.: Phonocardiography and venous pulsations. The use of the jugular pulse in the diagnosis of atrial septal defect. Dis. Chest, *54:* 544, 1968.

185. Tavel, M. E., Baugh, D., Fisch, C., and Feigenbaum, H.: Opening snap of the tricuspid valve in atrial septal defect; a phonocardiographic and reflected ultrasound study of sounds in relationship to movements of the tricuspid valve. Am. Heart J., *80:* 550, 1970.

186. Ting, Y. M.: Ultrasound cardiography in diagnosis of mitral insufficiency. Radiology, *109:* 253, 1973.

187. Troy, B. L., Pombo, J., and Rackley, C. E.: Measurement of left ventricular wall thickness and mass by echocardiography. Circulation, *45:* 602, 1972.

188. Ultan, L. B., Segal, B. L., and Likoff, W.: Echocardiography in congenital heart disease; preliminary observations. Am. J. Cardiol., *19:* 74, 1967.

189. Van Der Hauwaert, L. G.: The effect of the Valsalva maneuver on the splitting of the second sound. Acta Cardiol., *19:* 518, 1964.

190. Van Praagh, R.: What is the Taussig-Bing malformation? Circulation, *38:* 445, 1968.

191. Van Praagh, R., Corwin, R. D., Dahlquist, E. H., Freedom, R. M., Mattioli, L., and Nebesar, R. A.: Tetralogy of Fallot with severe left ventricular outflow tract obstruction due to anomalous attachment of the mitral valve to the ventricular septum. Am. J. Cardiol., *26:* 93, 1970.

192. Victoria, B. E., Gessner, I. H., and Schiebler, G. L.: Phonocardiographic findings in persistent truncus arteriosus. Br. Heart J., *30:* 812, 1968.

193. Wayne, H. H.: *Noninvasive Technics in Cardiology; the Phonocardiogram, Apexcardiogram, and Systolic Time Intervals.* Chicago: Year Book Medical Publishers, 1973.

194. Wesselhoeft, H., Fawcett, J. S., and Johnson, A. L.: Anomalous origin of the left coronary artery from the pulmonary trunk; its clinical spectrum, pathology, and pathophysiology, based on a review of 140 cases with seven further cases. Circulation, *38:* 403, 1968.

195. Weyman, A. E., Dillon, J. C., Feigenbaum, H., and Chang, S.: Echocardiographic patterns of pulmonic valve motion in pulmonic stenosis. Am. J. Cardiol., *33:* 178, 1974.
196. Williams, R. G., and Rudd, M.: Echocardiographic features of endocardial cushion defects. Circulation, *49:* 418, 1974.
197. Winsberg, F., Gabor, G. E., Hernberg, J. G., and Weiss, B.: Fluttering of the mitral valve in aortic insufficiency. Circulation, *41:* 225, 1970.
198. Winsberg, F., and Mercer, E. N.: Echocardiography in combined valve disease. Radiology, *105:* 405, 1972.
199. Womersley, J. R.: An elastic tube theory of pulse transmission and oscillatory flow in mammalian arteries. Wright Air Development Center Technical Report, WADC-TR, *56:* 614, 1957.
200. Zakrzewski, T. K., Slodki, S. J., and Luisada, A. A.: The first heart sound in atrial septal defect. Am. Heart J., *78:* 476, 1969.
201. Zoneraich, S. (Ed.): *Non-invasive Methods in Cardiology.* Springfield, Ill.: Charles C Thomas, 1974.
202. Zuberbuhler, J. R., Bauersfeld, S. R., and Pontius, R. G.: Paradox splitting of the second sound with transposition of the great vessels. Am. Heart J., *74:* 816, 1967.

chapter 10

Primary Myocardial Disease

The etiology of primary myocardial disease, a pathologic state involving the heart muscle, is unknown. Many names have been given to this entity such as diffuse myocardial disease, idiopathic cardiomyopathy, and others. Several etiologic factors have been implicated such as toxic, infectious metabolic, and congenital lesions. Primary myocardial disease is commonly classified as obstructive or non-obstructive. Obstructive disease is associated with abnormal hypertrophy of the myocardium as seen in patients with idiopathic hypertrophic subaortic stenosis and is described in Chapter 5. In this chapter only non-obstructive disease will be discussed.

Non-obstructive cardiomyopathies are classified as (1) restrictive and (2) congestive. Restrictive disease is associated with marked restriction of ventricular filling. Its features are similar to those seen in patients with constrictive pericarditis (see Chapter 11). The congestive type is most frequently associated with early onset of congestive heart failure and cardiomegaly. The auscultatory, phonocardiographic, and pulse wave abnormalities seen in both types of disease have few features in common. Unfortunately, symptoms do not occur in the early stages of the disease process. They are manifest late in the natural history of the disease when congestive heart failure develops.

HEART SOUNDS AND MURMURS

The first heart sound is normal or diminished (fig. 10.1). The second heart sound may be normal providing that pulmonary artery pressures are in the normal range. Most patients present with a picture of advanced heart failure and pulmonary hypertension, and the second heart sound may be single and accentuated due to increased intensity of the pulmonary component (fig. 10.2). Conduction defects of the right and left bundle branch block variety are a frequent finding. Wide and fixed splitting of the second heart sound is heard if a right bundle branch block

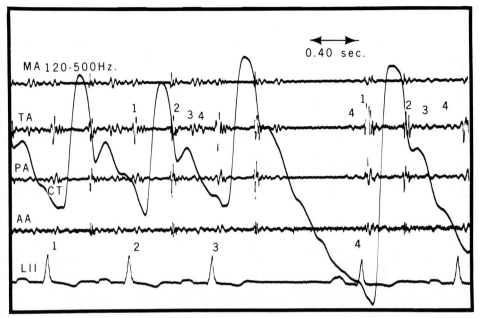

Fig. 10.1 Simultaneously recorded phonocardiogram at the mitral (MA), tricuspid (TA), pulmonic (PA), and aortic areas (AA), carotid pulse tracing (CT), and lead II (LII) of the electrocardiogram in a 42-year-old patient with severe congestive primary myocardial disease. Note marked diminution of the first and second heart sounds. Third and fourth heart sounds, well recorded at the mitral, tricuspid and aortic areas, are prominent. Beats 1–3 are sinus beats. Beat 4 is preceded by a long diastolic pause which is probably related to the preceding blocked atrial extrasystole. The post-extrasystolic beat 4 shows increased amplitude of the first heart sound. During the first three beats, the carotid pulse shows rapid upstroke time, a conspicuous dicrotic notch, and marked diminution of the ejection time. The electorcardiogram shows first degree atrioventricular block.

is present, or reversed splitting in the presence of left bundle branch block. A fourth heart sound is usually heard, particularly in patients with congestive myocardial disease, indicating decreased ventricular compliance and large ventricular end-diastolic volume. A third heart sound is almost uniformly present in this condition. It occurs 0.08–0.16 sec after the aortic valve closure sound. In restrictive disease, this sound has characteristics of the early diastolic pericardial "knock" heard in patients with constrictive pericarditis. Alternation of heart sounds is frequently observed in patients who also have pulsus alternans as demonstrated in the carotid pulse tracing (fig. 10.2).

Regurgitant systolic murmurs of mitral and/or tricuspid insufficiency are heard frequently in congestive myocardial disease due to dilatation of

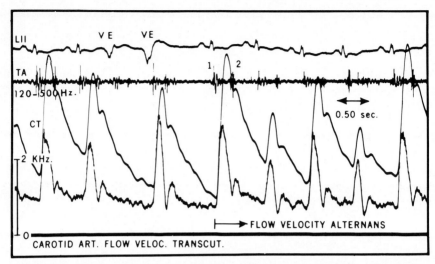

Fig. 10.2. Simultaneously recorded phonocardiogram, lead II (LII) of the electrocardiogram, carotid pulse tracing (CT) and transcutaneous Doppler carotid artery flow velocity in a 56-year-old patient with congestive myocardial disease. Two ventricular extrasystoles precipitate the appearance of typical pulsus alternans on both the carotid pulse tracing and Doppler carotid artery blood flow velocity tracing (see text).

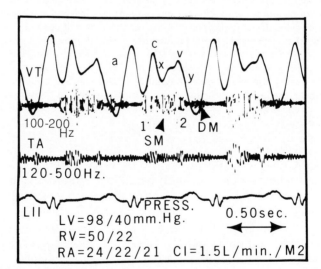

Fig. 10.3 Simultaneously recorded phonocardiogram at the mitral (MA) and tricuspid (TA) areas, jugular venous tracing (VT), and lead II (LII) of the electrocardiogram in a 42-year-old patient with primary myocardial disease and tricuspid insufficiency. A prominent, high frequency systolic regurgitant murmur is recorded at the tricuspid area. The jugular venous tracing shows a prominent A wave, sustained systolic wave, small x descent, prominent v wave and a rapid y descent. Note the marked elevation of left ventricular end-diastolic (LV), right ventricular (RV) and right atrial (RA) pressures, and diminished cardiac index (CI).

the mitral or tricuspid annulus (fig. 10.3). A soft, high frequency, systolic ejection murmur is present in both restrictive and constrictive disease due to turbulent flow across the pulmonic and aortic valves. Diastolic murmurs are not usually recorded in this condition.

CAROTID PULSE TRACING

The carotid pulse tracing shows a rapid ascending limb with a rapid downward systolic wave and diminished ejection time, usually associated with diminished left ventricular stroke volume (figs. 10.1 and 10.2). Since most patients are in heart failure, pulsus alternans is a common finding (figs. 10.2, 10.4, and 10.5). It may occur in the left or right heart circulation, or simultaneously in both circulations. If pulsus alternans is not present at rest, a mild degree of exercise stress will precipitate the appearance of this abnormality. It may also be induced by cardiac arrhythmias (fig. 10.2) or cardiac pacing (fig. 10.4). The presence of pulsus alternans in this disease state implies a poor prognosis since it is usually seen in the end stage of the natural history of cardiomyopathies.

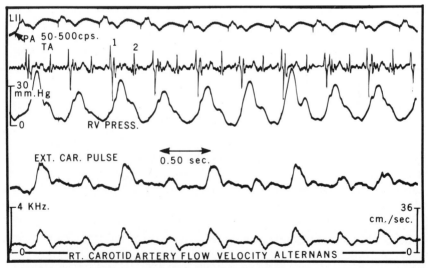

Fig. 10.4 Simultaneously recorded lead II (LII) of the electrocardiogram, tricuspid (TA) area phonocardiogram, right ventricular pressure (RV), carotid pulse tracing (EXT. CAR. PULSE) and transcutaneous carotid Doppler flow velocity curve recorded during right ventricular pacing in a 61-year-old woman. Note alternation of the right ventricular pressure, transcutaneous carotid artery velocity curve, carotid pulse tracing, and first and second heart sounds during ventricular pacing. It is apparent that pulsus alternans is present in the right and left heart circulations. PA = pacemaker artifacts.

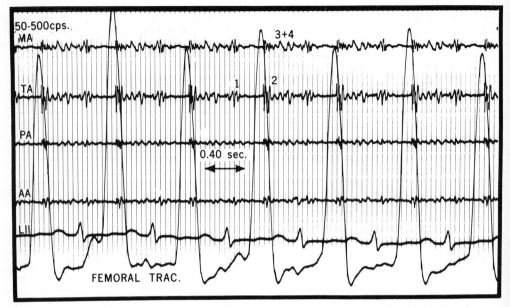

Fig. 10.5 Simultaneously recorded mitral (MA), tricuspid (TA), pulmonic (PA) and aortic (AA) area phonocardiogram, lead II (LII) of the electrocardiogram, and transcutaneous femoral artery pulse tracing in a 41-year-old patient with congestive primary myocardial disease. The first (1) and second (2) heart sounds are diminished on the phonocardiogram and the third (3) and fourth (4) sounds are prominent. Due to the rapid heart rate the two diastolic sounds (3 and 4) are summated (summation gallop). Note pulse alternation of the transcutaneous femoral artery pulse tracing.

JUGULAR VENOUS PULSE TRACING

The jugular venous pulse tracing shows a conspicuous A wave with a normal C wave and a normal or sustained systolic X descent (fig. 10.6). The V wave is large, with a rapid Y descent followed by a quick rise in early diastole. On the jugular venous tracing, it may be difficult to differentiate between cardiomyopathy and constrictive pericarditis (see Chapter 11). Alternation of the jugular venous pulse indicates the presence of associated severe right ventricular disease (fig. 10.7).

APEXCARDIOGRAM

The apexcardiogram shows a large A wave and a sustained systolic contraction (figs. 10.8 and 10.9). Late systolic bulges are common and indicate left ventricular dyskinesis (fig. 10.9). The rapid filling wave is prominent. Pulsus alternans can also be seen on the apexcardiogram as shown in figure 10.10.

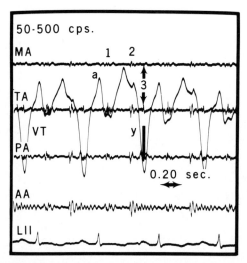

Fig. 10.6 Simultaneously recorded phonocardiogram at the mitral (MA), tricuspid (TA), pulmonic (PA) and aortic areas (AA) with a jugular venous pulse tracing (VT) and lead II (LII) of the electrocardiogram in a 27-year-old patient with restrictive primary myocardial disease. Amplitude of the A wave on the jugular venous tracing is slightly increased. This is followed by a sustained systolic wave and obliterated by the x descent. The v wave is slightly prominent, followed by a rapid y descent. A prominent, early third heart sound on the phonocardiogram coincides with the bottom of the y descent. Following the y descent, there is a rapid rise. The first and second heart sounds have decreased amplitude.

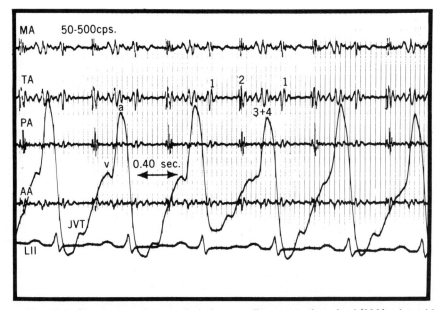

Fig. 10.7 Simultaneously recorded phonocardiogram at the mitral (MA), tricuspid (TA), pulmonic (PA), and aortic (AA) areas, lead II (LII) of the electrocardiogram, and jugular venous pulse tracing (JVT) in a 41-year-old patient with congestive primary myocardial disease. There is overall diminution of the first and second heart sounds recorded at several precordial areas on the phonocardiograms. The jugular venous pulse tracing shows typical features of pulsus alternans (see text).

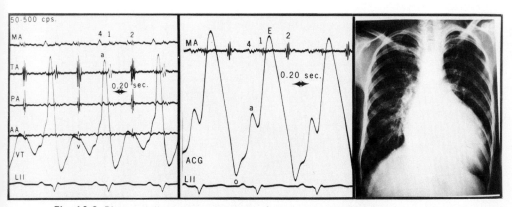

Fig. 10.8 Phonocardiographic and pulse wave abnormalities in a 15-year-old male patient with primary myocardial disease. Mitral (MA), tricuspid (TA), pulmonic (PA) and aortic (AA) area phonocardiograms recorded simultaneously with a jugular venous pulse tracing (VT), and lead II (LII) of the electrocardiogram are shown in the left panel. Marked exaggeration of the A wave on the jugular venous tracing is indicative of severe right ventricular hypertension and marked accentuation of the second heart sound is indicative of pulmonary hypertension. Mean pulmonary artery pressure was 75 mm Hg. In the middle panel the phonocardiogram at the mitral area (MA) was recorded simultaneously with the apexcardiogram (ACG) and lead II of the electrocardiogram. The marked exaggeration in amplitude of the A wave coincides with a prominent fourth heart sound on the phonocardiogram. The chest x-ray in the right panel shows a markedly enlarged cardiac silhouette.

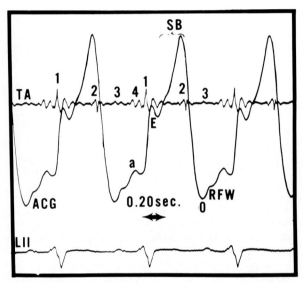

Fig. 10.9 Simultaneously recorded tricuspid area (TA) phonocardiogram, apex-cardiogram (ACG), and lead II (LII) of the electrocardiogram in a 49-year-old patient with congestive myocardial disease. The phonocardiogram was recorded in a frequency range of 50–500 Hz. The E point of the apexcardiogram is followed by a small systolic retraction and a late systolic bulge (SB). The third and fourth heart sounds on the phonocardiogram coincide with the peak of the rapid filling wave (RFW) and A wave on the apexcardiogram (see text).

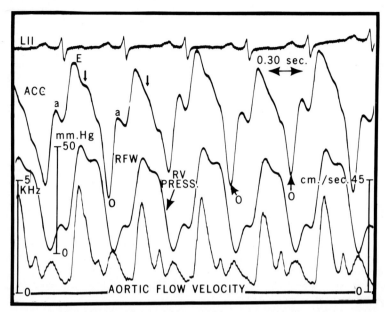

Fig. 10.10 Simultaneously recorded lead II (LII) of the electrocardiogram, apexcardiogram (ACG), right ventricular (RV) pressure, and aortic flow velocity curve using the Doppler flowmeter technique in a 38-year-old patient with severe congestive myocardial disease. Pulsus alternans is present in all three recordings. Stronger cardiac beats are associated with a large aortic velocity curve, high right ventricular pressure, and large deflection on the apexcardiogram. Observe the alternation of the E and O points and the rapid filling (RFW) and A waves in the apexcardiogram.

SYSTOLIC TIME INTERVALS

The ejection time (ET) is short and the pre-ejection period (PEP) is prolonged. Several reports have indicated that the ratio of PEP/ET is a good indicator of abnormal left ventricular function which is almost always present in primary myocardial disease. This ratio is above the normal value of 0.40 and seems to correlate well with diminished cardiac output, stroke volume and left ventricular ejection fraction.

ECHOCARDIOGRAM

The echocardiogram in patients with primary myocardial disease shows diminished excursion of the interventricular septum (fig. 10.11) and the posterior wall of the left ventricle (fig. 10.12). True paradoxical motion of the interventricular septum is rare. When right and/or left ventricular end-diastolic pressures are elevated, abnormal motion of the mitral and/or tricuspid valve is frequently seen, especially at the time of atrial contraction (tall A wave or in addition, the A-C interval is

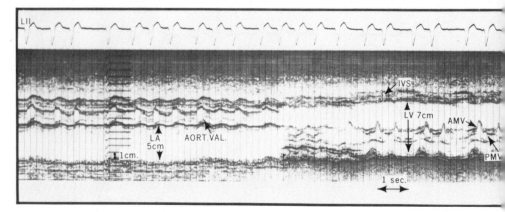

Fig. 10.11 Echocardiogram recorded in a 73-year-old patient with heart failure of unknown etiology showing flat motion of the interventricular septum (IVS). Note marked increase of the intracavity diameter of the left atrium to 5 cm and of the left ventricle (LV) to 7 cm. The electrocardiogram shows atrial fibrillation with variable ventricular rate. LA = left atrium, AMV and PMV = anterior and posterior mitral valve, respectively.

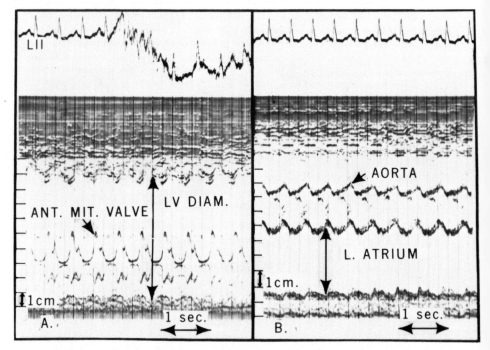

Fig. 10.12 Echocardiogram recorded in a 16-year-old patient with severe, congestive primary myocardial disease. The left panel shows marked increase in left ventricular internal dimension (LV DIAM) to 8.3 cm. The right panel shows marked increase in left atrial size (4.5 cm). Excursion to the posterior wall of the left ventricle is diminished (see text).

prolonged and the PR interval minus the A-C interval is short). The aortic valve is small, reflecting diminished cardiac output and stroke volume. Abnormal motion of the pulmonic valve (flat motion without an A dip) may also be seen indicating the presence of severe pulmonary hypertension. Measurements of intracavitary structures almost always demonstrate increased left atrial and left ventricular internal diameters, and right ventricular diameter.

REFERENCES

1. Abbasi, A. S., Chahine, R. A., MacAlpin, R. N., and Kattus, A. A.: Ultrasound in the diagnosis of primary congestive cardiomyopathy. Chest, *63:* 937, 1973.
2. Abbasi, A. S., MacAlpin, R. N., Eber, L. M., and Pearce, M. L.: Echocardiographic diagnosis of idiopathic hypertrophic cardiomyopathy with outflow obstruction. Circulation, *46:* 897, 1972.
3. Abbasi, A. S., MacAlpin, R. N., Eber, L. M., and Pearce, M. L.: Left ventricular hypertrophy diagnosed by echocardiography. N. Engl. J. Med., *289:* 118, 1973.
4. Anger, L. E.: Mitral and aortic valve incompetence in endocardial fibroelastosis; diagnostic and hemodynamic significance. Am. J. Cardiol. *28:* 309, 1971.
5. Andreini, A.: The rehophonocardiogram in myocardiopathy. Boll. Soc. Ital. Cardiol., *2:* 618, 1966.
6. Barritt, D. W., and al-Shammas, M.: Heart failure from unexplained cardiomyopathy. Br. Heart J., *28:* 674, 1966.
7. Bonnet, F., and Guebelle, F.: Value of phonocardiography in the diagnosis of cardiopathies in the young child. Rev. Med. Liege, *13:* 843, 1958.
8. Calzavara, G., Maschino, G., and Poli, D.: Phonocardiographic findings in obstructive hypertrophic myocardiopathy. Boll. Soc. Ital. Cardiol., *11:* 792, 1966.
9. Cheng, T. O.: Prompt squatting and systolic murmurs. Am. Heart J., *77:* 433, 1969.
10. Cueto, J., Toshima, H., Armijo, G., Tuna, N., and Lillehei, C. W.: Vectorcardiographic studies in acquired valvular disease with reference to the diagnosis of right ventricular hypertrophy. Circulation, *33:* 588, 1966.
11. Dower, G. E., and Horn, H. E.: The polarcardiograph; diagnosis of left ventricular hypertrophy. Am. Heart J., *74:* 368, 1967.
12. Epstein, E. J., Coulshed, N., Brown, A. K., and Doukas, N. G.: The "A" wave of the apex cardiogram in aortic valve disease and cardiomyopathy. Br. Heart J., *30:* 591, 1968.
13. Falcone, D. M., Moore, D., and Lambert, E. C.: Idiopathic hypertrophic cardiomyopathy involving the right ventricle. Am. J. Cardiol., *19:* 735, 1967.
14. Feigenbaum, H.: Newer aspects of echocardiography. Circulation, *47:* 833, 1973.
15. Fort, M. L., Chitty, J., Meadows, W. R., and Sharp, J. T.: The effect of ventricular alternation on a summation gallop sound; report of a case with left atrial and left ventricular intracardiac phonocardiograms. Am. J. Cardiol., *23:* 748, 1969.
16. Goodwin, J. F.: The non obstructive cardiomyopathies. Acta Cardiol., *21:* 272, 1966.
17. Goodwin, J. F., and Oakley, C. M.: The cardiomyopathies. Br. Heart J., *34:* 545, 1972.
18. Gould, L., and Lyon, A. F.: Pulsus alternans. An early manifestation of left ventricular dysfunction. Angiology, *19:* 103, 1968.
19. Hanby, R. I.: Primary myocardial disease; a prospective clinical and hemodynamic evaluation in 100 patients. Medicine (Baltimore), *49:* 55, 1970.
20. Harris, L. C., and Nghiem, Q. X.: Cardiomyopathies in infants and children. Prog. Cardiovasc. Dis., *15:* 255, 1972.
21. Harvey, W. P.: Clinical recognition and treatment of primary myocardial disease; introduction. Circulation, *32:* 830, 1965.
22. Harvey, W. P., and Perloff, J. K.: The auscultatory findings in primary myocardial disease. Am. Heart J., *61:* 199, 1961.
23. Harvey, W. P., Segal, J. P., and Gurel, T.: The clinical spectrum of primary myocardial disease. Prog. Cardiovasc. Dis., *7:* 17, 1964.

24. Harvey, W. P., and Segal, J. P.: Primary myocardial disease. Postgrad. Med., *42:* 144, 1967.
25. Hill, C. A., Harle, T. S., and Gaston, W.: Cardiomyopathy: A review of 59 patients with emphasis on the plain chest roentgenogram. Am. J. Roentgenol. Radium Ther. Nucl. Med., *104:* 433, 1968.
26. Hudson, R. E.: The cardiomyopathies: Order from chaos. Am. J. Cardiol., *25:* 70, 1970.
27. Ino, T.: Study of the idiopathic cardiomyopathy. Diagnostic value of the apexcardiogram, 131 scintiscanning of the heart and plasma hydroxyproline. Jap. Circ. J., *35:* 731, 1971.
28. Karatzas, N. B., Hamill, J., and Sleight, P.: Hypertrophic cardiomyopathy. Br. Heart J., *30:* 826, 1968.
29. Lundstrom, N. R., and Edler, I.: Ultrasound cardiography in infants and children. Acta Paediatr. Scand., *60:* 117, 1971.
30. McDonald, I. G., and Hobson, E. R.: A comparison of the relative value of noninvasive techniques—echocardiography, systolic time intervals, and apexcardiography—in the diagnosis of primary myocardial disease. Am. Heart J., *88:* 454, 1974.
31. Mercier, G., and Patry, G.: Quebec beer drinkers' cardiomyopathy; clinical signs and symptoms. Can. Med. Assoc. J., *97:* 884, 1967.
32. Morrow, A. G., Fisher, R. D., and Fogarty, T. J.: Isolated hypertrophic obstruction to right ventricular outflow; clinical, hemodynamic and angiographic findings before and after operative treatment. Am. Heart J., *77:* 814, 1969.
33. Nagle, R. E., Boicourt, O. W., Gillam, P. M., and Mounsey, J. P. D.: Cardiac impulse in hypertrophic obstructive cardiomyopathy. Br. Heart J., *28:* 419, 1966.
34. Nellen, M., Gotsman, M. S., Vogelpoel, L., Beck, W., and Schrire, V.: Effects of prompt squatting on the systolic murmur in idiopathic hypertrophic obstructive cardiomyopathy. Br. Med. J., *3:* 140, 1967.
35. Oakley, C. M.: Clinical recognition of the cardiomyopathies. Circ. Res., (Suppl.) *35:* 152, 1974.
36. Obeyesekere, I.: Idiopathic cardiomegaly in Ceylon; congestive cardiac failure, cardiomegaly, hepatomegaly, and portal fibrosis associated with malnutrition. Br. Heart J., *30:* 226, 1968.
37. Pietras, E. J., Meadows, W. E., Fort, M., and Sharp, J. T.: Hemodynamic alterations in idiopathic myocardiopathy including cineangiography from the left heart chambers. Am. J. Cardiol., *16:* 672, 1965.
38. Popp, R. L., and Levine, R.: Left atrial mass simulating cardiomyopathy. J. Clin. Ultrasound, *1:* 96, 1973.
39. Ramsey, H. W., Shar, S., Elliott, L. P., and Eliot, R. S.: The differential diagnosis of restrictive myocardiopathy and chronic constrictive pericarditis without calcification; value of coronary arteriography. Am. J. Cardiol., *25:* 635, 1970.
40. Reid, J. V. O.: The second heart sound in biventricular failure due to African cardiomyopathy. Am. Heart J., *68:* 38, 1964.
41. Rittenhouse, E. A., and Barnes, R. W.: Cardiac tamponade vs acute myocardial failure; differentiation by ultrasonic assessment of jugular venous velocity. Surg. Forum, *25:* 168, 1974.
42. Shabetal, R.. and Davidson, S.: Asymmetrical hypertrophic cardiomyopathy simulating mitral stenosis. Circulation, *45:* 37, 1972.
43. Shah, P. M., Gramiak, R., Kramer, D. H., and Yu, P. N.: Determinants of atrial (S_4) and ventricular (S_3) gallop sounds in primary myocardial disease. N. Engl. J. Med., *278:* 753, 1968.
44. Sheldon, W. C., Johnson, C. D., and Favaloro, R. G.: Idiopathic enlargement of the right atrium; report of four cases. Am. J. Cardiol., *23:* 278, 1969.
45. Storstein, O.: Primary myocardial disease in middle age. Geriatrics, *23:* 170, 1968.
46. Sumner, R. G., Segal, J. P., Harvey, W. P., and Gurel, T.: Diagnosis and treatment of primary myocardial disease. Circulation, *32:* 837, 1965.
47. Terman, D. S., Alfrey, A. C., Hammond, W. S., Donndelinger, T., Ogden, D. A., and

Holmes, J. H.: Cardiac calcification in uremia; a clinical, biochemical and pathologic study. Am. J. Med., *50:* 744, 1971.
48. Williams, J. F., Jr., Childress, R. H., Boyd, D. L., Higgs, L. M., and Behnke, R. H.: Left ventricular function in patients with chronic obstructive pulmonary disease. J. Clin. Invest., *47:* 1143, 1968.
49. Zuckermann, R.: The heart sound in special cardiopathies. Arch. Kreislaufforsch., *50:* 293, 1961.

chapter 11

Pericardial Disease

Diseases of the pericardium are classified as (1) acute pericarditis and (2) chronic pericarditis, with or without constriction. The disease may be due to primary infection of the pericardial membrane. It may, rarely, be secondary to a chronic or recurrent systemic disease process, such as recurrent viral, fungal, or bacterial pericarditis or involvement of the pericardium secondary to malignant tumor whose primary site may be in the pericardium. More commonly, it is secondary to involvement of the pericardium. Pericarditis following open heart surgery is fairly common and is usually of no major clinical significance. Detailed discussion regarding the etiologic factors is beyond the scope of this book.

ACUTE PERICARDITIS

Heart Sounds, Friction Rubs, and Murmurs

The first and second heart sounds are normal in acute pericarditis without significant effusion. The most characteristic feature of acute pericarditis without constriction is the presence of a pericardial friction rub which has three major components. The first occurs during mid- or late systole, the second during early or mid-diastole at the time of rapid filling of the ventricles or shortly thereafter and the third during atrial contraction (fig. 11.1). If the patient's rhythm is atrial fibrillation, the third component is absent. The triphasic rub consists of high frequency vibrations, variable in amplitude. It is best heard at the tricuspid and/or mitral areas. The friction rub varies with respiration, being loudest during expiration and when the patient is in the left lateral decubitus position (fig. 11.2). Mid- or late systolic clicks may be present but they are uncommon, found in only 10–15% of patients with this disease state.

PERICARDIAL EFFUSION

Pericardial effusion may result from a multitude of pathologic conditions involving the pericardium as the primary site, or it can be secondary to a systemic disease process. Abnormalities in cardiac

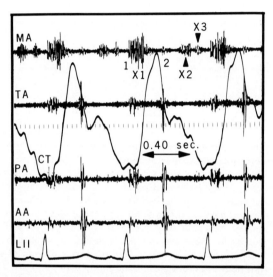

Fig. 11.1. Simultaneously recorded phonocardiogram at the mitral (MA), tricuspid (TA), pulmonic (PA) and aortic areas (AA), carotid pulse tracing (CT), and lead II (LII) of the electrocardiogram in a 17-year-old patient with rheumatic pericarditis. The phonocardiograms were taken at the setting of 500–2000 Hz. The first (1) and second (2) heart sounds have normal amplitude. The characteristic finding is the triphasic pericardial friction rub. The first component occurs in early or mid-systole. The mid- or early diastolic component (X2) is inscribed in mid-diastole. The atrial systolic component (X3) is recorded during atrial contraction and follows the P wave of the electrocardiogram. Note the "noisy" (vibrations or transients which have varying size, amplitude and duration) characteristics of these vibrations which are best recorded at the mitral and tricuspid areas.

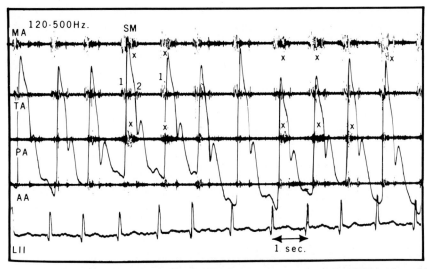

Fig. 11.2. Simultaneously recorded phonocardiogram at the mitral (MA), tricuspid (TA), pulmonic (PA) and aortic areas (AA), carotid pulse tracing, and lead II (LII) of the electrocardiogram in a 63-year-old patient who had post-operative pericarditis following aortic coronary saphenous bypass operation for coronary artery disease. The tracing was taken at a paper speed of 50 mm/sec in an attempt to record several cardiac cycles during various phases of the respiratory cycle. Several beats (X) were recorded during expiration. Note the marked variation in amplitude of the systolic component of the pericardial friction rub during various phases of the respiratory cycle. The noisy vibrations are more prominent during expiration (X). The first (1) and second (2) heart sounds have normal amplitude. In addition, there are marked changes in the total amplitude of the carotid pulse tracing. During expiration (X), the carotid pulse tracing has large amplitude and during inspiration it decreases (see text). **SM** = systolic murmur.

hemodynamics resulting from pericardial effusion are present when the amount of fluid exceeds 300 ml, causing significant impairment of ventricular filling.

Heart Sounds and Murmurs

The first heart sound is diminished in amplitude because late ventricular filling is decreased at the time of atrial contraction and the atrioventricular valves are in a semiclosed position. As a result, the rate of excursion of the atrioventricular valves is short. The second heart sound has diminished amplitude because stroke volume, pulmonary artery and aortic pressures are low (fig. 11.3). Third and fourth heart sounds are rarely present, particularly in younger patients. High frequency, low amplitude systolic regurgitant murmurs due to mitral and/or tricuspid insufficiencies are present in approximately 5–10% of patients.

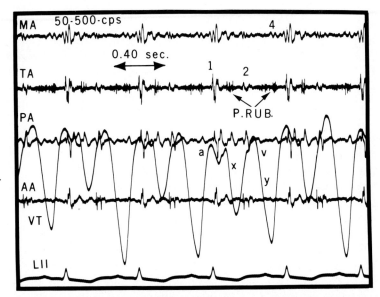

Fig. 11.3. Simultaneously recorded phonocardiogram at the mitral (MA), tricuspid (TA), pulmonic (PA) and aortic areas (AA), jugular venous pulse tracing (VT), and lead II (LII) of the electrocardiogram in a 45-year-old patient with uremic pericarditis and pericardial effusion with mild-to-moderate restriction of ventricular filling. The first (1) and second (2) heart sounds have normal amplitude. There is also a fourth (4) heart sound recorded best at the mitral area (MA). The pericardial friction rub (P RUB) only has a systolic and atrial systolic component. The early diastolic component is inconspicuous, probably due to a rapid heart rate. The jugular venous pulse tracing is abnormal showing a prominent A wave, small x descent followed by a rapid rise up to the peak of the v wave and a rapid y descent. Due to the rapid heart rate, the H wave is not recorded.

Carotid Pulse Tracing

The carotid pulse tracing has a normal contour or may show a rapid upstroke time and a short ejection time corresponding to the diminished stroke volume. Respiratory variations may occur in the amplitude of the carotid pulse tracing corresponding to so called "pulsus paradoxicus" (inspiratory fall in systolic arterial pressure exceeding 10–15 mm Hg). A great deal of care should be exercised in the clinical evaluation of pulsus paradoxicus, since it may be detected in patients without significant pericardial effusion. However, it is of clinical value if the auscultatory, phonocardiographic and pulse wave abnormalities are present. Pulsus alternans (see Chapter 10) may be seen, particularly in patients with large effusion, and is usually indicative of major impairment in left ventricular function.

Jugular Venous Pulse Tracing

The jugular venous pulse tracing may be normal when the amount of pericardial fluid is less than 150–300 ml. In the presence of significant right ventricular restriction, the jugular venous pulse tracing shows a prominent A wave, a sustained systolic wave and a rapid Y descent followed by a rapid early diastolic rise. The tracing is identical to that of patients with constrictive pericarditis (fig. 11.3), and resembles the square root symbol ($\sqrt{\ }$). The contour of the jugular venous pulse tracing reflects changes of pressure and flow in the right atrium and right ventricle. In patients with constrictive pericarditis, perciardial effusion with restriction of venticular filling or restrictive myocardial disease, right atrial, right ventricular early end-diastolic, and pulmonary artery pressures are elevated.

Apexcardiogram

The precordial pulsations are diminished and a technically satisfactory apexcardiogram is rarely recorded. However, if a good recording is obtained, it may show a marked retraction during systole indicating the presence of left ventricular dyskinesis (fig. 11.4) and may exhibit a large

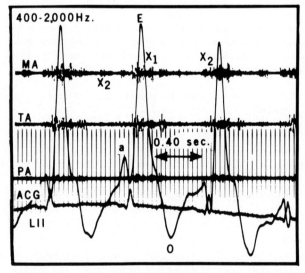

Fig. 11.4. Simultaneously recorded phonocardiogram at the mitral (MA), tricuspid (TA) and pulmonic areas (PA), apexcardiogram (ACG), and lead II (LII) of the electrocardiogram in a 53-year-old patient with post-operative pericarditis following aortic coronary artery bypass operation with mild-to-moderate restriction of ventricular filling. A typical triphasic pericardial friction rub with all three components is present: (X_1) during systole, (X_2) early diastole, and (X_3) during atrial contraction. The apexcardiogram shows a sharp E point with a short duration. It is followed by a rapid systolic retraction. The A wave is slightly prominent.

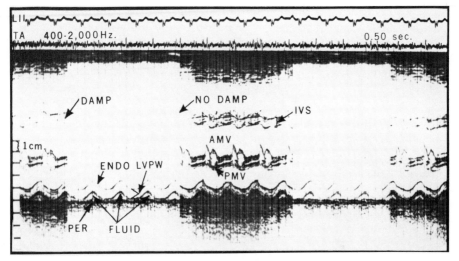

Fig. 11.5. Simultaneously recorded echocardiogram, phonocardiogram at the tricuspid area (TA), and lead II (LII) of the electrocardiogram in a 42-year-old patient with pericardial effusion due to uremic pericarditis. The tracings were taken at different damping settings. For proper identification of pericardial (PERIC) fluid, the best recording is obtained by increasing the damping setting as shown on the left and right sides of this figure. The diagnosis of pericardial effusion in this case could have been missed if the damping setting had not been adjusted properly. Paradoxical motion of the interventricular septum (IVS) is present (anterior instead of the normal posterior motion). This is frequently seen in this condition. The right ventricular dimension at end-diastole is enlarged to approximately 4.0 cm. The left ventricular internal dimension, at end-diastole is 5 cm, which is normal. There is 0.6 cm of posterior pericardial fluid representing a relatively small effusion. The interventricular septum measures 1 cm as does the left ventricular posterior wall. Both are of normal thickness. AMV = anterior mitral valve, PMV = posterior mitral valve, ENDO LVPW = endocardium of the left ventricular posterior wall.

A wave indicating the presence of a forceful left atrial contraction during late left ventricular diastolic filling.

Systolic Time Intervals

Ejection time is normal or diminished and varies with respiration. This is probably secondary to decreased stroke volume and decreased aortic pressure during respiration. These changes occur, however, only in patients with large effusion.

Echocardiogram

One of the first clinical applications of echocardiography was evaluation of patients with pericardial effusion. It gave great impetus to this diagnostic technique. The echocardiogram detects the presence of pericardial effusion and grossly quantitates the amount of pericardial fluid in the anterior and/or posterior aspects of the heart. Pericardial fluid is recognized by an "echo free" space separating the epicardial surface of the heart from the pericardium, (figs. 11.5–11.8). Tracings should be taken at multiple damping settings. By using too much damping, false effusion can be induced (fig. 11.7) in patients who do not have effusion. Additional findings on the echocardiogram include the presence of paradoxical motion of the interventricular septum (fig. 11.5) and an increase in thickness of the parietal pericardium. This technique is also of use in the evaluation of the removal of pericardial fluid as shown in figure 11.9.

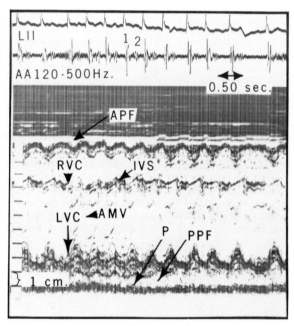

Fig. 11.6. Simultaneously recorded echocardiogram, phonocardiogram at the aortic area (AA) and lead II (LII) of the electrocardiogram in a 50-year-old patient with large anterior-posterior pericardial effusion (APF) and pleural effusion (PPF). The first (1) and second (2) heart sounds have varying amplitude because of changes in cycle length due to atrial fibrillation. The anterior pericardial effusion is approximately 1 cm and the posterior pericardial effusion is 1.7 to 2 cm. The left ventricular end-diastolic internal dimension is 5 cm. Right ventricular end-diastolic dimension is approximately 2.4 cm. Both chambers are within normal limits. Accurate left ventricular posterior wall measurements cannot be made. RVC = right ventricular cavity, IVS = interventricular septum, LVC = left ventricular cavity, AMV = anterior mitral valve, P = pleura.

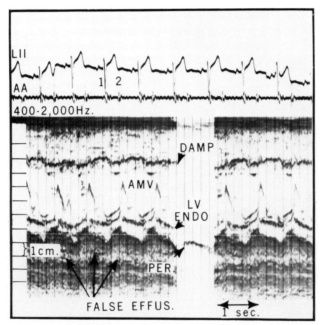

Fig. 11.7. Simultaneously recorded echocardiogram, lead II (LII) of the electrocardiogram, and phonocardiogram at the aortic area (AA) in a 19-year-old patient
illustrating the importance of using the proper technique to detect pericardial effusion
by means of echocardiography. On the left, a clear "echo free" space can be
misinterpreted as posterior pericardial effusion (false effusion). This may be
artifactually produced in normal subjects by directing the echocardiographic transducer too far medially or by using the wrong damping settings. Note that by increasing the damping, the recording of the pericardial (PER) and left ventricular
endocardial (LV ENDO) structures become clearly identifiable indicating the absence
of pericardial effusion. The first (1) and second (2) heart sounds are normal in the
phonocardiogram. There is a systolic ejection murmur in the phonocardiogram
representing turbulent flow across the aortic valve.

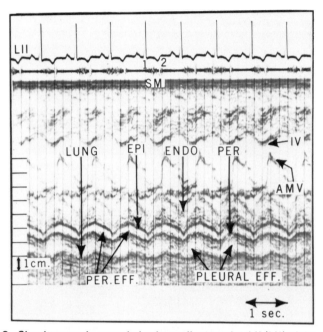

Fig. 11.8. Simultaneously recorded echocardiogram, lead II (LII) of the electrocardiogram, and phonocardiogram at the aortic area (AA) in a 20-year-old patient with severe arterial hypertension, renal failure, pleural and pericardial effusions. Note the "echo free" space behind the epicardium of the left ventricle (EPI) and the second "echo free" area behind the pericardium corresponding to a large pleural effusion (PLEURAL EFF) (see text). This tracing shows an abnormally large septum at 2 cm. The left ventricular posterior wall is equally thick, typically seen in patients with chronic renal disease and associated hypertension. There is a small (0.6 cm) posterior pericardial effusion. The right ventricular dimension at end-diastole is approximately 1.6 cm which is normal. The left ventricular internal dimension at end-diastole is 5.8 cm. The pleural effusion, not usually evaluated echocardiographically, measures approximately 1.5 cm. **ENDO** = endocardium, **AMV** = anterior mitral valve, **IV** = interventricular septum, **SM** = systolic murmur.

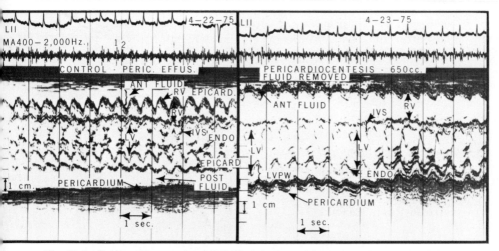

Fig. 11.9. Echocardiogram, lead II (LII) of the electrocardiogram, and mitral (MA) area phonocardiogram in a patient with a very large pericardial effusion. The left panel shows both anterior (ANT) and posterior (POST) pericardial fluid. The right panel shows a tracing taken 24 hours later, after removal of 650 cc of fluid via pericardiocentesis. IVS = interventricular septum, ENDO = endocardium, LVPW, left ventricular posterior wall, RV = right ventricle, LV = left ventricle.

CONSTRICTIVE PERICARDITIS

Constrictive pericarditis (Pick's disease) is due to marked fibrosis with or without calcification of the pericardium around the epicardial surface of the heart. Constriction is usually present on the surface of the left ventricle but it may involve multiple cardiac chambers.

Heart Murmurs and Sounds

The first heart sound is normal. The second heart sound is usually widely split with marked variations during respiration. One of the most striking features in patients with constrictive pericarditis is the presence of an early diastolic sound called a "pericardial knock" (fig. 11.10). This early "third heart sound" occurs within the range of 0.04–0.12 sec after the aortic valve closure sound and has high amplitude and low frequency characteristics. At times, on auscultation, it is difficult to differentiate this from a split second heart sound. However, with simultaneous recording of a phonocardiogram and apexcardiogram, this early diastolic sound should coincide with the peak of the rapid filling wave on the apexcardiogram, and if there is a split second sound both components should precede the O point of the apexcardiogram. The production mechanism for "pericardial knock" is not well known but is probably related to increased rapid filling of the non-distensible ventricles in the early diastolic phase of the cardiac cycle. This sound is best heard at the mitral and tricuspid areas. Prominent fourth heart sounds are frequently heard in constrictive pericarditis due to forceful atrial contraction against a non-distensible ventricle which also has poor compliance during the late diastolic phase of the cardiac cycle.

No definite characteristic murmurs can be detected. Low frequency atrioventricular diastolic murmurs resembling mitral and/or tricuspid stenosis have been described, but are rare. They may be the result of constriction around the atrioventricular valve rings causing a decrease in size of the mitral and/or tricuspid orifices, thus simulating mitral or tricuspid stenosis (see Chapters 4 and 6).

Carotid Pulse Tracing

The carotid pulse tracing has normal contour.

Jugular Venous Pulse Tracing

Inspection of the jugular venous pulsation should make the observer suspect the presence of constrictive pericarditis. If a jugular venous pulse tracing is recorded, it will show a large A wave, small X descent, sustained systolic and large H and V waves (fig. 11.10), reflecting abnormalities of right ventricular functions.

Apexcardiogram

In constrictive pericarditis, the apexcardiogram shows a large A wave representing a forceful atrial contraction against a non-distensible left ventricle during late diastole. The E point is sharp. During systole, there is a systolic retraction, followed by a late systolic wave, indicating the presence of left ventricular dyskinesis. A prominent and sharp rapid filling wave is present because most of the left ventricular filling occurs during that phase of diastole. The peak of the rapid filling wave coincides with the prominent early "third heart sound."

Systolic Time Intervals

Ejection time is usually diminished, corresponding to decreased stroke volume, ejection fraction, and aortic pulse pressures.

Echocardiogram

No definite patterns have been described outlining the use of echocardiography in patients with constrictive pericarditis. However, in this condition, one may find decreased diastolic motion of the posterior left ventricular wall. A rapid E-F slope of the anterior mitral valve may be present, probably representing an increased rapid rate of flow in the left ventricle during early diastole. However, these findings should be interpreted with caution since they may also be seen in patients with

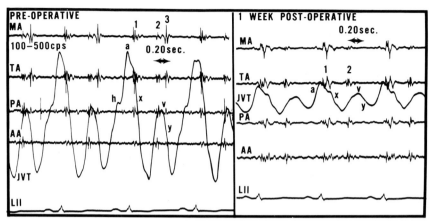

Fig. 11.10. Pre- and post-operative phonocardiograms at the mitral (MA), tricuspid (TA), pulmonic (PA) and aortic (AA) areas, jugular venous tracing (JVT) and lead II (LII) of the electrocardiogram in a 61-year-old patient with constrictive pericarditis. The pre-operative phonocardiogram shows an abnormal early third heart sound (3) and the A2-third heart sound interval measures 0.09 sec. This sound is well recorded in all precordial areas including the aortic area. The early third heart sound follows the peak of the v wave of the jugular venous pulse tracing. The first (1) and second (2) heart sounds are normal. The jugular venous pulse tracing shows prominent a and v waves, a rapid y descent, and a conspicuous h wave. One week following total pericardectomy, the third heart sound is no longer present. The jugular venous pulse tracing shows a decrease in the amplitude of both a and v waves, and slower x and y descents. The first (1) and second (2) heart sounds are normal.

primary myocardial disease. The interventricular septum has a paradoxical motion (anterior motion instead of normal posterior motion) during systole, as shown in figure 11.10.

REFERENCES

1. Abbasi, A. S., Ellis, N., and Flynn, J. J.: Echocardiographic M-scan technique in the diagnosis of pericardial effusion. J. Clin. Ultrsound, *1:* 300, 1973.
2. Boicourt, O. W., Nagle, R. E., and Mounsey, J. P.: The clinical significance of systolic retraction of the apical impulse. Br. Heart J., *27:* 379, 1965.
3. Boone, J. A., and Marsh, C. B.: Diagnosis of adhesive constrictive pericarditis. Am. Heart J., *68:* 576, 1964.
4. Braunwald, E., and Ross, J. Jr.: Hemodynamic alterations in pericardial diseases. Natl. Conf. Cardiovasc. Dis., *2:* 508, 1964.
5. Christensen, E. E., and Bonte, F. J.: The relative accuracy of echocardiography, intravenous CO_2 studies, and blood-pool scanning in detecting pericardial effusions in dogs. Radiology, *91:* 265, 1968.
6. Clauss, R. H.: Pericardial disease. Cardiovasc. Clin., *3:* 45, 1971.
7. Cohen, M. B., Gral, T., Sokol, A., Rubini, M. E., and Blahd, W. H.: Pericardial effusion in chronic uremia. Detection by photoscanning. Arch. Intern. Med., *122:* 404, 1968.
8. DeLand, F. H., and Felman, A. H.: Pericardial tumor compared with pericardial effusion. J. Nucl. Med., *13:* 697, 1972.
9. Durant, T. M.: Pericardial disease: diagnostic procedures. Natl. Conf. Cardiovasc. Dis., *2:* 506, 1964.

10. Ellis, K., and King, D. L.: Pericarditis and pericardial effusion; radiologic and echocardiographic diagnosis. Radiol. Clin. North Am., *11:* 393, 1973.
11. el-Sherif, A., and el-Said, G.: Jugular, hepatic, and praecordial pulsations in constrictive pericarditis. Br. Heart J., *33:* 305, 1971.
12. Feigenbaum, H.: Echocardiographic diagnosis of pericardial effusion. Am. J. Cardiol., *26:* 475, 1970.
13. Feigenbaum, H.: Ultrasonic cardiology. Diagnostic ultrasound as an aid to the management of patients with pericardial effusion. Dis. Chest, *55:* 59, 1969.
14. Feigenbaum, H., Waldhausen, J. A., and Hyde, L. P.: Ultrasound diagnosis of pericardial effusion. J.A.M.A., *191:* 711, 1965.
15. Fontenelle, L. J., Cuello, L., and Dooley, B. N.: Subxiphoid pericardial window; a simple and safe method for diagnosing and treating acute and chronic pericardial effusions. J. Thorac. Cardiovasc. Surg., *62:* 95, 1971.
16. Glaser, J.: Echocardiographic diagnosis of septic pericarditis in infancy. J. Pediatr., *83:* 697, 1973.
17. Goldberg, B. B., Ostrum B. J., and Isard, H. J.: Ultrasonic determination of pericardial effusion. J.A.M.A., *202:* 927, 1967.
18. Holmes, J. C., and Fowler, N. O.: Diagnosis of pericarditis. Postgrad. Med., *44:* 92, 1968.
19. Holt, J. P.: The normal pericardium. Am. J. Cardiol., *26:* 455, 1970.
20. Horowitz, M. S., Schultz, C. S., Stinson, E. B., Harrison, D. C., and Popp, R. L.: Sensitivity and specificity of echocardiographic diagnosis of pericardial effusion. Circulation, *50:* 239, 1974.
21. Idriss, F. S., Hisashi, N., and Muster, A. J.: Constrictive pericarditis simulating liver disease in children. Arch. Surg., *109:* 223, 1974.
22. Kay, C. F., Joyner, C. R., Helwig, J. Jr., and Raymond, T. F.: The "late systolic heartbeat" of pericardial effusion. Am. Heart J., *72:* 7, 1966.
23. Kenner, H. M., and Wood, E. H.: Intrapericardial, interpleural, and intracardiac pressures during acute heart failure in dogs studied without thoracotomy. Circ. Res., *19:* 1071, 1966.
24. Kahn, A. M., Nejat, M., and Bloomfield, D. A.: The measurement of pericardial effusion volume. Chest, *63:* 762, 1973.
25. Klein, J. J., Raber, G., Shimada, H., Kingsley, B., and Segal, B. L.: Evaluation of induced pericardial effusion by reflected ultrasound. Am. J. Cardiol., *22:* 49, 1968.
26. Klein, J. J., and Segal, B. L.: Pericardial effusion diagnosed by reflected ultrasound. Am. J. Cardiol., *22:* 57, 1968.
27. Lange, R. L., Botticelli, J. T., Tsagaris, T. J., Walker, J. A., Gani, M., and Bustamante, R. A.: Diagnostic signs in compressive cardiac disorders; constrictive pericarditis, pericardial effusion, and tamponade. Circulation, *33:* 763, 1966.
28. Lundstrom, N. R., and Edler, I.: Ultrasoundcardiography in infants and children. Acta Paediatr. Scand., *60:* 117, 1971.
29. McHenry, M. M., Ord, J. W., Johnson, R. R., and Shoener, J. A.: Exercise performance and stroke volume changes in two patients with constrictive pericarditis. Am. Heart J., *70:* 180, 1965.
30. Madaras, J. S. Jr., Taber, R. E., and Lam, C. R.: Constrictive pericarditis; diagnosis and operative management. Dis. Chest, *52:* 746, 1967.
31. Maia, I. G., Neto, C. D., Romao, N., Santos, M. A., Filho, J. N., Murad, M., and Reis, N. B.: A contribution of intracavitary electrocardiography to the differential diagnosis of right ventricular diastolic restriction syndrome. Am. Heart J., *88:* 401, 1974.
32. Matin, P., Ray, G., and Kriss, J. P.: Combined superior vena cava obstruction and pericardial effusion demonstrated by radioisotopic angiocardiography. J. Nucl. Med., *11:* 78, 1970.
33. Miscia, V. G., Holsinger, J. W., Mathers, D. H., and Eliot, R. S.: Primary pericardial tumor masquerading as constrictive pericarditis. J.A.M.A., *230:* 722, 1974.
34. Moreyra, E., Knibbe, P., and Segal, B. L.: Constrictive pericarditis masquerading as mitral stenosis. Chest, *57:* 245, 1970.

35. Moscovitz, H. L.: Pericardial constriction versus cardiac tamponade. Am. J. Cardiol., *26:* 546, 1970.
36. Moss, A. J., and Bruhn, F.: The echocardiogram; an ultrasound technic for the detection of pericardial effusion. N. Engl. J. Med., *274:* 380, 1966.
37. Pate, J. W., Gardner, H. C., and Norman, R. S.: Diagnosis of pericardial effusion by echocardiography. Ann. Surg., *165:* 826, 1967.
38. Pieroni, D. R., Park, S. C., Holbrook, P. R., and Houghton, P. B.: Echocardiographic diagnosis of septic pericarditis in infancy. J. Pediatr., *82:* 689, 1973.
39. Potter, D. J., and Cohen, A. I.: Diagnosis and management of uremic constrictive pericarditis. Ariz. Med., *28:* 302, 1971.
40. Pridie, R. B., and Turnbull, T. A.: Diagnosis of pericardial effusion by ultrasound. Br. Med. J., *3:* 356, 1968.
41. Ramsey, H. W., Sbar, S., Elliott, L. P., and Eliot, R. S.: The differential diagnosis of restrictive myocardiopathy and chronic constrictive pericarditis without calcification; value of coronary arteriography. Am. J. Cardiol., *25:* 635, 1970.
42. Ratshin, R. A., Smith, M., and Hood, W. P. Jr.: Possible false-positive diagnosis of pericardial effusion by echocardiography in presence of large left atrium. Chest, *65:* 112, 1974.
43. Rothman, J., Chase, N. E., Kricheff, I. I., Mayoral, R., and Beranbaum, E. R.: Ultrasonic diagnosis of pericardial effusion. Circulation, *35:* 358, 1967.
44. Samuels, L. D., and Stewart, C.: Rapid diagnosis of pericardial effusion with Tc-99m pertechnatate. J. Pediatr., *76:* 125, 1970.
45. Schlesinger, Z., Kraus, K. Y., and Neufeld, H. N.: Rapidly developing constrictive pericarditis in an infant simulating mitral valve obstruction. Acta Paediatr. Scand., *58:* 87, 1969.
46. Shabetai, R., Fowler, N. O., and Fenton, J. C.: Restrictive cardiac disease; pericarditis and the myocardiopathies. Am. Heart J., *69:* 271, 1965.
47. Shapiro, E., and Salick, A. I.: A clarification of the paradoxic pulse. Adolf Kussmaul's original description (A. Kussmaul). Am. J. Cardiol., *16:* 426, 1965.
48. Simcha, A., and Taylor, J. F. N.: Constrictive pericarditis in childhood. Arch. Dis. Child., *46:* 515, 1971.
49. Soulen, R. L., Lapayowker, M. S., and Gimenez, J. L.: Echocardiography in the diagnosis of pericardial effusion. Radiology, *86:* 1047, 1966.
50. Spodick, D. H.: Acoustic phenomena in pericardial disease. Am. Heart J., *81:* 114, 1971.
51. Spodick, D. H.: Electrocardiogram in acute pericarditis; distributions of morphologic and axial changes by stages. Am. J. Cardiol., *33:* 470, 1974.
52. Spodick, D. H.: Pericardial friction; characteristics of pericardial rubs in fifty consecutive, prospectively studied patients. N. Engl. J. Med., *278:* 1204, 1968.
53. Stein, L., Shubin, H., and Weil, M. H.: Recognition and management of pericardial tamponade. J.A.M.A., *225:* 503, 1973.
54. Tornaria, M., Cortes, R., and Fiandra, O.: Auscultation and phonocardiography in diseases of the pericardium. Thorax, *13:* 330, 1964.
55. Weiss, A., and Luisada, A. A.: The friction rubs of pericarditis. Chest, *60:* 491, 1971.
56. Weiss, E. R., Blahd, W. H., Winston, M. A., and Krishnamurthy, G. T.: Rapid diagnosis of pericardial effusion utilizing the scintillation camera. Am. J. Cardiol., *30:* 258, 1972.
57. Wright, F. W.: The diagnosis of free and loculated pericardial effusions during haemodialysis by diagnostic radiology, isotope scintiscanning and ultrasound. Br. J. Clin. Pract., *26:* 143, 1972.

chapter 12

Other Non-Invasive Diagnostic Techniques

In addition to the techniques described in previous chapters there are a number of non-invasive diagnostic techniques in cardiology which have not been covered. Some of them do play an important role in the diagnostic approach to patients with cardiovascular diseases and are utilized in several medical centers and others are gaining increasing importance. In this chapter, we will summarize some of them and indicate their diagnostic value in the study of patients with cardiovascular diseases.

VECTORCARDIOGRAPHY AND ELECTROCARDIOGRAPHY

It is beyond the scope of this book to describe the usefulness of resting or exercise electrocardiograms in the diagnosis of cardiovascular diseases. However, the increasing value of vectorcardiography must be emphasized. Renewed interest in vectorcardiography has been made possible through the development of vectorcardiographic criteria for the diagnosis of atrial and ventricular hypertrophies, myocardial infarction, and conduction defects which have been validated by invasive techniques such as coronary arteriography, right and left heart catheterization and cardiac angiography, His bundle electrograms, and necropsy findings. These studies have shown the vectorcardiogram is a superior technique as compared to the electrocardiogram in recognition of these disease states.

Correlation of the vectorcardiogram with coronary arteriograms and biplane left ventricular angiograms demonstrating akinetic segments, which subsequently have been removed at the time of open heart surgery, has established the validity of this non-invasive technique in the study of patients with coronary artery disease and ventricular asynergy. Vectorcardiograms are especially useful in patients with inferior and posterior wall myocardial infarctions, right and/or left atrial hypertrophy, certain types of right ventricular overloading, and in the recognition of myocardial infarction in the presence of conduction defects. Although vectorcardiography using time display (running loops) can detect most cardiac arrhythmias recognized on the electrocardiogram, as yet there is no proof that it will add significantly to the diagnosis of arrhythmias, as recorded on the electrocardiogram.

BALLISTOCARDIOGRAPHY

Ballistocardiography has been used for many years by several investigators to evaluate cardiovascular performance. Ballistocardiography, by definition, is a recording of the motions of the body caused by the shift in the center mass of blood caused by cardiac contraction. Due to multiple problems related to recording devices, this technique has not become popular. The ballistocardiographic wave form consists of numerous vibrations. A normal ballistocardiogram is shown in figures 12.1 and 12.2.

Attempts have been made to utilize the ballistocardiogram for determination of cardiac output and stroke volume; however, large discrepancies have been found between measurements obtained with ballistocardiograms as compared with other techniques. This technique has not proven to be a good indicator for assessment of left ventricular performance.

Abnormal wave form patterns have been described in some patients with congenital heart disease but no definite reproducible, characteristic abnormalities have been demonstrated. Reports have shown that this technique is of some value in the evaluation of patients with aortic stenosis and/or insufficiency. Patients with mitral stenosis and mitral insufficiency show abnormal notching, particularly during the first part of the pre-ejection period and in the first third of left ventricular systole. However, this is difficult to record and reproducibility of these findings has not been consistent enough to be of routine clinical usefulness. In patients with coronary artery disease and angina pectoris, there are some wave form abnormalities, however none of these abnormalities are characteristic for that disease state. In addition, this technique has been used on patients recovering from acute myocardial infarction (figs. 12.3 and 12.4) in patients with abdominal aortic aneurysm, hypertensive cardiovascular diseases and in studies on the influence of pharmacological agents in cardiovascular performance.

KINETOCARDIOGRAPHY

Kinetocardiography, by definition, is the recording of the low frequency vibrations over the precordium in the range of 30–40 Hz. The instrumentation uses a series of bellows with a sensing device and a probe at one end. A flat head, at the end of the probe (approximately 7 cm in

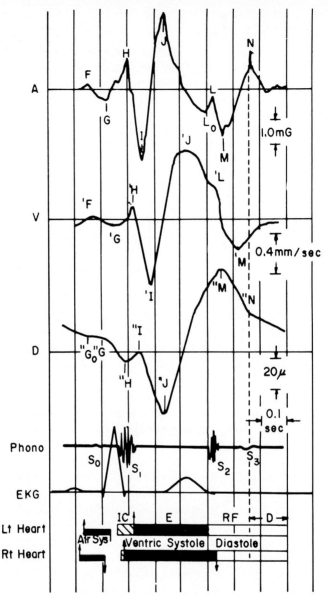

Fig. 12.1 Simultaneously recorded normal ultra-low frequency acceleration (A), velocity (V), and displacement (D) ballistocardiograms with the phonocardiogram and electrocardiogram. The various phases of the cardiac cycle are indicated at the bottom of this illustration. Observe the complexity of the wave form of the ballistocardiogram. All waves, as related to the cardiac cycle, are indicated. The H, I, and J waves are most important. The L wave (acceleration) is equivalent to the K wave of the high frequency ballistocardiographic recording system. This wave is usually not so prominent in the ultra-low frequency ballistocardiogram. (From W. R. Scarborough, E. F. Folk, P. M. Smith, and J. H. Condon: The nature and records from ultra-low frequency ballistocardiographic systems and their relation to circulatory events. Am. J. Cardiol., 2: 613–641, 1958, with permission.)

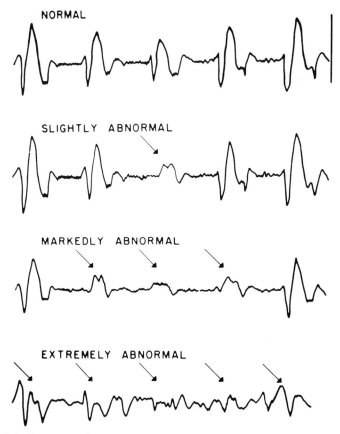

Fig. 12.2. Representative ballistocardiograms of four groups of patients according to the Starr qualitative classification based upon the proportion of normal to
abnormal complexes. The tracings from top to bottom were recorded simultaneously
and adjusted to permit vertical alignment of the respiratory cycle. Arrows point to the
complex of normal, slightly, markedly, and extremely abnormal wave forms. (From I.
Starr: *Proceedings of the First Congress Ballistocardiography and Cardiovascular
Dynamics*, pp. 7–20. Amsterdam: Karger, 1966, with permission.)

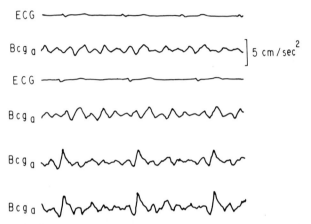

Fig. 12.3. Series of ballistocardiograms (Bcg) in a 43-year-old patient with coronary artery disease who underwent 6 months of training following a myocardial infarction. The top tracing, taken at the beginning of the training period, is grossly abnormal. The simultaneously recorded electrocardiogram (ECG) is important for identification of the proper complexes. Records 2, 3, and 4 (bottom of illustration) taken after 2, 4, and 6 months of training show a progressive increase in the force and normalization of the wave form. Record 4 falls within the normal range. (From J. O. Holloszy, J. S. Skinner, A. J. Barry, and T. K. Cureton: Effect of physical conditioning on cardiovascular function; a ballistocardiographic study. Am. J. Cardiol., *14:* 761-770, 1964, with permission.)

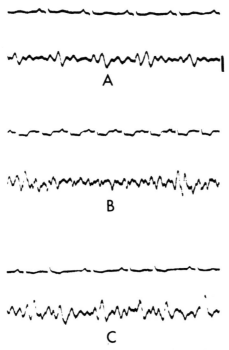

Fig. 12.4. Electrocardiogram and high frequency ballistocardiogram recorded before, during and following an episode of angina pectoris in a 63-year-old patient with coronary artery disease. Tracing A illustrates a usual record for this patient when he was not having angina pectoris and the blood pressure was 120/80 mm Hg. Tracing B was recorded during an episode of angina pectoris and the blood pressure at that time was 110/80 mm Hg. Tracing C was recorded approximately 5 minutes after sublingual administration of 0.6 mg of nitroglycerin when the pain subsided and the blood pressure at that time was 120/80 mm Hg. Note the disorganized wave form in the middle record during an episode of coronary insufficiency and marked changes in tracing C following relief of angina pectoris. (From I. Starr and A. Noordergraaf: *Ballistocardiography in Cardiovascular Research*, p. 235. Philadelphia: Lippincott, 1967, with permission.)

diameter) is placed against the chest wall. The system is then connected to a PM5-0.20-350 Statham strain-gauge transducer (fig. 12.5). The bellows are placed perpendicular against the chest wall to record pulsations at any given point. The major difference between the kinetocardiogram and the apexcardiogram is that the kinetocardiographic transducer records absolute displacement of the movements of the precordium, and the transducer is placed at several positions on the chest and not necessarily at the point of maximal apical impulse.

The nomenclature used in the kinetocardiogram to define the wave form and placement of the transducer uses the initial K for kinetocardiogram. The first number that follows the K represents the standard

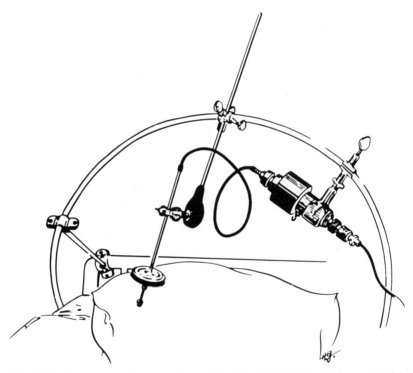

Fig. 12.5. Diagram of kinetocardiographic instrumentation used to record low frequency precordial movements. The bellows in the center of the figure is connected by tubing to a PM5-0.2-350 Statham transducer mounted on a crossbar. The probe on the other end of the bellows can be placed perpendicular to any area of the chest wall to record precordial movements. (From **W. H. Bancroft, Jr., and E. E. Eddleman, Jr.: Methods and physical characteristics of the kinetocardiographic and apexcardiographic systems for recording low frequency precordial motion. Am. Heart J.,** *73:* **756–764, 1967, with permission.)**

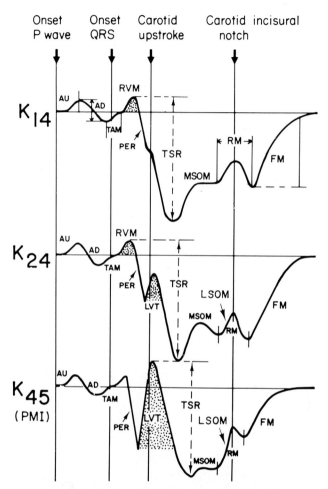

Fig. 12.6. Diagrammatic representation of normal kinetocardiograms recorded at three different precordial positions (K-14, K-24, and K-45). The nomenclature used is based upon the origin of movements and location within the cardiac cycle. Various phases of cardiac cycle are indicated by onset of the P wave and QRS complex of the electrocardiogram, and by the beginning of the upstroke and the dicrotic notch of the carotid pulse tracing. AU = atrial upstroke, AD = atrial downstroke, TAM = terminal atrial movement, RVM = right ventricular movement or initial outward movement, PER = pre-ejection retraction, LVT = left ventricular thrust, TSR = total systolic retraction, MSOM = mid-systolic outward movement, RM = relaxation movement, FM = filling movement, and LSOM = late systolic movement. (From E. E. Eddleman, Jr.: Kinetocardiography; in *Noninvasive Cardiology*, p. 238, A. M. Weissler (ed.). New York: Grune & Stratton, Inc., 1974, with permission.)

electrocardiographic precordial position and the second number identifies the interspaces from which the recording is made. The most commonly used locations are K-14, K-24, K-45, K-55, and Kem. A typical, normal kinetocardiogram from positions K-14, K-24, and K-45 is shown in figure 12.6. For example, K-14 as shown in figure 12.6 is ob-

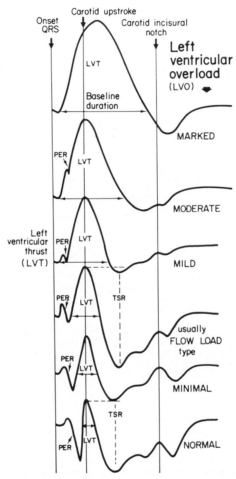

Fig. 12.7. Diagrammatic representation of abnormalities seen on the kinetocardiogram in patients with left ventricular overload. A normal kinetocardiographic curve is shown at the bottom of this illustration. As the abnormalities in the wave form of the kinetocardiogram increase, amplitude of the apex impulse becomes exaggerated and there is an increase in duration along the baseline. Eventually there is an absence of the pre-ejection retraction (PER) which occurs prior to onset of the rapid rise of the carotid pulse tracing. (From E. E. Eddleman, Jr.: Kinetocardiography; In *Noninvasive Cardiology*, p. 247, A. M. Weissler (ed.). New York: Grune & Stratton, Inc., 1974, with permission.)

tained from the electrocardiographic V_1 position or in the right parasternal line at the fourth left intercostal space; K-24 is at the fourth intercostal space at the left sided parasternal area; K-45 is at the mid-clavicular line at the fifth intercostal space and the recording closely resembles the wave form of the apexcardiogram. In the K-55 position, the transducer is placed at the anterior axillary line at the left, fifth intercostal space. Kem represents a record obtained with the transducer positioned at the mid-epigastric area below the xyphoid area.

The kinetocardiogram has been shown to be of value in the study of left ventricular function, particularly using tracings obtained at K-45 and K-55 positions (fig. 12.7). Abnormal records have been found in patients with mitral stenosis (fig. 12.8) at position K-24 which usually detects abnormal precordial motion in patients with right ventricular pressure overloading (fig. 12.9). Left ventricular impulses which can be obtained in positions K-43, K-44, and K-45 appear to be useful in the recognition of abnormal left ventricular contractions in patients with mitral insufficiency (fig. 12.10), aortic stenosis (fig. 12.11), and aortic insufficiency (fig. 12.7) or idiopathic hypertrophic subaortic stenosis (fig. 12.12).

The value of this technique in evaluating patients with coronary artery disease (fig. 12.13) and myocardial infarction has been demonstrated.

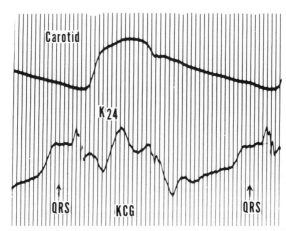

Fig. 12.8. Kinetocardiogram from position K-24 and carotid pulse tracing in a patient with mitral stenosis and mild elevation of pulmonary artery pressure. At cardiac catheterization, this patient was found to have a mean pulmonary artery pressure of 24 mm Hg and mean pulmonary "wedge" pressure of 16 mm Hg. Left ventricular stroke volume was 61 ml per beat and a calculated mitral valve area was 2.1 cm. The kinetocardiogram shows a mild increase in amplitude of the initial and mid-systolic right ventricular outward movements. (From E. E. Eddleman, Jr.: Kinetocardiography; In *Noninvasive Cardiology*, p. 251, A. M. Weissler (ed.). New York: Grune & Stratton, Inc., 1974, with permission.)

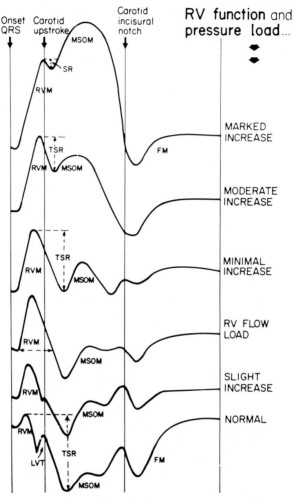

Fig. 12.9. Diagrammatic representation of various abnormalities seen in the kinetocardiogram in patients with various degrees of right ventricular overloading. Note that with progressive increase in the right ventricular function, the amplitude of the initial outward movement becomes larger. The mid-systolic retraction is markedly exaggerated in patients with right ventricular pressure load. A normal kinetocardiogram recording from that anatomical location is shown for comparison. Various times of the cardiac cycle are shown as related to the onset of the QRS complex of the electrocardiogram, and beginning of the upstroke and dicrotic notch of the carotid pulse tracing. **TAM** = terminal atrial movement, **RVM** = right ventricular movement or initial outward movement, **SR** = systolic retraction, **RV** = right ventricle, **PER** = pre-ejection retraction, **LVT** = left ventricular thrust, **TSR** = total systolic retraction, **MSOM** = mid-systolic outward movement, and **FM** = filling movement. (From E. E. Eddleman Jr.: Kinetocardiography; In *Noninvasive Cardiology*, p. 249, A. M. Weissler (ed.). New York: Grune & Stratton, Inc., 1974, with permission.)

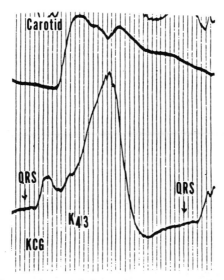

Fig. 12.10. Simultaneously recorded carotid pulse tracing and kinetocardiogram at position K-43 in a patient with pure mitral insufficiency. The hemodynamics on this patient demonstrated an elevated mean pulmonary artery pressure to 26 mm Hg; left ventricular end-diastolic volume, 240 ml; left ventricular end-systolic volume, 113 ml; left ventricular stroke volume, 127 ml; forward stroke volume, only 24 ml/beat and regurgitant flow calculated to be 103 ml/beat or 10 L/min (81%). Note the prominence of late systolic outward motion on this tracing. (From E. E. Eddleman, Jr.: Kinetocardiography; In *Noninvasive Cardiology*, p. 253, A. M. Weissler (ed.). New York: Grune & Stratton, Inc., 1974, with permission.)

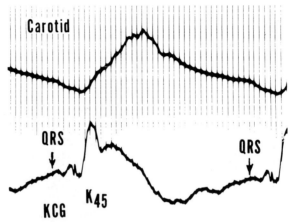

Fig. 12.11. Simultaneously recorded carotid pulse tracing and kinetocardiogram (KCG) at position K-45 in a patient with isolated aortic valvular stenosis with a gradient of 58 mm Hg across the aortic valve and a calculated aortic valve area of 0.9 cm^2. On the kinetocardiogram, amplitude of the left ventricular impulse is not markedly exaggerated but it is sustained throughout systole. The time of onset of the QRS complex in the electrocardiogram is indicated. The carotid pulse tracing shows a slow upstroke time and the other findings seen in patients with aortic valvular stenosis. (From E. E. Eddleman, Jr.: Kinetocardiography; In *Noninvasive Cardiology*, p.254, A. M. Weissler, (ed.). New York: Grune & Stratton, Inc., 1974, with permission.)

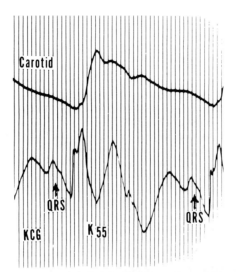

Fig. 12.12. Simultaneously recorded carotid pulse tracing and kinetocardiogram at position K-55 in a patient with proven idiopathic hypertrophic subaortic stenosis. The kinetocardiogram shows a double left ventricular impulse during systole. The gradient between the apex and the outflow tract of the left ventricle varied between 20 and 40 mm Hg. Onset of the QRS complex of the electrocardiogram is indicated. (From E. E. Eddleman, Jr.: Kinetocardiography; In *Noninvasive Cardiology*, p. 268, A M. Weissler (ed.). New York: Grune & Stratton, Inc., 1974, with permission.)

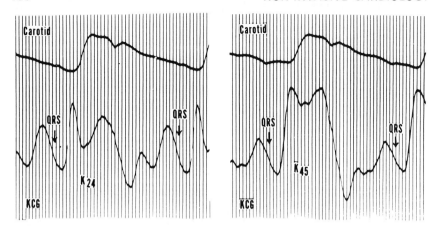

Fig. 12.13. Simultaneously recorded carotid pulse tracing and kinetocardiogram (KCG) at positions K-24 and K-45 in a patient with inferoposterior myocardial infarction. The coronary arteriogram revealed triple vessel coronary artery disease with complete occlusion of the left anterior descending and left circumflex arteries. In addition, the left diagonal branch was stenosed with an associated 80% lesion in the right coronary artery. The left ventriculogram shows a large area of akinesis of the left ventricular wall. The important feature on this kinetocardiogram is a large, sustained outward movement with a prominent A wave. (From E. E. Eddleman, Jr.: Kinetocardiography; In *Noninvasive Cardiology*, p. 257, A. M. Weissler (ed.). New York: Grune & Stratton, Inc., 1974, with permission.)

The best recording areas to detect the abnormalities in the kinetocardiogram in these patients are at positions K-44, K-35, K-34, and K-24. Paradoxical motions on these records have been detected as well as late systolic bulges representing left ventricular dyskinesis. Exaggerated A waves in some records are similar to the ones described for the apexcardiogram. Patients with congenital heart disease such as atrial and ventricular septal defects, pulmonary stenosis, tetralogy of Fallot, patent ductus arteriosus, and Ebstein's disease which are associated with right ventricular overloading can be detected in kinetocardiograms in the areas which record right ventricular movements.

RADIOLOGIC TECHNIQUES

The use of radiography for non-invasive evaluation of patients with cardiovascular disease is beyond the scope of this book. However, a brief description of techniques using x-ray image intensification systems will be given.

For many years, fluoroscopy of the heart has been used to study cardiac motion as well as to detect chamber enlargement. Recording cardiac motion on radiographic film, called roentgenkymography, provides a method for analysis of some segments of the external heart borders. The most important value of roentgenkymography is the detection of calcification of the cardiac valves and in evaluation of patients with pericardial disease.

ELECTROKYMOGRAPHY

Electrokymography is defined as a technique which records motion of the cardiac borders during various phases of the cardiac cycle. One of the most important applications of this technique, as described in the past, has been in patients with coronary artery disease and in the follow-up of patients who sustained acute myocardial infarction so that segments of left ventricular dyskinesis can be followed at time intervals demonstrating improvement in the left ventricular wall motion.

RADARKYMOGRAPHY

This technique records continuous movements of the cardiac border through an electronic tracing system connected to a televised video system used during fluoroscopy of the heart. It is of value in studying the motion of the left ventricle, left atrium, aorta, etc., and various segments of the cardiac silhouette in different projections. This technique has been shown to be of some value in evaluating patients with aortic valvular disease and left ventricular dyskinesis.

NUCLEAR CARDIOLOGY

The use of radionuclides has gained increasing popularity during the past few years as a non-invasive approach to evaluate patients with cardiovascular diseases. It is beyond the scope of this book to describe the technique in great detail. The instrumentation used to detect the presence of radiation is fairly complex. It consists of a gamma radiation detector having a scintillation crystal. The scintillation camera produces an image of injected tracer. Although there are a number of cameras available, the most commonly used is the Anger camera. It is also possible to obtain a simultaneous electrocardiogram with the image data, thus allowing the capability of timing the various segments of the cardiac cycle. This technique has been found useful in detecting cardiac enlargement of the atrial and ventricular chambers, areas of ventricular dyskinesis, ventricular aneurysm and in other conditions. Detection and gross quantitation of shunts in patients with congenital heart disease and the study of left ventricular volume with ejection fractions is also possible (figs. 12.14–12.18).

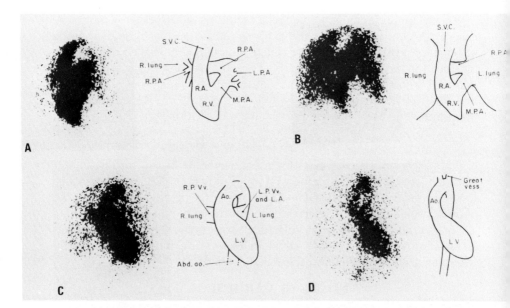

Fig. 12.14. Normal nuclear angiocardiogram. Serial frames taken 0.3 sec apart in the anterior position. Filling activity of the superior vena cava (SVC), right atrium (RA), right ventricle (RV), pulmonary outflow tract and main pulmonary artery (MPA) are shown in panel A. In panel B, nuclear activity is no longer present in the superior vena cava but has moved into the lungs. A space which is occupied by the left ventricle is not yet filled. Panel C shows activity in the left atrium (LA), left ventricle (LV) and aorta (Ao). In Panel D note aortic activity which extends below the diaphragm. The total time sequence from A to D is 9 sec. (From P. J. Hurley, H. W. Strauss and H. N. Wagner: Radionuclide angiography in cyanotic congenital heart disease. Johns Hopkins Med. J., *127:* 46, 1970, with permission.)

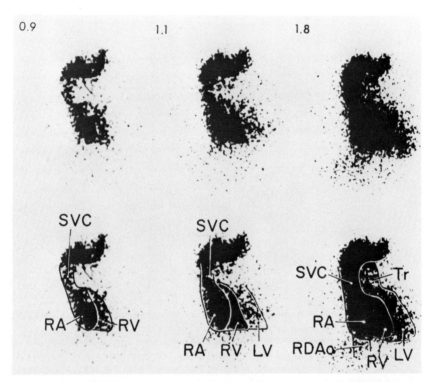

Fig. 12.15. Nuclear angiocardiogram in a patient with truncus arteriosus and associated ventricular septal defect. The tracer was injected into the left arm and the subclavian vein is seen emptying into the superior vena cava (SVC), right atrium (RA), and right ventricle (RV). In the following frames, the left ventricle (LV) fills, followed by the truncus (Tr) and aorta which is located on the right side. RDAo = right descending aorta. (From J. Wesselhoeft, P. J. Hurley, H. N. Wagner, and R. D. Rowe: Nuclear angiocardiography in the diagnosis of congenital heart disease in infants. Circulation, *45*: 77, 1972, with permission.)

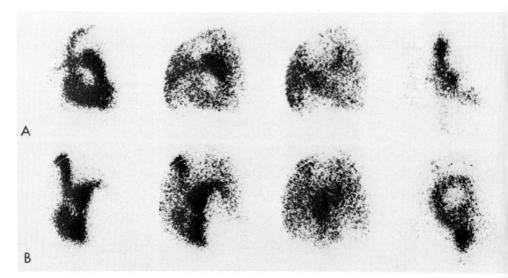

Fig. 12.16. Nuclear angiocardiogram in a patient with mitral stenosis. The apparent break in the superior vena cava (SVC) in the right anterior oblique position (Panel A) corresponds to the innominate vein emptying unlabeled blood into the superior vena cava. The enlarged left atrium fills in the third frame in both views and persists through the left ventricular phase of this cycle. Panel B is from a left anterior oblique position. (From H. W. Strauss and B. Pitt: Nuclear cardiology; In *Noninvasive Cardiology*, p. 385, A. M. Weissler (ed.). New York: Grune & Stratton, 1974, with permission.)

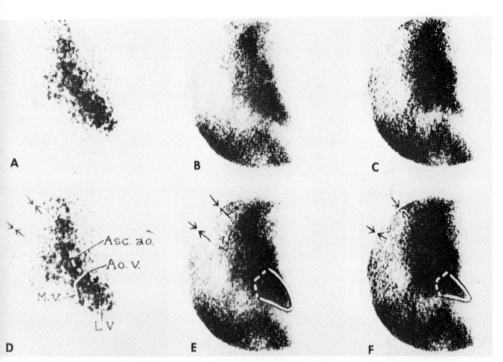

Fig. 12.17. Complete left ventricular outline obtained at end-systole and end-diastole by combining data from A, left ventricular phase of the nuclear angiocardiogram; B, end-diastolic gated image; C, end-systolic gated image. The mitral (M.v.) and aortic valve (Ao.v.) planes, determined from frame A, are superimposed on the scintiphoto. The recticule, indicated by an arrow, is a constant reference. The valve planes are then superimposed on frame B and C. The outline of the left ventricle (L.V.) at end-diastole and end-systole is traced and valve planes are superimposed as shown. Asc. Ao. = ascending aorta. From H. W. Strauss, B. L. Zaret, P. J. Hurley, T. K. Natarajan, and B. Pitt: A scintiphotographic method for measuring left ventricular ejection fraction in man without cardiac catheterization. Am. J. Cardiol., *28:* 575, 1971, with permission.)

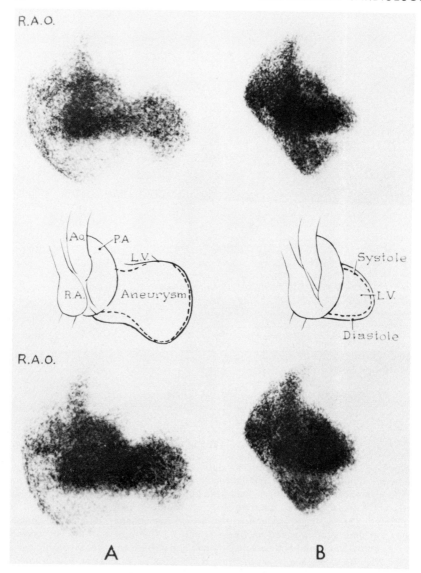

R.A.O.

R.A.O.

A   B

Fig. 12.18. Nuclear angiocardiogram showing cardiac blood pool scans with the patient in a right anterior oblique position (RAO). The patient has an anterior apical left ventricular aneurysm. End-systolic images are shown at the top and end-diastolic images on the bottom. Panel A, tracing taken pre-operatively, reveals location of the aneurysm at the apex which has a very small movement. Panel B, post-operative tracing, shows a poorly contracting ventricle without evidence of the aneurysm. RA = right atrium, Ao = aorta, PA = pulmonary artery, and LV = left ventricle. (From H. W. Strauss and B. Pitt: Nuclear cardiology; In *Noninvasive Cardiology*, p. 393, A. M. Weissler (ed.). New York: Grune & Stratton, Inc., 1974, with permission.)

REFERENCES

Ballistocardiography

1. Burger, H. C., Noordergraaf, A., and Verhagen, A. M. W.: Physical basis of the low-frequency ballistocardiograph. Am. Heart J., 46: 71, 1953.
2. Hamilton, W. F.: Measurement of the cardiac output, in Handbook of Physiology. Circulation, 1(2): 575, 1962.
3. Hamilton, W. F., and Dow, P.: Cardiac and aortic contributions to the human ballistocardiogram. Am. J. Physiol., 133: 313, 1941.
4. Holloszy, J. O., Skinner, J. S., Barry, A. J., and Cureton, T. K.: Effect of physical conditioning on cardiovascular function; a ballistocardiographic study. Am. J. Cardiol., 14: 761, 1964.
5. Noordergraaf, A., and Pollack, G. H.: Ballistocardiography and cardiac performance. Bibl. Cardiol., 19: 1, 1967.
6. Scarborough, W. R.: Current status of ballistocardiography. Prog. Cardiovasc. Dis., 2: 263, 1959.
7. Scarborough, W. R., Folk, E. F., Smith, P. M., and Condon, J. H.: The nature and records from ultra-low frequency ballistocardiographic systems and their relation to circulatory events. Am. J. Cardiol., 2: 613, 1958.
8. Starr, I.: Proceedings of the First Congress Ballistocardiography and Cardiovascular Dynamics, p. 7. Amsterdam: Karger, 1966.
9. Starr, I.: Progress towards a physiological cardiology—a second essay on the ballistocardiogram. Ann. Intern. Med., 63: 1079, 1965.
10. Starr, I., Horwitz, O., Mayock, R. L., and Kumbhaar, E. B.: Standardization of the ballistocardiogram by simulation of the heart's function at necropsy; with a clinical method for the estimation of cardiac strength and normal standards for it. Circulation, 1: 1073, 1950.
11. Starr, I., and Noordergraaf, A.: Ballistocardiography in Cardiovascular Research, p. 235. Philadelphia: J. B. Lippincott, 1967.
12. Starr, I., and Noordergraaf, A.: Ballistocardiography in Cardiovascular Research, p. 347. Philadelphia: J. B. Lippincott, 1967.
13. Starr, I., and Noordergraaf, A.: Ballistocardiography in Cardiovascular Research, p. 438. Philadelphia: J. B. Lippincott, 1967.
14. Starr, I., and Schnabel, T.G.: Studies made by simulating systole at necropsy; III. On the genesis of the systolic waves of the ballistocardiogram. J. Clin. Invest., 33: 10, 1954.
15. Trefny, Z., and Wagner, J.: A quantitative ballistocardiograph. Bibl. Cardiol., 19: 19, 1967.

Kinetocardiography

1. Bancroft, W. H. Jr., and Eddleman, E. E. Jr.: Methods and physical characteristics of the kinetocardiographic and apexcardiographic systems for recording low-frequency precordial motion. Am. Heart J., 73: 756, 1967.
2. Eddleman, E. E. Jr.: Kinetocardiographic changes as the result of mitral commissurotomy. Am. J. Med., 25: 733, 1958.
3. Eddleman, E. E. Jr.: Kinetocardiography, In A. M. Weissler (Ed.), Noninvasive Cardiology, p. 238. New York, Grune & Stratton, 1974.
4. Eddleman, E. E. Jr., Hughes, M. L., and Thomas, H. D.: Estimation of pulmonary artery pressure and pulmonary vascular resistance from ultra-low frequency precordial movements (kinetocardiograms). Am. J. Cardiol., 4: 662, 1959.
5. Eddleman, E. E. Jr., and Thomas, H. D.: The recognition and differentiation of right ventricular pressure and flow loads; a correlative study of kinetocardiograms, electrocardiograms, fluoroscopy, and cardiac catheterization data in patients with mitral stenosis, septal defect, pulmonic stenosis and isolated pulmonary hypertension. Am. J. Cardiol., 4: 652, 1959.
6. Eddleman, E. E. Jr., Yoe, R. H., Tucker, W. T., Knowles, J. L., and Willis, K.: The dynamics of ventricular contraction and relaxation in patients with mitral stenosis as studied by the kinetocardiogram and ballistocardiogram. Circulation, 11: 774, 1955.
7. Eddleman, E. E. Jr., Willis, K., Reeves, T. J., and Harrison, T. R.: The kinetocardio-

gram; I. Method of recording precordial movements. Circulation, *8:* 269, 1953.

8. Eddleman, E. E. Jr., Willis, K., Christianson, L., Pierce, J. R., and Walker, R. P.: The kinetocardiogram; II. The normal configuration and amplitude. Circulation, *8:* 370, 1953.

9. Eddleman, E. E. Jr., and Willis, K.: The kinetocardiogram; III. The distribution of forces over the anterior chest. Circulation, *8:* 569, 1953.

10. Harrison, T. R., and Hughes, L.: Precordial systolic bulges during anginal attacks. Trans. Assoc. Am. Physicians, *71:* 174, 1958.

11. Skinner, N. S. Jr., Leibeskind, R. S., Phillips, H. L., and Harrison, T. R.: Angina pectoris; effect of exertion and of nitrites on the precordial movements. Am. Heart J., *61:* 250, 1961.

Electrokymography and Radarkymography

1. Bartley, O.: Electrokymographic changes in myocardial infarction. Acta Radiol., *54:* 81, 1960.

2. Cohen, L. S., Simon, A. L., Whitehouse, W. C., Schuette, W. H., and Braunwald, E.: Heart motion video-tracking (radarkymography) in diagnosis of congenital and acquired heart disease. Am. J. Cardiol., *22:* 678, 1968.

3. Dack, S., Paley, D. H., and Sussman, M.D.: A comparison of electrokymography and roentgenkymography in the study of myocardial infarction. Circulation, *1:* 551, 1950.

4. Henny, G. C., and Boone, B. R.: Electrokymograph for recording heart motion utilizing the roentgenoscope. Am. J. Roentgenol. Radium Ther. Nucl. Med., *54*(3): 217, 1945.

5. Kazamias, T. M., Gander, M. P., Ross, J. Jr., and Braunwald, E.: Detection of left-ventricular-wall motion disorders in coronary artery disease by radarkymography. N. Engl. J. Med., *285*(2): 63, 1971.

6. Zinsser, H. F. Jr., Kay, C. F., and Benjamin, J. M. Jr.: The electrokymograph; studies in recording fidelity. Circulation, *2:* 197, 1950.

Nuclear Cardiology

1. Blumgart, H. E., and Weiss, S.: Studies on the velocity of blood flow; III. The velocity of blood flow and its relation to other aspects of the circulation in patients with rheumatic and syphilitic heart disease. J. Clin. Invest., *4:* 149, 1927.

2. Carr, E. A., Gleason, G., Shaw, J., and Krontz, B.: The direct diagnosis of myocardial infarction by photoscanning after administration of cesium-131. Am. Heart J., *68:* 627, 1964.

3. Donato, L., Holmes, R. A., and Wagner, H. N.: The circulation, in H. N. Wagner (Ed.), *Principles of Nuclear Medicine*, p. 563. Philadelphia: W. B. Saunders, 1968.

4. Graham, T. P., Goodrich, J. K., Robinson, A. E., and Harris, C. C.: Scintiangiocardiography in children; rapid sequence visualization of the heart and great vessels after intravenous injection of radionuclide. Am. J. Cardiol., *25:* 387, 1970.

5. Hurley, P. J., Strauss, H. W., and Wagner, H. N.: Radionuclide angiography in cyanotic congenital heart disease. Johns Hopkins Med. J., *127:* 46, 1970.

6. Kriss, J. P., Enright, L. P., Hayden, W. G., Wexler, L., and Shumway, N. E.: Radioisotopic angiocardiography; wide scope of applicability in diagnosis and evaluation of the therapy in diseases of the heart and great vessels. Circulation, *43:* 792, 1971.

7. Parker, J. A., Secker-Walker, R. H., Hill, R., Siegel, B. A., and Potchen, E. J.: Calculation of left ventricular ejection fraction. J. Nucl. Med., *13:* 81, 1972.

8. Prinzmetal, M., Corday, E., Spritzler, R. J., and Fleig, W.: Radiocardiography and its clinical applications. J.A.M.A., *139:* 617, 1949.

9. Strauss, H. W., Zaret, B. L., Hurley, P. J., Natarajan, T. K., and Pitt, B.: A scintiphotographic method for measuring left ventricular ejection fraction in man without cardiac catheterization. Am. J. Cardiol, *28:* 575, 1971.

10. Wesselhoeft, H., Hurley, P. J., Wagner, H. N., and Rowe, R. D.: Nuclear angiocardiography in the diagnosis of congenital heart disease in infants. Circulation, *45:* 77, 1972.

11. Zaret, B. L., Hurley, P. J., and Pitt, B.: Noninvasive scintiphotographic diagnosis of left atrial myxoma. J. Nucl. Med., *13:* 81, 1972.

12. Zaret, B. L., Strauss, H. W., Martin, N. D., Wells, H. P., and Flamm, M.D.: Noninvasive evaluation of regional myocardial perfusion with potassium-43; study of patients at rest, exercise, and during angina pectoris. N. Engl. J. Med., *288:* 809, 1973.

chapter 13

Illustrative Cases

The purpose of this chapter is to demonstrate the use of non-invasive techniques in the diagnosis of certain disease states which have not been covered in the previous chapters.

Illustrative phonocardiograms, echocardiograms, and pulse waves will be related to the patient's clinical and hemodynamic findings whenever appropriate.

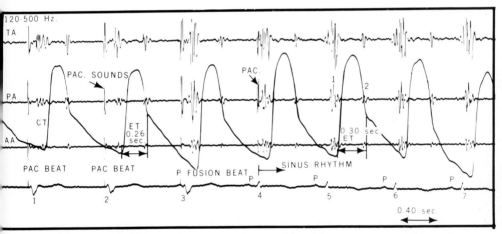

Fig. 13.1. Simultaneously recorded phonocardiogram at the tricuspid (TA), pulmonic (PA,) and aortic areas (AA), lead II of the electrocardiogram and carotid pulse tracing (CT) in a 69-year-old patient with a transvenous pacemaker implanted in the apex of the right ventricle. The first two beats are pacemaker (PAC) beats. Beat 3 is a fusion beat, and beats 4–7 are sinus beats. In the first four beats, there is a high frequency vibration occurring before the first heart sound representing the so called "pacemaker sounds." This vibration is not present in the sinus beats. In the carotid pulse tracing, ejection time (ET) is decreased to 0.26 sec in the pacemaker beats as compared to 0.30 sec in the sinus beats. The origin of the pacemaker sounds is not clear but they are recorded in approximately 40% of patients with implanted pacemakers and they may have an extracardiac origin.

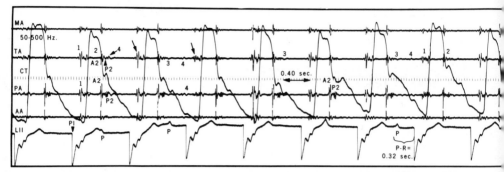

Fig. 13.2. Simultaneously recorded phonocardiogram at the mitral (MA), tricuspid (TA), pulmonic (PA) and aortic areas (AA), lead II (LII) of the electrocardiogram, and carotid pulse tracing (CT) in a 20-year-old patient with a permanently implanted pacemaker in the epicardial surface of the left ventricle (PI = pacemaker impulse). The rhythm is complete heart block. Note varying amplitude of the first heart sound which correlates with the timing of inscription of the P wave of the electrocardiogram. The fourth heart sound is recorded in proximity to the QRS complexes whenever the P wave occurs during the diastolic period of the cardiac cycle. The second heart sound shows fixed splitting due to the presence of complete right bundle branch block.

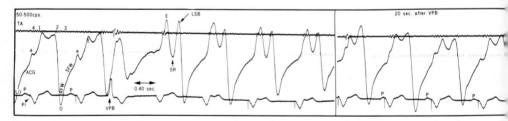

Fig. 13.3. Simultaneously recorded tricuspid area (TA) phonocardiogram, apexcardiogram (ACG), and lead II (LII) of the electrocardiogram in a 62-year-old patient with coronary artery disease and a transvenous pacemaker implanted in the apex of the right ventricle. The first two pacemaker beats are preceded by P waves. In these beats note the presence of an A wave in the apexcardiogram and a small systolic bulge. A ventricular premature beat (VPB) is inscribed. Following this beat, there is a marked increase in systolic retraction (SR) followed by a large, late systolic bulge (LSB) which progressively decreases in the subsequent cardiac cycle. Twenty seconds after inscription of the ventricular premature beat, the configuration of the apexcardiogram is quite similar to the first two beats recorded on the left side. PI = pacemaker impulse, RFW = rapid filling wave, and SFW = short filling wave.

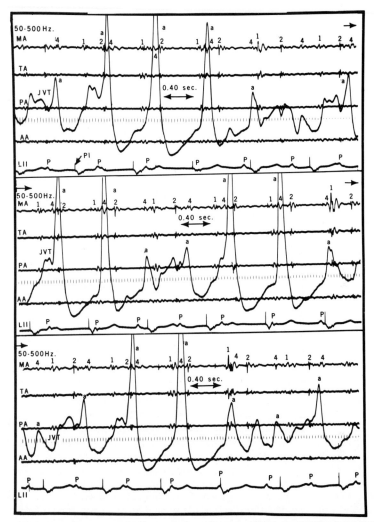

Fig. 13.4. Continuous recording of the phonocardiogram at the mitral (MA), tricuspid (TA), pulmonic (PA) and aortic areas (AA), jugular venous pulse tracing (JVT), and lead II (LII) of the electrocardiogram in a 68-year-old patient with complete heart block and a pacemaker implanted in the right ventricle (PI = pacemaker impulse). Note the varying configuration of the jugular venous tracing. When the P wave is inscribed during the QRS complex and consequently during ventricular systole, the right atrium contracts against a closed tricuspid valve causing quite prominent A waves. These large magnitude A waves are called cannon waves and represent regurgitant flow into the jugular veins secondary to atrial contraction against a closed tricuspid valve. Also note the varying amplitude of the A waves when atrial contraction occurs in the diastolic interval. The magnitude of the A wave (atrial contraction) during diastole depends upon the timing of the P wave in relation to the QRS complex. When the P wave just precedes the QRS, there is a normal A/V ratio. Note the "wandering" nature of the recorded fourth heart sound.

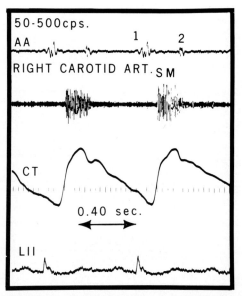

Fig. 13.5. Simultaneously recorded aortic area (AA) phonocardiogram with another microphone placed over the right carotid artery, carotid pulse tracing (CT), and lead II (LII) of the electrocardiogram in a 62-year-old patient with carotid artery stenosis. Note the presence of a systolic bruit over the right carotid area where a stenotic lesion was found in the carotid arteriogram. The systolic bruit starts in mid-systole with maximal intensity near the second heart sound. The bruit has a high frequency, noisy characteristic. **SM** = systolic murmur.

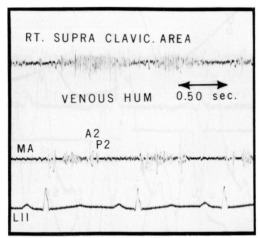

Fig. 13.6. Simultaneously recorded mitral area (MA) phonocardiogram with another microphone placed at the right supraclavicular area (RT. SUPRA CLAVIC. AREA) over the right jugular vein and lead II (LII) of the electrocardiogram in a 4-year-old patient with a venous hum. The typical configuration of a venous hum consists of a high frequency, high amplitude continuous murmur having a maximal peak at the level of the second heart sound. This type of murmur is frequently heard in children due to turbulent flow through the jugular vein.

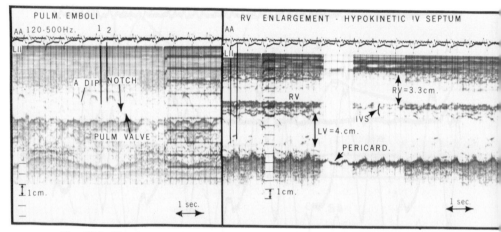

Fig. 13.9. Simultaneously recorded aortic area (AA) phonocardiogram, lead II (LII) of the electrocardiogram and echocardiogram in a 49-year-old patient with pulmonary emboli. (Left panel) Note abnormal motion of the pulmonary valve consisting of the absence of an A dip. There is also systolic notching of this valve as seen in patients with pulmonary hypertension. (Right panel) Echocardiogram on the same patient demonstrating an increase in right ventricular diameter to 3.3 cm. The interventricular septal thickness is 1.1 cm. It exhibits flat motion as seen on the right panel. The left ventricular posterior wall thickness measures 1 cm. The right panel echocardiogram was taken at varying damping settings for better identification of the various cardiac structures. RV = right ventricle, LV = left ventricle, and IVS = interventricular septum.

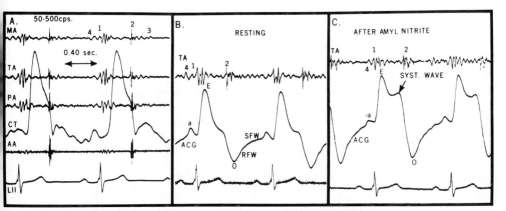

Fig. 13.10. (Panel A) Simultaneously recorded phonocardiogram at the mitral (MA), tricuspid (TA), pulmonic (PA) and aortic areas (AA), carotid pulse tracing (CT), and lead II (LII) of the electrocardiogram in a 31-year-old patient with athletic heart syndrome. The first and second heart sounds are normal. Third and fourth heart sounds are best recorded at the mitral area. The carotid pulse tracing is normal. (Panel B) Simultaneously recorded tricuspid area (TA) phonocardiogram, apexcardiogram (ACG), and lead II of the electrocardiogram at rest. The A wave in the apexcardiogram coincides with the fourth heart sound. Note the absence of any systolic bulge on this record. (Panel C) Shortly after inhalation of amyl nitrite, the apexcardiogram shows a prominent and late systolic bulge (SYST. WAVE). Late systolic bulges have been described in patients with athletic heart syndrome and do not correlate with the presence of abnormalities of left ventricular function. The etiology of these graphic abnormalities remains obscure in this syndrome. RFW = rapid filling wave and SFW = slow filling wave.

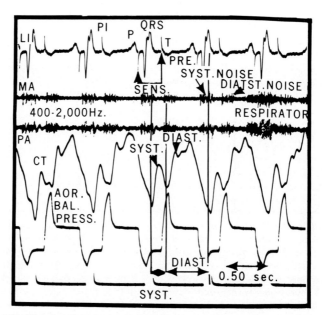

Fig. 13.11. Simultaneously recorded lead II (LII) of the electrocardiogram, phonocardiogram at the mitral (MA) and pulmonic areas (PA), carotid pulse tracing (CT), and the aortic balloon pressure recording (AOR. BAL. PRESS.) in a 48-year-old patient. The recordings were made during the post-operative period in a patient with assisted circulation from the intra-aortic balloon functioning at a 1:1 ratio. The sensing (SENS.) spikes of the counterpulsation unit are indicated (PI). Note the diastolic wave in the carotid pulse tracing which corresponds to high frequency, high amplitude diastolic vibrations in the phonocardiogram as the intra-aortic balloon inflates and deflates. Respiratory artifacts are recorded on the last beat of the tracing.

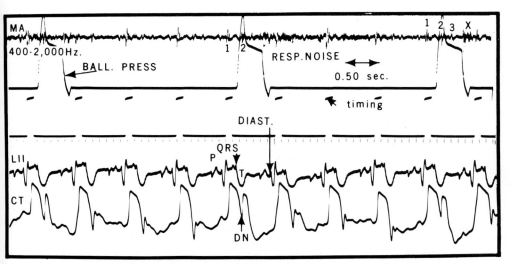

Fig. 13.12. Simultaneously recorded mitral area (MA) phonocardiogram, lead II (LII) of the electrocardiogram, intra-aortic balloon pressure (BALL. PRESS), and carotid pulse tracing (CT) in a 65-year-old patient. The tracings were recorded during the post-operative period in a patient who had aortocoronary artery bypass and assisted circulation with an intra-aortic balloon functioning at a 4:1 ratio. As noted on the carotid pulse tracing, every fourth beat is accompanied by a diastolic wave corresponding to the time (arrow) that the intra-aortic balloon is inflated, causing the diastolic augmentation of the blood pressure. The diastolic wave immediately follows the dicrotic notch (DN) of the carotid pulse tracing. Also, observe the high frequency, high amplitude sound on the phonocardiogram (X) at the time when the balloon deflates. Third and fourth heart sounds are also recorded.

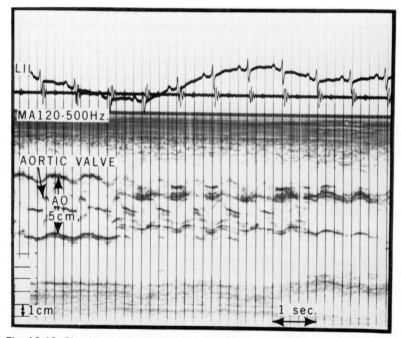

Fig. 13.13. Simultaneously recorded echocardiogram, mitral area (MA) phonocar-diogram and lead II (LII) of the electrocardiogram in a 67-year-old patient with an aneurysm of the ascending aorta (AO). Note significant increase in the size of the aortic root which measures 5 cm. The aortic valve opening measures 2 cm which is within the normal range. The aortic root diameter becomes smaller as the ultrasonic beam is directed toward the outflow tract of the left ventricle (right side of the recording).

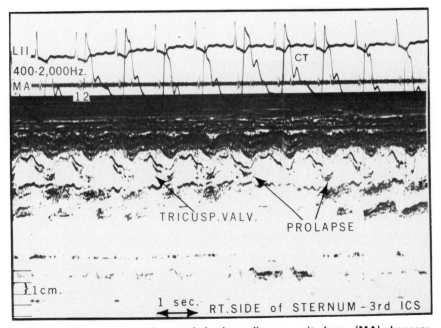

Fig. 13.14. Simultaneously recorded echocardiogram, mitral area (MA) phonocardiogram, carotid pulse tracing (CT), and lead II (LII) of the electrocardiogram in a 58-year-old patient with prolapse of the tricuspid valve documented by right and left cardiac catheterization and angiography.

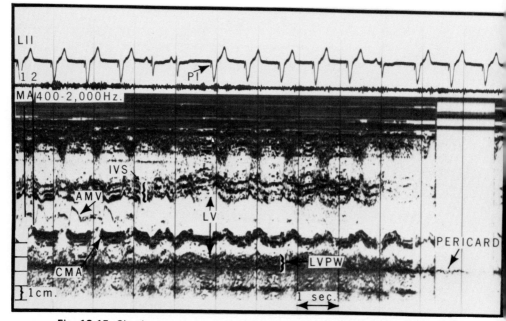

Fig. 13.15. Simultaneously recorded lead II (LII) of the electrocardiogram, mitral area (MA) phonocardiogram, and echocardiogram in a 80-year-old patient with calcified mitral annulus (CMA). Note heavy and disorganized echoes behind the posterior leaflet of the mitral valve representing calcification of the mitral annulus. The septum (IVS) measures approximately 1.1 cm and moves paradoxically. The left ventricular posterior wall thickness (LVPW) measures about 1 cm. The left (LV) ventricular internal dimension is 4.3 cm. Right ventricular dimension measures 3.1 cm. AMV = anterior mitral valve and PI = pacemaker impulse.

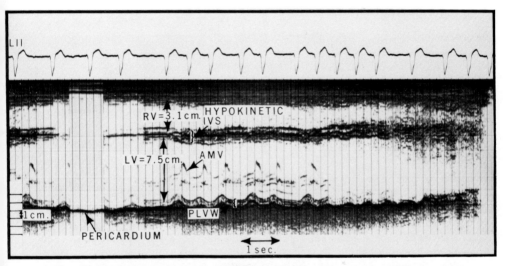

Fig. 13.16. Simultaneously recorded lead II (LII) of the electrocardiogram and echocardiogram in a 73-year-old patient with congestive heart failure due to coronary artery disease and dilatation of the left ventricle. Note flat motion of the interventricular septum (IVS) which measures 1.3 cm. The left ventricular posterior wall (PLVW) measures 1.2 cm. There is a marked increase in left ventricular (LV) internal diameter to 7.5 cm. The pericardium has flat motion. The right ventricular (RV) diameter is 3.1 cm. AMV = anterior mitral valve.

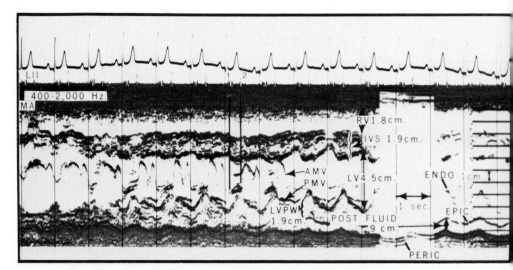

Fig. 13.17. Simultaneously recorded lead II (LII) of the electrocardiogram, mitral area (MA) phonocardiogram, and echocardiogram in a 73-year-old patient with severe hypertension due to renal vascular disease, left ventricular hypertrophy and posterior pericardial effusion. Note the presence of an echo free space behind the epicardium. In addition, note thickening of the pericardium (PERIC) as well as increased thickness of the interventricular septum (IVS) and left ventricular posterior wall (LVPW) of the type seen in patients with concentric left ventricular hypertrophy particularly in patients with long standing arterial hypertension. The left ventricular (LV) internal diameter is within the normal limits at 4.5 cm. The left atrium measures 4 cm and the aortic root is 3 cm. The recordings were taken at various damping settings for proper identification of the pericardium. AMV = anterior mitral valve, PMV = posterior mitral valve, RV = right ventricle, ENDO = endocardial surface of the left ventricle, and EPIC = epicardial surface of the left ventricle.

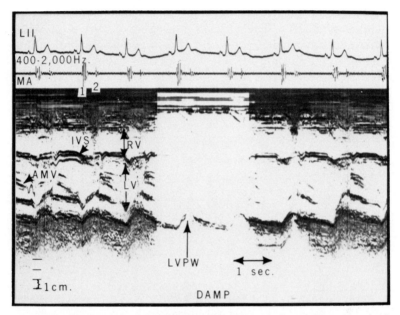

Fig. 13.18. Simultaneously recorded lead II of the electrocardiogram, mitral area (MA) phonocardiogram and echocardiogram in a 41-year-old patient with congenital absence of the left pericardium documented by right and left heart catheterization and angiocardiography. The echocardiogram demonstrates absence of the pericardium with good motion of the left ventricular posterior wall (LVPW). IVS = interventricular septum, AMV = anterior mitral valve, RV = right ventricle, and LV = left ventricle.

APPENDIX

The normal values for measurements of intracavitary diameters and wall or septal thickness obtained from the echocardiogram in infants, children, and adults are shown in Table 1–7. Each table indicates the range and mean values for these measurements as related to body weight in infants and children. Table 8 shows the effect of various physiological and pharmacological maneuvers on the configuration and amplitude of heart sounds and murmurs. Table 9 shows the systolic time intervals in diseases of the heart.

Appendix Table 1. Right Ventricular Anterior Wall Thickness (Diastolic) (in cm)—Neonates

	Hagan $n = 200$	Solinger				
		$n = 21$	$n = 28$	$n = 25$	$n = 22$	$n = 23$
Weight	m = 7.6 lb	2.27 kg	2.73 kg	3.18 kg	3.64 kg	4.09 kg
Range	0.20–0.47	0.11–0.29	0.13–0.31	0.16–0.34	0.18–0.36	0.20–0.38
Mean	0.30 ± 0.01	0.20	0.22	0.25	0.27	0.29

Appendix Table 2. Right Ventricular Cavity (Diastolic) (in cm)

(A) Neonates and Infants

	Hagan n = 200	Meyer n = 50	Solinger					Feigenbaum n = 26
			n = 21	n = 28	n = 25	n = 22	n = 23	
Weight	m = 7.6 lb	m = 3.2 kg	2.27 kg	2.73 kg	3.18 kg	3.64 kg	4.09 kg	0-25 lb m = 17 lb
Range	0.61-1.50	1.0-1.7	1.04-1.46	1.10-1.52	1.16-1.58	1.23-1.65	1.29-1.71	0.3-1.5
Mean	1.14 ± 0.04	1.3	1.25	1.31	1.37	1.44	1.50	0.9

(B) Older Children

	Feigenbaum				
	n = 26	n = 20	n = 15	n = 11	n = 5
Weight	25-50 lb m = 39 lb	50-75 lb m = 62 lb	75-100 lb m = 89 lb	100-125 lb m = 113 lb	125-200 lb m = 165 lb
Range	0.4-1.5	0.7-1.8	0.7-1.6	0.8-1.7	1.2-1.7
Mean	1.0	1.1	1.2	1.3	1.3

Appendix Table 3. Septal Thickness (Diastolic) (in cm)
(A) Neonates and Infants

| | Hagan n = 200 | Solinger | | | | | Feigenbaum n = 26 |
		n = 21	n = 28	n = 25	n = 22	n = 23	
Weight	m = 7.6 lb	2.27 kg	2.73 kg	3.18 kg	3.64 kg	4.09 kg	0–25 lb m = 17 lb
Range	0.18–0.40	0.21–0.33	0.24–0.36	0.26–0.38	0.29–0.41	0.31–0.43	0.4–0.6
Mean	0.27 ± 0.004	0.27	0.30	0.32	0.35	0.37	0.5

(B) Older Children

| | Feigenbaum | | | | |
	n = 26	n = 20	n = 15	n = 11	n = 5
Weight	25–50 lb m = 39 lb	50–75 lb m = 62 lb	75–100 lb m = 89 lb	100–125 lb m = 113 lb	125–200 lb m = 165 lb
Range	0.5–0.7	0.6–0.7	0.7–0.8	0.7–0.8	0.7–0.8
Mean	0.6	0.7	0.7	0.7	0.8

From S. J. Goldberg: *Pediatric & Adolescent Echocardiography—A Handbook.* Copyright 1975 by Year Book Medical Publishers, Inc., Chicago. with permission.

Appendix Table 4. Aortic Root Diameter (Diastolic) (in cm)

(A) Neonates and Infants

	Hagan n = 200	Meyer n = 50	Solinger n = 21	n = 28	n = 25	n = 22	n = 23	Feigenbaum n = 26
Weight	m = 7.6 lb	m = 3.2 kg	2.27 kg	2.73 kg	3.18 kg	3.64 kg	4.09 kg	0-25 lb m = 17 lb
Range	0.81-1.2	0.7-1.2	0.93-1.13	0.97-1.17	1.02-1.22	1.07-1.27	1.11-1.31	0.7-1.7
Mean	1.0 ± .006	1.0	1.03	1.07	1.12	1.17	1.21	1.3

(B) Older Children

	Feigenbaum n = 26	n = 20	n = 15	n = 11	n = 5
Weight	25-50 lb m = 39 lb	50-75 lb m = 62 lb	75-100 lb m = 89 lb	100-125 lb m = 113 lb	125-200 lb m = 165 lb
Range	1.3-2.2	1.7-2.3	1.9-2.7	1.7-2.7	2.2-2.8
Mean	1.7	2.0	2.2	2.3	2.4

Appendix Table 5. Left Atrial Dimension (End Ventricular Systole) (in cm)

(A) Neonates and Infants

	Hagan n = 200	Meyer n = 50	Solinger n = 21	Solinger n = 28	Solinger n = 25	Solinger n = 22	Solinger n = 23	Feigenbaum n = 26
Weight	m = 7.6 lb	m = 3.2 kg	2.27 kg	2.73 kg	3.18 kg	3.64 kg	4.09 kg	0–25 lb m = 17 lb
Range	0.5–1.0	0.6–1.3	0.68–1.05	0.74–1.11	0.80–1.17	0.86–1.23	0.92–1.29	0.7–2.3
Mean	0.7 ± 0.01	0.9	0.87	0.93	0.99	1.05	1.11	1.7

(B) Older Children

Feigenbaum

	n = 26	n = 20	n = 15	n = 11	n = 5
Weight	25–50 lb m = 39 lb	50–75 lb m = 62 lb	75–100 lb m = 89 lb	100–125 lb m = 113 lb	125–200 lb m = 165 lb
Range	1.7–2.7	1.9–2.8	2.0–3.0	2.1–3.0	2.1–3.7
Mean	2.2	2.3	2.4	2.7	2.8

From S. J. Goldberg: *Pediatric & Adolescent Echocardiography—A Handbook.* Copyright 1975 by Year Book Medical Publishers, Inc., Chicago, with permission.

Appendix Table 6. Mitral Valve Depth, Amplitude and Velocity (E-F Slope)—Neonates

	Hagan n = 200	Meyer n = 50	Solinger				
			n = 21	n = 28	n = 25	n = 22	n = 23
Weight	m = 7.6 lb	m = 3.2 kg	2.27 kg	2.73 kg	3.18 kg	3.64 kg	4.09 kg
Depth (cm)							
Range	—	3.1–4.7	—	—	—	—	—
Mean	—	3.8	—	—	—	—	—
Amplitude (cm)							
Range	0.60–1.20	0.6–1.2	.85–1.11	.89–1.15	.93–1.19	.97–1.23	1.01–1.27
Mean	0.81 ± 0.01	1.0	.98	1.02	1.06	1.10	1.14
Velocity (mm/sec)							
Range	60–130	38–80	—	—	—	—	—
Mean	80 ± 1	53	—	—	—	—	—

From S. J. Goldberg: *Pediatric & Adolescent Echocardiography—A Handbook.* Copyright 1975 by Year Book Medical Publishers, Inc., Chicago, with permission.

Appendix Table 7. Normal Adult Values

	Mean	Range	No. of Subjects
Age	27 yrs	13–54 yrs	75
BSA	1.79 m²	1.45–2.22 m²	74
RVD:			
Supine	1.5 cm	0.7–2.3 cm	39
Left lateral	1.7 cm	1.0–2.6 cm	44
Change	0.2 cm	0.0–0.6 cm	8
LVID	4.6 cm	3.5–5.6 cm	73
LV wall thickness	0.9 cm	0.7–1.1 cm	75
IV septal wall thickness	0.9 cm	0.7–1.1 cm	73
LA dimension	2.9 cm	1.9–4.0 cm	72
Aortic root	2.7 cm	2.0–3.7 cm	64
Aortic valve opening	1.9 cm	1.6–2.6 cm	44

From H. Feigenbaum: *Echocardiography*. Copyright 1972 by Lea & Febiger, Philadelphia, with permission.

Appendix Table 8. Physiological and Pharmacological Maneuvers Utilized in Analysis of Heart Sounds and Murmurs

Sounds and Murmurs	Respiration		Valsalva maneuver	Postural Changes				Isometric handgrip exercise	Drugs	
	Inspiration	Expiration		Lying	Sitting	Standing	Squatting		Vasodilator drugs (amyl nitrite)	Vasoactive drugs (phenylephrine)
Mitral stenosis: Opening snap	—	—	—	—	—	—	—	—	—	A_2-OS interval widens
Mitral diastolic murmur	—	—	—	↑ Left lateral pos.	—	—	—	↑	↑	→
Mitral insufficiency: Systolic murmur	—	—	→	—	—	→	↑	↑	↓	↑
Mitral valvular prolapse Systolic click	—	—	↓	↑→	↑→ or ↔	↓←	↑↑*	↑↑*	↓	↑↑*
Systolic murmur	—	—	→	↑ Leg raise	← ↔	↑→	←→	↑↑*	←	←↑ (Isoprenaline)
Aortic stenosis: Systolic murmur	—	—	←	↓ Leg raise	←	←	→	←	→	←↑ (Isoprenaline)
Idiopathic hypertrophic subaortic stenosis: Systolic murmur	—	—	←	↑ Sitting + leaning	—	—	—	←	←	←
Aortic insufficiency: Diastolic murmur	—	—	—	—	—	→	←	—	→	→
Austin flint murmur	—	—	—	—	—	←	←	—	←	↕
Tricuspid insufficiency: Systolic murmur	←	→	—	—	—	—	—	—	—	—
Tricuspid stenosis: Mid-diastolic murmur	←	→	—	—	—	—	—	—	—	—
Pulmonary stenosis: Systolic murmur	→	—	—	—	—	—	—	←	←	—

Appendix Table 8 (Continued)

Sounds and Murmurs	Respiration		Valsalva maneuver	Postural Changes					Isometric handgrip exercise	Drugs	
	Inspiration	Expiration		Lying	Sitting	Standing	Squatting			Vasodilator drugs (amyl nitrite)	Vasoactive drugs (phenylephrine)
Pulmonary insufficiency: Diastolic murmur	↑	—	—	—	—	—	—	—	←	↔
Atrial septal defect: S₂	A₂-P₂ fixed Splitting	A₂-P₂ fixed Splitting	A₂-P₂ fixed Splitting							
—						—		—		
Systolic murmur	—	—	—	—	—	—	—		↔	↔
Ventricular septal defect: Systolic murmur	A₂-P₂ fixed Splitting	—	—	—	—	—	—	←	↔ *	↕ *
Tetralogy of Fallot: Systolic murmur	—	—	—	—	←	—	—	—	→→	→←→
PDA	←	—	{Earlier phase III ↑} ↑ Leg raise ↑	←	→	←		↑	—	—
S₃ + S₄ (right)	—	—	↓ {Earlier phase III ↑}	←	→	→		—	—	—
S₃ + S₄ (left)	—	←	↓ {Earlier phase III ↑} ←	→				—	—	—

Ventricular septal defect = small defect with pulmonary hypertension systolic murmur ↓ with amyl nitrite and ↑ phenylephrine.
Ventricular septal defect = large defect with hyperkinetic pulmonary hypertension systolic murmur ↑ **with amyl nitrite and ↓ with phenylephrine.**
↑ = increased, ↓ = decreased, ↔ = unchanged, →→ = click or murmur is moving toward A₂-OS, →*→ = ... S₂ = second heart sound, S₃ = third heart sound, S₄ = fourth heart sound.

Appendix Table 9. Systolic Time Intervals in Diseases of Heart

	Pre-Ejection Period	Left Ventricular Ejection Time	Total Electro-mechanical Systole	PEP/LVET Ratio
Chronic non-valvular heart disease: Primary myocardial disease	↑	↓	↔	↑
Chronic coronary artery disease	↑	↓	↓	↑
Acute myocardial infarction	↑↓ ↔	↓	↓	↔↑
Myocardial revascularization	↓	↑	↔	↓
Hypertensive heart disease:				
Compensated	↔	↔	↔	↔
Decompensated	↑	↓	↑	↑
Constrictive pericarditis:	↔	↔	↔	↔
With myocardial involvement	↑	↓		↑
Pericardial effusion with cardiac tamponade	Variable with respiration and blood pressure			
Valvular heart disease:				
Aortic stenosis	↓	↑	↑↔	↓
With heart failure	↑↔	↓↔		↑↔
Idiopathic hypertrophic subaortic stenosis	↓	↑	↓	↓
Aortic insufficiency	↓	↑		↓
Aortic insufficiency with heart failure	↑↔	↓↔		↑↔
Mitral stenosis	↑	↓		↑
Mitral insufficiency: Mitral valve replacement	↑	↓		↑
Conduction defects:				
Right bundle branch block with left anterior	↔	↔		↔
Left bundle branch block	↑	↔↓	↑	
Right bundle branch block wit left anterior hemiblock	↑	↔		
Cardiac arrhythmias, atrial fibrillation:				
Long R-R cycle	↓	↑		↓
Short R-R cycle	↑	↓		↑
Ventricular premature contraction	↑	↓		
Post-extrasystolic beats	↓	↑		
Ventricular tachycardia	↑	↓		
Atrial pacing	↔			
Ventricular pacing		↑		
Pulsus alternans during weak beats	↑	↓	↔	
Drugs:				
1. *Amyl nitrite inhalation*				
Normals	↓	↑		
Coronary Artery Disease	↔	↔		
2. Sympathomimetic drugs				
Isoprenaline	↓	↓		
Epinephrine	↓	↔↓		
Phentolamine	↓	↑		
3. Propanolol	↑	↓	↔	
4. Digitalis	↓	↓	↓	

↑ = Increase, ↓ = decrease, ↔ = unchanged.

Index